The Computing Neuron

COMPUTATION AND NEURAL SYSTEMS SERIES

SERIES EDITOR

Christof Koch
California Institute of Technology

EDITORIAL ADVISORY BOARD MEMBERS

Recent advances in the mathematical theory of nonlinear feedback networks, combined with new methods in neurophysiology and the development of digital/analog VLSI and optical computing technologies, have led to the emergence of a new paradigm in information processing: 'Neural Networks'.

The Addison-Wesley Series in *Computation and Neural Systems* attempts to reflect the diversity of this new field by publishing textbooks, course materials and monographs, including the following topics:

- Biophysical Modelling of Synapses, Dendrites and Neurons
- Modelling Neurophysiological and Psychophysical Data at the Network and System Levels
- Computational Theories of Vision, Audition, Olfaction, Language Understanding, and Motor Control
- Cybernetics and System Theory
- Pattern Recognition
- Theory of Neural Networks (e.g. Learning)
- Theory of Dynamic Systems
- Hardware Implementation of Networks (e.g. VLSI, Optics)

The series editor, Dr Christof Koch, is Assistant Professor of Computation and Neural Systems at the California Institute of Technology. Dr Koch works at both the biophysical level, investigating information processing in single neurons and in networks such as the visual cortex, as well as studying and implementing simple resistive networks for computing motion, stereo and colour in biological and artificial systems.

The Computing Neuron

Edited by

Richard Durbin
Stanford University

Christopher Miall
King's College, Cambridge

Graeme Mitchison
King's College, Cambridge

ADDISON-WESLEY
PUBLISHING
COMPANY

Wokingham, England · Reading, Massachusetts · Menlo Park, California
New York · Don Mills, Ontario · Amsterdam · Bonn
Sydney · Singapore · Tokyo · Madrid · San Juan

Cover designed by Crayon Design of Henley-on-Thames and printed by The Riverside Printing Co. (Reading) Ltd.
Printed in Great Britain by T.J. Press (Padstow), Cornwall.

First printed 1989.

British Library Cataloguing in Publication Data

The computing neuron.
   1. Animals. Information processing. Role of nervous system
   I. Durbin, Richard   II. Miall, Christopher   III. Mitchison, Graeme   IV. Series
   591.1'88

   ISBN 0–201–18348–X

Library of Congress Cataloging in Publication Data

The Computing neuron.

   (Computation and neural systems)
   Based on papers presented at a meeting held in Cambridge in the summer of 1988, sponsored by King's College Research Centre and others.
   Includes bibliographies and index.
   1. Neural circuitry – Congresses.   2. Neural computers – Congresses.   I. Durbin, Richard.   II. Miall, Christopher.   III. Mitchison, Graeme.   IV. King's College (University of Cambridge). Research Centre.
   V. Series.   [DNLM: 1. Models, Neurological – congresses. 2. Neurons – physiology – congresses.   WL 102.5 C738 1988]
   QP363.3.C66   1989   591.1'88   89-14979

   ISBN 0–201–18348–X

Foreword

The brain computes! This idea was anything but a truism at the time of Aristotle or Galen, when the very concept of information and computing had not yet even entered the language. Descartes might have had an inkling of what could be implied by this statement, while to us, living at the end of the second millennium in a culture being increasingly dominated by computers, the idea appears commonplace. This 'brain-as-computer' metaphor provided one of the main driving forces behind cybernetics in the 1940s and fueled the excitement with which perceptrons and other simple networks were studied in the 1960s. In contrast to those research efforts, however, the current 'computational neuroscience' paradigm has strong roots among both theoreticians and experimentalists. Their principal motivation is the realization that while biophysical, anatomical and physiological data are necessary to understand the brain, they are, unfortunately, not sufficient.

The present volume brings together some of the best researchers within computational neuroscience and connectionism, unified by their desire to understand nervous systems, ranging from very simple animals such as the nematode *C. elegans* with 302 neurons *in toto* or the lobster stomatogastric ganglion with 30 neurons to the mammalian visual system and hippocampus with up to a hundred million neurons. The intent of the conference on which these papers are based was to study biological networks, leaving out the applied side of neural networks. One of the areas of special emphasis represented at the workshop – and reflected in this volume – are neural networks in invertebrates, in particular those generating temporal patterns. If we are to come to an understanding of how information is processed in higher mammals, we had better first understand how these anatomically and neurophysiologically well-characterized networks function. Learning, development and memory have provided much of the impetus behind theoretical work in the neural network field; here a number of new neurobiologically-inspired approaches are presented and discussed. The volume concludes with two contributions studying the problem of computing optical flow.

When reading the individual chapters, it is frequently difficult to decide unequivocally whether the authors are experimentalists or theoreticians, or indeed both. This, better than anything else, documents the progress we have made over the last few years.

The *Computation and Neural Systems Series* – Over the past 600 million years, biology has solved the problem of processing massive amounts of noisy and highly redundant information in a constantly changing environment by evolving networks of billions of highly interconnected nerve cells. It is the task of scientists – be they mathematicians, physicists, biologists, psychologists, or computer scientists – to understand the principles underlying information processing in these complex structures. At the same time, researchers in machine vision, pattern recognition, speech understanding, robotics, and other areas of artificial intelligence can profit from understanding features of existing nervous systems. Thus, a new field is emerging: the study of how computations can be carried out in extensive networks of heavily interconnected processing elements, whether these networks are carbon- or silicon-based. Addison-Wesley's new *Computation and Neural Systems Series* will reflect the diversity of this field with textbooks, course materials, and monographs on topics ranging from the biophysical modelling of dendrites and neurons, to computational theories of vision and motor control, the implementation of neural networks using VLSI or optics technology, and the study of highly parallel computational architectures.

Christof Koch
Pasadena, California

Preface

This book includes a selection of work presented to a meeting on *The Neuron as a Computational Unit* held in Cambridge in the summer of 1988. The aim of the meeting was to discuss the computational role of the neuron and to relate its properties to those of the 'neurally-inspired' units that form computational elements in connectionist networks. These networks have undergone a rapid increase in popularity recently, following developments in learning algorithms that allow multi-layer networks to solve quite complex tasks. These developments have been captured in the connectionist 'bible', the two volume PDP book edited by Rumelhart and McClelland. However, as widely acknowledged by exponents of connectionism, the units in these networks are generally simple threshold devices, quite unlike most biological neurons, whilst the algorithms used are not always biologically plausible. It would be fair to say that neuroscientists' interest in this field of computer modelling is tempered by some scepticism.

We therefore aimed to assemble a group of connectionists and neurobiologists to address the relationship between these two fields. We chose neuroscientists working on both vertebrate systems (the visual cortex, retina and hippocampus), and on invertebrates (principally those working on the networks underlying pattern generation). The latter group were chosen because of the detailed knowledge of some invertebrate networks, generally unmatched in the vertebrate field (although we include here an honorary invertebrate, the frog tadpole). These were balanced by more theoretical work on learning algorithms, on artificial visual systems, and on temporal pattern detection and storage.

In collecting together these rather diverse chapters we have striven to bring out as much interdisciplinary discussion as possible. We have also summarized our own thoughts on the discussion at the meeting and on the work presented in this book in the form of three introductory chapters. We have tried to avoid as much overlap as possible; each editor approaches the central theme of the book from a rather different angle. In the spirit of this interdisciplinary endeavour, we have not divided the book into separate parts, so there is no clear split between the theoretical and biological work. Rather, there is a gradual shift of emphasis, from the early chapters on learning and cognitive functions, into the central section on biological networks, and into the final section on networks for visual processing. To retain the style and spontaneity of each contribution, we have retained the idiosyncrasies of the trans-Atlantic divide. You will find neurones and neurons here, some exhibiting behaviour and others behavior.

The meeting was supported by King's College Research Centre, the National Science Foundation, the Wellcome Trust, Addison-Wesley Publishers Limited, and IBM (United Kingdom) Trust, and we would like to acknowledge their financial assistance. We would also like to acknowledge the help of the college staff who made the meeting so enjoyable and easy to organize. We are grateful to the managers of the Research Centre for their support of this project, and we thank Catherine Marinković for her valuable assistance in all matters. Production of the book was made possible with the facilities of King's College Research Centre. The drawing of a local non-spiking locust interneuron used in the design on the front cover was kindly provided by Malcolm Burrows.

Finally, when planning the meeting earlier in the year, we felt it was important to provide a brief introduction to neural network models for those biologists unfamiliar with this work. This took the form of a two-day workshop preceding the main meeting, at which we gave an overview of some common models and algorithms. We also provided a number of computer demonstrations, running on Apple Macintosh computers, to allow participants hands-on experience of these models. These programs proved to be popular, and successful in demonstrating the main features of network models. They were written to be as clear and straightforward as we could manage: they are interactive and have displays showing the operation of the network. They are available on a single Macintosh disk, which includes 10 demonstrations and some explanatory notes. To cover the distribution and copying costs, we charge £12 or $20 for each copy of the disk. If you want a copy, please send a cheque or money order to one of us, at the King's College Research Centre, King's College, Cambridge, CB2 1ST, UK.

Richard Durbin, Chris Miall and Graeme Mitchison
King's College, Cambridge
March 1989

Contributors

Atwell, D.
> Department of Physiology, University College, Gower Street, London
> WC1E 6BT, UK

Barlow, H.B.
> Department of Physiology, Cambridge University, Cambridge CB2 3EG, UK

Barto, A.G.
> Department of Computer and Information Science, University of Massachusetts
> at Amherst, Massachusetts MA 01003, USA

Burrows, M.
> Department of Zoology, University of Cambridge, Downing Street, Cambridge
> CB2 3EJ, UK

Chattarji, S.
> Laboratory for Computational Neurobiology, The Salk Institute, P.O. Box
> 85800, San Diego, California CA 92138, USA

Cottrell, G.W.
> Department of Computer Science and Engineering, University of California, San
> Diego, La Jolla, California CA 92093, USA

Durbin, R.M.
> Department of Psychology, Stanford University, Palo Alto, California CA 94305,
> USA

Földiák, P.
> Department of Physiology, Cambridge University, Cambridge CB2 3EG, UK

Hsu, A.
> Computation and Neural Systems Program, Divisions of Biology and
> Engineering and Applied Science 216-76, California Institute of Technology,
> Pasadena, California CA 91125, USA

Jack, J.J.B.
    University Laboratory of Physiology, University of Oxford, Parks Road,
    Oxford OX1 3PT, UK

Kammen, D.M.
    Divisions of Biology and Engineering 216-76, California Institute of Technology,
    Pasadena, California CA 91125, USA

Koch, C.
    Computation and Neural Systems Program, Divisions of Biology and Engineering
    and Applied Science 216-76, California Institute of Technology, Pasadena,
    California CA 91125, USA

Kristan Jr., W.B.
    Department of Biology, University of California, San Diego, La Jolla,
    California CA 92093, USA

Kullmann, D.M.
    University Laboratory of Physiology, University of Oxford, Parks Road,
    Oxford OX1 3PT, UK

Larkman, A.U.
    University Laboratory of Physiology, University of Oxford, Parks Road,
    Oxford OX1 3PT, UK

Laughlin, S.
    Department of Zoology, University of Cambridge, Downing Street,
    Cambridge CB2 3EJ, UK

Laurent, G.J.
    Department of Zoology, University of Cambridge, Downing Street,
    Cambridge CB2 3EJ, UK

Lockery, S.R.
    Department of Biology, University of California, San Diego, La Jolla,
    California CA 92093, USA

Longuet-Higgins, H.C.
    Centre for Research in Perception and Cognition, Laboratory of Experimental
    Psychology, University of Sussex, Brighton BN1 9QG, UK

McLaren, I.P.L.
    Department of Experimental Psychology, University of Cambridge, Downing
    Street, Cambridge CB2 3EB, UK

Major, G.M.
    University Laboratory of Physiology, University of Oxford, Parks Road,
    Oxford OX1 3PT, UK

Mason, A.J.R.
University Laboratory of Physiology, University of Oxford, Parks Road,
Oxford OX1 3PT, UK

Mathur, B.
Science Center, Rockwell International, Thousand Oaks, California CA 91360,
USA

Mazzoni, P.
Department of Biology B-022, University of California, San Diego, La Jolla,
California CA 92093, USA

Miall, R.C.
King's College Research Centre, King's College, Cambridge CB2 1ST, UK

Mitchison, G.J.
King's College Research Centre, King's College, Cambridge CB2 1ST, UK

Poggio, T.
Artificial Intelligence Laboratory, Massachusetts Institute of Technology,
Cambridge, Massachusetts MA 02139, USA

Roberts, A.
Department of Zoology, University of Bristol, Bristol BS8 1UG, UK

Robertson, R.M.
Department of Biology, Queen's University, Kingston, Ontario K71 3N6,
Canada

Rolls, E.T.
Department of Experimental Psychology, University of Oxford, South Parks
Road, Oxford OX1 3UD, UK

Sejnowksi, T.J.
Laboratory for Computational Neurobiology, The Salk Institute, P.O. Box 85800,
San Diego, California CA 92138, USA

Selverston, A.I.
Department of Biology B-022, University of California, San Diego, La Jolla,
California CA 92093, USA

Stanton, P.K.
Departments of Neuroscience and Neurology, Albert Einstein College of
Medicine, 1410 Pelham Parkway South, Bronx, New York NY 10461, USA

Stratford, K.J.
University Laboratory of Physiology, University of Oxford, Parks Road,
Oxford OX1 3PT, UK

Tessier-Lavigne, M.
    Howard Hughes Medical Institute, Columbia University, New York, USA

Torre, V.
    Dipartimento di Fisica, Università di Genova, Via Dodecaneso 33, CAP 16146,
    Genova, Italy

Wang, H.T.
    Science Center, Rockwell International, Thousand Oaks, California CA 91360,
    USA

Wittenberg, G.
    Department of Biology, University of California, San Diego, La Jolla,
    California CA 92093, USA

Yang, W.
    Artificial Intelligence Laboratory, Massachusetts Institute of Technology,
    Cambridge, Massachusetts MA 02139, USA

Yuille, A.L.
    Division of Applied Science, Harvard University, Cambridge,
    Massachusetts MA 02138, USA

Contents

1
On the Correspondence Between Network Models and the Nervous System

Richard Durbin

1.1 Introduction

The aim of this brief introductory chapter is to discuss the correspondence between model networks and the neural systems they purport to model. There is a wide variety of opinion and much confusion over this issue, leading to inappropriate attacks on, and defences of, neural models. As I see it, our knowledge about true neural computation is very sparse, and therefore the critical issue is, how weak can the correspondence be and still give worthwhile information? Clearly a less precise model can provide less information, but if formulated wisely it will have more chance of permanence at a time when there are many basic neurobiological facts still to be learnt. Rather than give a general review of the issue of correspondence in neural modelling, I will argue here for a particular theoretical framework in which there is no precise identification of model units with real neurons, but in which the models still provide valid information about real neural circuitry.

For the purposes of this chapter I am only interested in models that reveal something about the function or organization of real nervous systems. There is a legitimate artificial intelligence interest in neural network models, arising from their potential ability to perform interesting computational tasks, but the goal of neural modelling should be to help indicate how functionally meaningful neural behaviour is produced by the nervous system. It may at times be useful to consider a model that is in fact wrong and will later be replaced. Such a model can draw attention to critical phenomena and direct experimental research. However it is clearly desirable to study models that perform some processing in the same way as it is done in the nervous system, and are therefore valid in the long term. Here I want to consider what is necessary for a model to be valid in this sense. I will suggest that a model can be valid even when elements of the model network circuitry are not directly identified with neural cells and synapses. In fact this seems to be the appropriate level to consider most current network models of complex neural circuitry.

Following Miall (Chapter 2), I will always refer to units in model networks as 'units', and real nerve cells as 'neurons' or 'cells'. In addition I will refer to the subregion of the brain that is being modelled as the 'neural system', in contrast to the 'model' or 'network'.

1.2 Problems of correspondence between networks and nervous systems

Because the units in model networks normally resemble simplified neurons, it is natural to equate them with real nerve cells, and therefore to equate the connection weights between units with synapses between neurons. This suggests a one-to-one correspondence between the model and the neural system. However there is an immediate problem with this: in most cases there are many more neurons involved in the true circuit than in the model, they are of several clearly different types, and the circuitry is almost invariably much more complex than in the model, involving different types of connections between different cell types, feedback loops, etc. I think it is fair to say that there is no model of a part of the vertebrate brain, such as the hippocampus, cerebellum or neocortex, that accurately mirrors the computational process at the level of cellular activity. A precise detailed model is hard to achieve even for invertebrate neural systems (Robertson, Chapter 14). This only highlights the problems faced by vertebrate neural models, since it suggests that standard model units require extra features even when the connection circuitry is known precisely (Selverston & Mazzoni, Chapter 11). There are several possible responses to the criticism that model circuitry is at best incomplete, and, if taken literally, most likely incorrect. After considering direct interpretations in which units and weights are identified with true cells and synapses in the brain, I will argue that it is more realistic to avoid such literal identification, but that we can still relate unit activity levels to single cell recordings.

The most direct approach (having abandoned one-to-one correspondence) is to claim that units do correspond to real cells, but only to a subset of them; that they are the subset of neurons that really count for the computation, and that the rest of the neuronal circuitry and additional cellular complexities are irrelevant to the particular properties being considered in this simplified model. Such an approach is powerful when it is valid, as it is potentially with Selverston & Mazzoni's model of central pattern generation in the lobster stomatogastric ganglion (Chapter 11). It allows one to explore which of the vast array of anatomical and cellular properties are important in the various functional phenomena of the whole system. In their case a simple temporal adaptation of the cellular output function appeared to be sufficient to explain the basic oscillatory behaviour. However they are modelling an extremely well characterized system, in which they know which cells are critical, and can measure the properties they want to include in their model. Even then they are circumspect about the model's physiological relevance. It seems certain that we do not yet know enough about brain circuitry in higher animals, except perhaps in the retina (Attwell & Tessier-Lavigne, Chapter 18), to make the correct assumptions necessary for this type of model. Even in invertebrates such as the nematode *Caenorhabditis elegans*, whose entire cellular neuroanatomy is known in great detail, accurate cellular modelling seems currently unrealistic (White *et al.*, 1986; Durbin, 1987).

A variant of this approach is to suggest that other cells are important, but that their effects are included by incorporating extra connections that really represent polysynaptic chains of connections. An example of this would be the frequent suggestion that units with both positive and negative outputs can be justified by assuming that there are interposed inhibitory cells that change the sign of the connection. To suggest that there is a dedicated 'sign changer' per synapse is clearly ridiculous, but various schemes using shared inhibitory neurons can be envisaged. Other examples are provided by local excitation, long range inhibitory interactions in self-organizing models of cortical map development (von der Malsburg, 1973; Swindale, 1980, 1982) where the inhibition presumably takes place via local interneurons. Justifications for cortical models are often made at this level, with units corresponding to pyramidal cells. However most neuroscientists remain sceptical that the effects of 'all those other funny types of neurons' can be subsumed into some bland linear connections. There are also clearly more complex interactions among and within pyramidal cells than are allowed for in most models.

However, what is the alternative? It would be possible to ignore any correspondence between the insides of the model and the workings of the nervous system, and only claim that the algorithm embodied in the model reflects that used in the brain, so that outputs are comparable. This is basically the position taken in psychophysical models, which might show that the model will respond in the same way as the brain to test stimuli, but which do not worry about implementation. It also corresponds to Marr's algorithmic level of explanation (Marr, 1982), and the level of the discussion by Poggio *et al.* (Chapter 19) of visual motion detection algorithms. This is a worthwhile approach in itself, but it reveals nothing about the way the nervous system works, which I described as the goal for neural modelling, and it seems an admission of defeat for models specifically based on neuron-like units and architecture. In contrast, when Wang *et al.* (Chapter 20) describe a neural network implementation of one of the motion algorithms discussed by Poggio *et al.*, they do so with the explicit aim of suggesting a correspondence between neurons in various visual cortical areas and components of the algorithm.

1.3 A less precise level of correspondence

I believe that there is a middle way between the black-box approach of the previous paragraph and the one-to-one labelled correspondence discussed before. As an example of this approach, consider the use of feedforward networks to model neural systems performing a particular task (Lehky & Sejnowski, 1988; Wang *et al.*, Chapter 20; Zipser & Andersen, 1988). As direct models these are subject to the criticisms expressed above. However they may still reflect in a less precise fashion the way that the task is carried out in the neural system. The suggestion is that there can be a large class of computational systems which operate in a similar way, and which include both network models and the neural system they model. The similarities that we require are that all the systems in the class use comparable representations, and that they derive the representations in sequence from each other in a comparable fashion. This does not necessarily imply that the systems have equivalent connectivity diagrams and computational details. In particular, the circuitry of the neural system may be much more complicated than that of the model systems. This level of correspondence will be referred to as the analogy level in the following, and models viewed in this way as analogy level models, or imprecise models.

By 'representations' I mean the firing patterns over the units for particular inputs and the joint unit response characteristics of units over a range of inputs. These are the phenomena that can be measured by neurophysiological techniques, and it at this level that the models are compared to data. I am claiming that it may be legitimate to compare the response properties of units in some section of the model network with those of cells in a corresponding subregion of the neural system, even when the respective circuitry is not directly equivalent. There is still a correspondence, but now at the level of regions or layers, not individual cells. The feedforward models mentioned above all contain (and/or generate) units that show similar receptive field properties to those of cells in the corresponding brain area, satisfying the first of the proposed requirements.

The second requirement, that computations between representations are carried out in a comparable fashion, is not so clearly established. The obvious similarities between model and neural system are that the computation is carried out by layers of parallel units receiving distributed input from other layers, and that the output of each unit is only marginally affected by any one input, so that information is carried in a distributed fashion by joint action of many units. It appears that these facts are quite constraining, since the network considered by Zipser & Andersen, which aligns two maps dynamically, requires a large number of units to perform a calculation that is in principle fairly simple. It is significant that the equivalent neural system in the brain seems to require a similarly extensive system. In part the potential value of the models of Lehky & Sejnowski (1988) and Wang *et al.* (Chapter 20) is that they make predictions about how particular computations are carried out. They consequently may give insight into the functional relevance of visual cortical cells with particular response properties, suggesting how those properties might be generated, and what they may be used for.

In Chapter 10 Kristan *et al.* consider a feedforward network model of the leech circuitry for responding to touch. In this case the cells at the input and output stages of the neural system are reproducibly identifiable and well characterized. They are connected via an unknown number of interneurons using polysynaptic as well as disynaptic connections. The model is a three-layer network, of the same type as considered above (Lehky & Sejnowski, 1988; Zipser & Andersen, 1988). The aim of the model is to suggest possible patterns of activity on the interneurons over a variety of different tasks for which the input and output representations are known. The authors are cautious about the correspondence between the model and neural circuitry, and state that their purpose was to suggest testable hypotheses about interneuron activity patterns. However, any correspondence that there is must be at the analogy level considered above, because the interneuronal circuitry is known to be more complex than that modelled.

1.3.1   *Simple associative networks as neural models*

The relationship of basic associative learning networks, such as those of Rosenblatt (1962), Longuet-Higgins *et al.* (1970) and Hopfield (1982), to learning in the brain can also best be analysed at the analogy level. In no case do these models purport to accurately model memory storage in a particular area of the brain. However there is a strong argument that they share certain properties that are typical of neural memory, such as robustness, completion and generalization. These properties arise from similarities of operation, i.e. distributed representation of information in synaptic connections set by local interactions. It seems likely that information storage in various places in the brain may well depend on similar operating principles (cerebellum: Ito, 1984; spinal cord: Kullmann, Chapter 15; hippocampus: Rolls, Chapter 8), and therefore fall into the same class of computational systems as the models. If this is true, then in an important sense the models capture a key feature of information storage for those neural systems, even if in the different neural systems the actual cellular mechanisms used may be quite different, and may involve distinct types of cells. Clearly, more detailed information about the biological mechanisms used in a specific neural system could restrict the class of possible computational systems to a particular subclass, which would lead to stronger predictions about the types of representation used (for example simple Hebbian algorithms work best with uncorrelated patterns; see Mitchison, Chapter 3).

1.3.2   *Self-organizing models for neural maps*

A third example of the value of considering models at the analogy level is provided by a series of models for the spatial self-organization of brain areas that contain sensory or motor maps (Willshaw & von der Malsburg, 1976; Swindale, 1980, 1982; Durbin & Willshaw, 1987; Kohonen, 1987). There are many examples of neural maps in different regions of the nervous system; in most cases properties are mapped on a surface, such as the retino-tectal map on the tectum, and sensory maps on cortex. The models all operate by training a sheet of units, representing the neural surface, on stimuli which sample the mapped properties. For each presented stimulus there is some form of competition between activities of units on the sheet. For example Kohonen (1987) assumes a 'winner take all' competition, while Durbin & Willshaw (1987) assume normalization of responses, and Willshaw & von der Malsburg (1976) and Swindale (1980, 1982) consider a centre-surround operation. There is substantial evidence for competition playing an important role during map formation in many different neural mapping situations. After competition has taken place, the response properties of the remaining active units are changed so as to respond better to the presented stimulus. This is achieved by some form of Hebbian or error-correcting learning term. When averaged over a large number of stimulus presentations the competition and learning phases ensure that all the range of stimuli are well represented on the sheet of units.

In addition to the Hebbian learning term, there is in each model an additional term to make neighbouring units in the sheet tend to represent similar stimuli. This can be effected either by a 'leakage' of activity to neighbours (either during competition, Willshaw & von der Malsburg, 1976, or afterwards, Kohonen, 1987), or by direct adaptation of the response properties of neighbouring units so as to make them more similar (Durbin & Willshaw, 1987). Both strategies could correspond to some form of local excitatory interaction, which would be neurally quite reasonable. One important point is that self-organization does not have to start from a completely disordered representation; in fact the models operate best in refining a crude pre-established map. This corresponds well with the development of many neural maps, which show some initial spatial organization arising from order in the afferent projections. An additional feature is that the models tend to operate better when the local interactions are initially more extended, then refine as the map sharpens its structure. Again this reflects what is seen during development of maps, that receptive field sizes narrow as the map sharpens up.

We have seen that all these map-making models, which superficially appear quite different, have similar underlying principles; empirically they all produce similar results, which are also similar to real neural maps (Ritter & Schulten, 1986). I would argue that the worth of the models is reflected in the extent to which the development of real neural maps depends on these principles, perhaps instantiated by different mechanisms in different areas of the brain, rather than by the degree of detailed correspondence of the mechanism proposed. This is precisely the analogy level of correspondence described above.

1.4 Discussion

In a sense, in suggesting that the correspondence between most current network models and the nervous system should be considered at the analogy level, I am arguing for robustness in neural models. In addition to insensitivity to parameter changes, I am suggesting that it is important that there is also robustness to changes in unit properties, architectures and interaction rules. It will often be the common ground between a collection of models and the neural system that is important, rather than the detailed properties of any one model. This approach is necessary because of our lack of basic knowledge about the brain areas being modelled. Conversely, it means that many detailed criticisms, that particular properties of modelling units are not seen in real neurons, are less relevant. For instance it would be inappropriate to criticize a feedforward layered network model for having both positive and negative output from each unit, because several studies have shown that when units are restricted to being all excitatory or all inhibitory a slightly larger network gives almost identical results, including comparable unit response properties (Parker, 1985).

Of course, in order to claim exemption from criticisms on the grounds of robustness, the robustness must be shown to be sufficiently strong such that the neural system is contained in the class of systems being considered. This is what is hard to establish. There are two possible approaches: comparison of the results of lots of variant models to data, and theoretical analysis showing generality of the phenomenon being modelled. The significance of basic associative nets as models of neural learning, outlined above, provides an example of the first approach; similarly for the self-organizing models. A good example of the theoretical approach is provided by Miller *et al.* (1986), who characterize the basic types of receptive field that arise in competitive Hebbian models such as described by Linsker (1986a, b, 1987), Yuille & Kammen (Chapter 21) and Miller & Stryker (1988). In these models a Hebbian weight modification rule, together with competition between the input weights to a unit, results in development of receptive field structures like those seen in visual cortex. The developmental update rule can be viewed as an operator whose behaviour is dependent on spatial correlations in the input. Whatever complex non-linear interactions are involved, the eigenfunctions of the linearized operator determine the basic forms of the receptive fields, which arise from symmetry-breaking of an undifferentiated field (Yuille & Kammen, Chapter 21). The basic form of the eigenfunctions can be calculated analytically (Miller *et al.*, 1986). The theory therefore covers a wide variety of models (including, in addition to those already mentioned, Swindale, 1980, and Pearson *et al.*, 1987) and possible biological situations.

Although it does not achieve the final reductionist goal, there are several ways in which an imprecise model can help us understand the nervous system. First, it suggests certain basic mechanisms that should have neural instantiations, for which neuroscientists can then search. An example is Hebbian synaptic modification, for which there now seems to be a plausible mechanism in the hippocampus involving NMDA receptors (Nicoll *et al.*, 1988). In this case the basic modelling idea of synaptic strength increase under concurrent pre- and post-synaptic activity is important, although the details of the learning rule and local circuitry used in the hippocampus are unknown. Second, it can help identify critical physiological properties for particular tasks. Testable hypotheses concerning the output responses to various stimuli can be generated in any algorithmic model. In addition, even imprecise neural models will also generate predicted cellular response properties at intermediate levels of computation (Kristan *et al.*, Chapter 10). These can then be compared with the recorded properties of cells presented with the equivalent more complex stimuli (Allman *et al.*, 1985). Third, it can lead to new psychological models, based on components and structures that are effective in modelling the physiological data (Rumelhart & McClelland, 1986).

In summary, I have sought to justify imprecise models on the basis of their belonging to a class of comparable systems that is sufficiently broad to contain the neural system being modelled. A consequence is that the relationship of a new model to other previous models is important, in addition to its relationship to neuronal data. The reason for this is that the more that a set of related models reflecting various known features of the neural system show the same basic property, the more likely it is that they are expressing a general truth also expressed in the nervous system. Another consequence is that it is probably unhelpful to include highly detailed representations of cellular properties in models of large scale computations over entire brain areas, whose local circuitry is largely a mystery. On the other hand, it can often be worthwhile to incorporate elements of more realistic neural processing into models; it is just such an approach that is likely to turn up new ideas which are valid even in incomplete models of neuronal circuitry. Overall, the analogy level approach is obviously not as satisfying as being able to directly follow the interactions of individual neurons via their synapses (Selverston & Mazzoni, Chapter 11), but this should not obscure its value in cases where a precise model is clearly overambitious. Meanwhile there is plenty of scope for both modelling and neuroscience to tighten up the correspondence, by establishing more facts about the neural systems that allow more restrictive classes of theoretical systems to be considered.

Acknowledgement

Although I take full responsibility for the views expressed here, I owe a significant debt to Graeme Mitchison for many stimulating conversations, and some sound advice on this manuscript. I also thank King's College, Cambridge, for a research fellowship. I am presently a Lucille P. Markey visiting fellow at Stanford University.

References

Allman J., Miezin F. & McGuiness E. (1985) Stimulus specific responses from beyond the classical receptive field: neurophysiological mechanisms for local-global comparisons in visual neurons. **Ann. Rev. Neurosci. 8**, pp. 407-430

Durbin R.M. (1987) **Studies on the organisation and development of the nervous system of *Caenorhabditis elegans*.** Ph.D. Thesis, Cambridge University.

Durbin R.M. & Willshaw D.J. (1987) An analogue approach to the travelling salesman problem using an elastic net method. **Nature 326**, pp. 689-691

Hopfield J.J. (1982) Neural networks and physical systems with emergent collective computational abilities. **Proc. Nat. Acad. Sci. USA 79**, pp. 2554-2558

Ito M. (1984) **The cerebellum and neural control**. Raven, New York.

Kohonen T. (1987) **Self-organisation and associative memory**. 2nd edition, Springer-Verlag, Berlin.

Lehky S.R. & Sejnowski T.J. (1988) Network model of shape-from-shading: Neural function arises from both receptive and projective fields. **Nature 333**, pp. 452-454

Linsker R. (1986a) From basic network principles to neural architecture: emergence of spatial-opponent cells. **Proc. Nat. Acad. Sci. USA 83**, pp. 7508-7512

Linsker R. (1986b) From basic network principles to neural architecture: emergence of orientation-selective cells. **Proc. Nat. Acad. Sci. USA 83**, pp. 8390-8394

Linsker R. (1987) From basic network principles to neural architecture: emergence of orientation columns. **Proc. Nat. Acad. Sci. USA 83**, pp. 8779-8783

Longuet-Higgins H.C., Willshaw D.J. & Buneman O.P. (1970) Theories of associative recall. **Quart. Rev. Biophys. 3**, pp. 223-244

von der Malsburg C. (1973) Self-organisation of orientation sensitive cells in the striate cortex. **Kybernetik. 14**, pp. 85-100

Marr D. (1982) **Vision**. W.H. Freeman, San Francisco.

Miller K.D., Keller J.B. & Stryker M.P. (1986) Models for the formation of ocular dominance columns solved by linear stability analysis. **Soc. Neurosci. Abstr. 12**, p. 1373

Miller K.D. & Stryker M.P. (1988) Models for the formation of ocular dominance columns: computational results solved by linear stability analysis. **Soc. Neurosci. Abstr. 14**, p. 1122

Nicoll R.A., Kauer J.A. & Malenka R.C. (1988) The current excitement in long-term potentiation. **Neuron 1**, pp. 97-103

Parker D.B. (1985) **Learning-Logic**, TR-47, Center for Computational Research in Economics and Management Science, MIT.

Pearson J.C., Finkel L.H. & Edelman G.M. (1987) Plasticity in the organization of adult cerebral cortical maps: a computer simulation based on neuronal group selection. **J. Neurosci. 7**, pp. 4209-4223

Rosenblatt F. (1962) **Principles of neurodynamics**. Spartan, New York.

Ritter H. & Schulten K. (1986) On the stationary state of Kohonen's self-organising sensory mapping. **Biol. Cybern. 54**, pp. 99-106

Rumelhart D.E. & McClelland J.L. (1986) **Parallel Distributed Processing: explorations in the microstructure of cognition**. Vols 1 & 2, MIT Press. Cambridge, Mass.

Swindale N.V. (1980) A model of the formation of ocular dominance stripes. **Proc. Roy. Soc. Lond. B. 208**, pp. 243-64

Swindale N.V. (1982) A model of the formation of orientation columns. **Proc. Roy. Soc. Lond. B. 215**, pp. 211-230

White J.G., Southgate E., Thomson J.N. & Brenner S. (1986) The structure of the nervous system of *Caenorhabditis elegans*. **Phil. Trans. R. Soc. Lond. B. 314**, pp. 1-340

Willshaw D.J. & von der Malsburg C. (1976) How patterned neural connections can be set up by self-organisation. **Proc. Roy. Soc. Lond. B. 194**, pp. 431-445

Zipser D. & Andersen R.A. (1988) A back-propagation programmed network that simulates response properties of a subset of posterior parietal neurons. **Nature 331**, pp. 679-684

2

The Diversity of Neuronal Properties

Christopher Miall

Summary

Neurons in biology adopt very diverse forms, both in their shape and in their range of physiological properties. The units in connectionist networks are much simpler, but how much of the simplification is justified? A clear answer is difficult to give because of our poor understanding of neuronal function when embedded in networks. To advance, it seems we will need methods to define the computational role of units in place within artificial and biological networks. We are probably safe in assuming that the very wide range of neuron types or classes identified on the basis of their morphological features does not reflect an equal range of operational types. However, a broad range of computational types is seen. In particular, time dependent properties of biological neurons are ubiquitous and varied, and are likely to be important to their computational abilities. I will argue that the current forms of neural networks, while suitable for some computational tasks, have an impoverished temporal repertoire and so are unsuited to many time dependent operations faced by animals.

2.1 Introduction

The recent widespread discussion of artificial neural networks may yet have a major impact on the way neurobiologists approach the real networks that they study. Some of the ways the two fields are beginning to influence each other are clearly shown in this book (Chapters 7 - 11). However, the current neural network models comprise units that are a very long way from real neurons in their behaviour (Chapters 11 - 14 & 16). It is not clear to what extent artificial networks will help in the analysis of biological networks, nor whether more biological data will aid computer scientists in designing more powerful computational systems. Certainly, the current generation of connectionist models are impoverished in the behaviour of their units: what we must now discover are the right properties to include into our simulations. Hillis (1988) has argued that if we get the *basic* features right, what emerges from massive parallelism may be an accurate model of neural operations; the details will be relatively unimportant. This argument is appealing. I believe that to continue to simulate neural systems, with the aid of learning algorithms coming from the connectionist models, will be as helpful to us in reaching these basic features as will be neurophysiological endeavours.

In this chapter, therefore, I want to present some arguments about the relationships between neurobiology and connectionism, mainly from a biological perspective, which can be roughly divided into four themes. I should say at the outset that the boundaries between these are not always sharp and so some points I raise may well relate to more than one 'theme'. I should also make clear the terminology that I will use. Unless quotation marks are used, the terms *neuron* or *cell* will refer only to biological neurons; the term *unit* will be reserved for artificial 'neural' networks.

The four themes to be addressed are framed around comments that have been made by neurobiologists against connectionist models as models of the nervous system. They are:

1) neurons have complex physiological properties that are important to their computational function; in particular their time dependent properties are missing in most model units;

2) neurons have more complex and variable connections to other neurons than do connectionist units;

3) the architecture of connectionist models is biologically unrealistic;

4) connectionist learning rules are biologically unrealistic.

Many points about the biology of neurons that could be included in a discussion of these topics have been made before (Crick & Asanuma, 1986; Selverston, 1988). In general I will try not to repeat these. Instead, I will discuss some ways progress may be made in modelling real neural networks, and what connectionist networks may be able to tell us about their biological counterparts. If some of the arguments listed above can be overcome then I think there is hope for fruitful interactions between neurobiology and connectionism. On this basis, I will go on to present some preliminary work on a 'hybrid' neural/connectionist network designed to produce oscillatory motor behaviour.

2.1.1 *The physiological properties of neurons*

The contrast between the simple units in neural nets and the electrophysiological properties of real neurons is prominent in this book. Can we define any properties of real neurons that should be included within the units of 'neurally-inspired' models? Bullock (1976) presented a list of 46 separate variable properties of neurons, of which 23 clearly have some temporal dependence, and another 7 are activity dependent. Surely many of these implement directly, or are involved indirectly with each neuron's computational abilities?

In general the units within connectionist networks mimic real neurons only in that they sum activity on their inputs, weighted by synaptic efficacies, and produce an output that is a linear or non-linear function of the input. The previous behaviour of the unit usually can only affect its current behaviour by influencing the synaptic weights, although there are some exceptions that I will discuss later (Sutton & Barto, 1981; Sompolinski & Kanter, 1986; Lapedes & Faber, 1986). Although the output of the constituent units is often described as representing the instantaneous firing frequency of a neuron, this is not really the case. The unit's output is independent of its previous state and can change instantly from one level to another. In contrast to these units, most real neurons are greatly affected by their recent history, and it is tempting to suggest that the recent behaviour of the cell is at least as important if not more important than the current inputs. This is because most interneurons require more than a single input spike to activate them from rest, and each input has an effect on the membrane potential of the interneuron that greatly outlasts the duration of the input spike. Once a cell is induced to spike by receiving sufficient excitatory inputs, it is refractory for a brief interval, so that further input is less effective. Moreover, neurons cannot recognize instantaneous firing frequencies at any one moment, but must integrate their inputs over some period. And furthermore, many neurons show changes in responses (for example adaptation and facilitation) that are time and activity dependent.

Can we say any more about neurons when they are put into context within a network? It seems that the neuroscientists with the most detailed knowledge of cells operating within biological networks are those studying simple motor pattern generation. Those studying early visual processing systems (in vertebrates and invertebrates) lie close behind. The main advantage in analysing pattern generating systems is that the network has a deceptively simple goal. It must produce an output rhythm in the presence of tonic inputs or even without any input. Furthermore, many of these systems have been found to produce an output that resembles to some degree the normal output even when deprived of all sensory feedback (Delcomyn, 1980). Therefore, the scientist has a network at his disposal that will produce a recognizable output, over and over again, even in highly constrained laboratory conditions. In invertebrates, these advantages have been amplified by the fact that most, if not all, of the interneurons involved are identifiable individuals that can be recognized and studied repeatedly (Selverston & Mazzoni, Chapter 11; Burrows & Laurent, Chapter 13; Robertson, Chapter 14). We are now threatened with being submerged by a rapidly growing mountain of detail from these motor systems, but few principles have yet emerged (see discussion by Selverston, 1980; Selverston & Moulins, 1985). Perhaps the two most common features are that most pattern generating circuits have some cells with special pacemaking properties and that mutual inhibition is widespread. In fact, an extraordinary range of dynamic and temporal neuronal properties can be found within these networks. This range of properties seen among invertebrate neurons is not atypical, and is likely to be found also in vertebrate nervous systems. However, as yet we have little idea how to understand the action of these networks *in situ*, nor whether physiological properties displayed by individual neurons in these systems will lead to a useful classification of cell types.

One can of course argue that the current network models address areas of neurophysiology in which temporal aspects of the neurons' behaviour are relatively unimportant. It seems plausible that much of the mammalian cortex is designed to process information quickly - it is difficult to see why this should not be so, as there can be little advantage in computing things more slowly than is possible. This may be particularly true of the visual cortex since vision is an important sense to most mammals, and in man delays in visual perception limit many of our behaviours (Poulton, 1974). The visual cortex may therefore be expected to operate rapidly, and its neurons to have short 'histories'. At the limit, one could argue, they may be represented as operating instantaneously. Other areas, for example the association cortex, might be equally rapid in operation. The success of connectionist models in matching some features of the visual (Linsker, 1986; Lehky & Sejnowski, 1988; Yuille & Kammen, Chapter 21) or parietal cortex (Zipser & Andersen, 1988) may reflect this lack of longer term 'temporal' processing. However, other cognitive processes, such as olfaction, audition and motor control, are constrained principally by external factors or by the time course of sensory sampling. So here, central neuronal computation may not be the rate-limiting step, and the cortical areas involved might be expected to display more obvious temporal features.

Even in visual perception there are many time-dependent processes, such that the exact timing of stimuli is critical to their interpretation. There must be serial operations that help process the temporal events as well as the obvious parallel mechanisms handling spatial features. This implies that physiological properties of the neurons may be important at both ends of the temporal spectrum: there may be long and short term features important to their operation. Rhythmic or reverberatory activity can be found in almost all brain areas - particularly the olfactory bulb, olfactory cortex, hippocampus, but also (via thalamic projections: Andersen & Andersson, 1968) much of the cortex, including the visual cortex (Gray & Singer, 1989). It is still unclear what purpose this activity serves, but it seems most unlikely that it is *not* involved in the information processing that goes on. Recent evidence from the visual cortex (Gray *et al.*, 1989) suggests that oscillations in cortical neurons are critical for the combination of separate attributes of stimuli. And in Chapter 7, Sejnowski *et al.* show how the temporal relationships between stimuli are important in learning (LTP and LTD) in the hippocampal neurons. This level of neuronal processing has yet to be modelled in connectionist networks. Indeed, it is still an open question to what degree a network requires its component units to have complex properties in order to generate temporal patterns. Networks of simple units can indeed display complex output patterns (Kauffman, 1969; see also Section 2.2.2), but these are generally the result of purely sequential activity of chains of neurons, rather than 'emergent' behaviour of the whole network.

The temporal nature of neurons is thus highly significant in all well studied circuits, and I believe is a feature that must soon be incorporated into 'neural' network models. It seems likely that if these models are to help us understand the networks underlying motor control, auditory processing or the perception of time, then they will have to have longer histories, and display some of the temporal features of real neurons.

To my knowledge there are few examples of networks that combine these more realistic temporal properties of neurons with the connectionist learning rules. One is the work of Buhmann & Schulten (1986), who used realistic 'neuronal' elements to solve associative problems, confirming the intuitive feeling that real neurons could replace the units in most connectionist networks without harm - except of course in the computer power needed to simulate them. However, their task was spatial and not temporal. Longuet-Higgens (Chapter 6) proposes a mechanism for the storage of temporal sequences using 'neurons' as simple delay lines. I have presented a scheme in which 'beat' interactions between groups of oscillating neurons can be used to store and recall temporal sequences (Miall, 1989). Tank & Hopfield (1987) used predetermined delay lines outside the adaptive part of a network that could respond to auditory signals. Likewise, Kawato *et al.* (1987) set up a range of dynamic sub-units that could be linked together through learning to match the unknown properties of an external motor system. Torras (1986) used a network of pacemaker cells with plastic firing rates but fixed synapses to detect and copy input rhythms. And Kurogi (1987) simulated temporal pattern recognition with units showing temporal integration and accommodation, but had no learning process in the network. Sutton & Barto (1981) use time in a somewhat different way to give their units a temporary record (an 'eligibility trace') of previous action, that allows the units to solve difficult learning problems without an external 'teacher'. None of these examples fully combines the learning aspects of neural networks with biologically realistic units.

There are at least three ways to integrate the dynamic properties of real neurons into connectionist models. The first would be to simulate known properties and connections of biological nets with the correct proportions of cell types and to employ learning algorithms to set the synaptic strengths. This might be appropriate for simulations of hippocampus (see Rolls, Chapter 8) or cerebellum. Here we know a lot about the individual units and connections but rather little about how information is processed within the network. Models could help in providing examples of how the constituent neurons can cooperate to store or transform the incoming activity patterns, and what changes in network behaviour we could expect during learning. The second technique would be again to simulate the neurons accurately, but initially to connect them randomly and use learning algorithms to teach the network to reproduce known temporal pattern(s) of output. The connections that develop could then be compared to the real networks, to test the uniqueness of the observed circuits and to understand the range of behaviours a given network can produce. This might also provide insights to the changes in networks as they switch from one output behaviour to another (Kristan *et al.*, Chapter 10, and Selverston & Mazzoni, Chapter 11). I see this as most useful in simulations of motor pattern generators, about which we have very detailed information on neuron types and connections. The third technique would be to develop algorithms that could alter the dynamic properties of the units, rather than just their synaptic weights. There is no reason to limit changes to the synapses and it would be equally possible to alter, for example, the time-constants for individual units. However, it might be difficult to control changes in more than one type of parameter at the same time, since there is usually only one measure of the network performance available. I imagine this process could be put to simulation of the networks underlying early visual processing (Laughlin, Chapter 17, and Attwell & Tessier-Lavigne, Chapter 18), where we can apply relatively time-constant stimuli, and know much about the dynamic behaviour of the neurons.

2.1.2 The anatomy of neurons

Real neurons are anatomically distinct: they have highly varied structures and connect to different (perhaps individual) sets of inputs and outputs. In a connectionist network the operational rules governing the behaviour and the changes in connection strengths are frequently the same for all units within the model. The units may even start out with identical synaptic weights. Therefore, an argument against network models is that all the units are 'anatomically' identical. It is not true, though, that a network contains identical units after training. The synaptic weights differentiate during training and some connections may even disappear (Section 2.1.3). Therefore the mature network contains many distinct units that connect to other units with different - and often unique - combinations of excitatory and inhibitory synapses.

Interestingly, in those areas of the vertebrate brain that appear most specialized for learning - the hippocampus and the cerebellum (Ito, 1984; Shepherd, 1979) - and also in the mushroom bodies of the honeybee (Mobbs, 1982), which are important for learning, neurons appear to be much less specialized (i.e. of more uniform morphology) than elsewhere. For example the cerebellar cortex has just 5 cell types and each Purkinje cell looks much the same as all the others. So biological tissue specialized for learning may be most comparable to connectionist networks, where all units are alike. In a similar vein, we should not regard the neocortex or the nervous system of invertebrates as a blank page or equivalent to an *untrained* network, but as one that through evolution or development has had many connections specified to facilitate its operation. In other words, most neuronal networks are more comparable with *trained* networks, specialized for a particular function. Their neurons have become individually distinct because they encompass some information processing capabilities. It is therefore not surprising that neurons are varied; the challenge is to relate the classes of cells in network models to those seen in biology.

Despite much effort by neuroscientists, it is not clear how many separate classes of neurons should be distinguished just on the basis of their anatomy and connections. In invertebrates it is clear that many neurons are identifiable individuals; it may turn out that *all* are uniquely identifiable. In vertebrates there are a number of obvious classes into which neurons can be grouped, for example pyramidal and stellate cells (for a classification see Shepherd, 1979), but how many sub-classes should be recognized? Anatomical classification has some justification, as it is clear that the *major* anatomically defined cell types in the brain have different physiological properties. For example, the pyramidal cells and spiny stellate cells seem only to be excitatory, while smooth stellate cells seem to be inhibitory (Shepherd, 1979). The electrophysiological properties of Purkinje cells are very different from those of granule cells (Ito, 1984). There are clearly functionally distinct cells in the retina (Dowling, 1987). There may be a morphological distinction between simple and complex cells in the visual cortex (see Gilbert, 1983). The list can be extended *ad infinitum*, but this argument can be taken too far: Lorente de Nó (1933) separated just the smooth stellate cells in the neocortex into over 60 sub-classes on the basis of their morphology. Subdivision to these lengths seems functionally meaningless at our current level of understanding.

Furthermore, it is not clear that all different types of neurons perform different computational operations. For example, while a cell may receive inputs from a unique set of sensory cells and output onto a unique pool of motor neurons, it may be performing exactly the same operations as many other cells with very different morphologies. What must be distinguished is its role in the computational problem being solved. A neuron's identity rests on its morphology and distribution of its inputs and outputs (presumably governed at least in part by its developmental history and lineage), but its function cannot be fully assessed without knowledge of the strengths and specificity of these connections, and of which are active in particular instances. Burrows & Laurent make just this point in Chapter 13 (see also Lehky & Sejnowski, 1988). This process - determining the function(s) of a cell - is of course difficult. In fact this point is very familiar to biologists. It forms a major obstacle when attempting to classify the properties of individual neurons from anatomical grounds or when studying their electrophysiology singly or at best in parallel with 3 or 4 other cells.

The goal of correctly identifying function is made all the more difficult as we learn more about neurons. For example, Laurent & Burrows (1989) suggest that separate integrative and output properties may occur in different branches of a non-spiking locust interneuron. Stratford *et al.* (Chapter 16) show that the synapses on different dendritic tufts of cells in the rat visual cortex could have significantly different effects at the spike initiation zone. Other dendrites may have localized integrative or 'veto' properties (Shepherd, 1978). These facts argue for localized preprocessing within neurons. Of course, such localized processing properties could be incorporated in connectionist networks by assuming that several units represent a single neuron. This would however need to be coupled with some hierarchical structure to preserve the distinction between *inter*-neuronal synapses and *intra*-neuronal connections. And, as if these weren't enough complications to cope with, connections in small biological networks can be radically 'rewired' by modulatory peptides (Selverston & Mazzoni, Chapter 11; reviews: Harris-Warrick & Flamm, 1986, and McCrohan, 1988), making further attempts at static wiring diagrams seem short-lived.

It is therefore rather a depressing thought that the plethora of network demonstrations that are currently being aired suffer just the same problems of classification of their hidden units as do biological networks (Yuille & Kammen, Chapter 21; Lehky & Sejnowski, 1988; Zipser & Andersen, 1988). What seems to be required, and what may emerge from studies of the types of hidden units found in a network repeatedly trained to solve a particular task, is a classification in terms of computational role rather than just morphology. What I have in mind is a distinction of units (and hopefully neurons, too) into operational classes such as filter, feature detector and perhaps, command cell that are essentially independent of the fine detail of their connections. For example, the hidden units in a network detecting shapes from their shading of light (Lehky & Sejnowski, 1988) can be grouped into three types on the basis of their output specificity (their 'projective fields'). These correspond to feature detectors or filters for orientation, direction of curvature, and relative magnitude. At this level, the function of each cell is context dependent, and I believe can only be truly assessed in as normal circumstances as possible. Hence, what appears to be a complicated multi-modal unit may be a rather precise feature detector in the normal behaviour of the organism (Barlow & Földiák, Chapter 4; Reichert *et al.*, 1985). Beyond this, the three types of unit in Lehky & Sejnowski's model could be classified further by consideration of their receptive field shapes, particularly as some units seem nearly identical to others. But if we continue to sub-divide the cell types, we rapidly lose sight of the processing capacity of the units and end up chasing down individual connections. So what is required is some idea of the variability of connections allowed within each computational class.

2.1.3 The architecture of networks

Another argument raised against connectionist models is that units often connect to all others in that layer or in the adjacent layers. Because this is not biologically reasonable (see Burrows & Laurent, Chapter 13, and Robertson, Chapter 14) it cannot hold as a general model for biological systems. However, not all connectionist models are fully interconnected. For example, in multi-layer networks the connections from one layer to another may be localized. Yuille & Kammen (Chapter 21) and Linsker (1986) employ a Gaussian distribution of connections from units on one layer to another in modelling the visual cortex (see Fukushima, 1988 or Frohn *et al.*, 1987 for other examples). And in modelling the hippocampus, Rolls (Chapter 8) has taken care to preserve the percentages of connections close to those found in mammalian hippocampus. (In an interesting comparison between neural networks and fluid dynamics, MacGregor & Tajchman (1988) warn that care should be taken in scaling down from the massive parallelism found in biology to computer models of a manageable size. They argue that properties equivalent to the Reynolds number for fluids must be conserved for realistic dynamic behaviour to emerge in the model system, and propose that one such property is the connection ratio between units. Strictly maintaining the percentages while scaling down the total number of cells may distort the network's behaviour.)

Furthermore, networks may start out fully interconnected before training, but in some cases connections are effectively sparse after training because many of the weights may be near to zero. In back-propagation, synapses do not continue to strengthen beyond the point where they are effective in a particular training task. But networks employing Hebbian learning rules often develop unmanageably powerful synapses, as the Hebbian rule is one of positive feedback. To overcome this problem, several schemes have been proposed to limit synaptic weights during training. Weights may be normalized such that the total of weights in the network is kept at a particular value, or weights exceeding a level may be inhibited from further increase. More interesting here are the schemes for synaptic weight decay, where synapses decay towards zero or towards a small percentage of their maximum strength, unless they are periodically restored by the learning procedure. All these schemes can therefore result in networks with many synaptic weights near zero. Such a network could presumably be cleared of these almost ineffective connections without degrading its performance (although a slight balancing of the remaining synapses might be required through a further period of training). Thus, individual units can become effectively isolated from others, and can no longer be said to be fully interconnected. Nor are they any longer 'anatomically' identical.

2.1.4   Rules for training networks

There is a stronger argument that connectionist models employ algorithms that are biologically unrealistic, and in this we can also include objections to units that have both excitatory and inhibitory outputs. Note, however, that such neurons do exist (Kandel, 1976) and so cannot be ruled out for all models. And while these arguments may be valid for particular nervous tissues, there are ways to get around them. For example, networks can be developed that have units that are only excitatory or inhibitory and still perform well (McLaren, Chapter 9; Lapedes & Faber, 1986). Likewise, there may be ways to implement error-correcting learning (of which back-propagation is one form) within the constraints of known neurophysiology - perhaps by using diffuse error signals of the kind discussed by Barto (Chapter 5) through neuromodulatory influences (e.g. from locus coeruleus, raphe nuclei or ventral tegumentum). Mitchison (Chapter 3) discusses alternative ways to implement back-propagation. However, to exactly mimic how the neocortex works (see Crick & Asanuma, 1986) - or any other bit of the brain - will be valuable but of less general use than a wider understanding of how biological networks operate.

More pertinent to biologists, I believe, is the argument that the solutions to the problems are an important feature of these networks rather than just the algorithms themselves. In other words, we should be using these techniques to test possible ways to solve problems and to generate hypothetical networks to test against our understanding of real networks (Kristan *et al.*, Chapter 10). We can create artificial networks by thinking out their operations in advance, which seems difficult (Hopfield & Tank, 1986); we can generate them by chance (through 'evolutionary' searches, Section 2.2.3); or we can use learning algorithms. There seems no reason to exclude the latter method just because the particular biological network we are simulating does not itself show learning. This argument for the solutions of the algorithms should not be taken to be wholly against the study of learning algorithms. Models of learning networks may be highly beneficial if they suggest mechanisms for learning in biological systems. Furthermore, we are still uncertain of the number of configurations of a network that can solve a particular problem. It is likely that different algorithms would suggest different solutions. For example, an algorithm seeking to economize on the number of connections might result in a different network to an algorithm economizing on the numbers of units, and different again from one limiting synaptic weights. Further progress on learning algorithms will be necessary to provide answers to these questions.

To continue the above argument, it is worth discussing the likely convergence of artificial and biological networks onto similar solutions to problems. Can we be sure that the networks that we artificially construct bear any relationship to real networks, particularly if we abstract such a limited set of neural properties to include in the connectionist units? Robertson argues that we cannot (Chapter 14). He quite rightly points out that the neurons in any biological system are highly constrained by their evolutionary history (Dumont & Robertson, 1986) and that they may not be optimally suited to their present task. However, as I have argued earlier (Section 2.1.3), I believe that much of the idiosyncrasy of neurons lies in their connections and not in their fundamental operations. If we can learn what are the basic forms of neurons necessary in a network to perform an operation, we may be able to successfully develop 'cartoons' (Stratford *et al.*, Chapter 16) that incorporate the important properties of the neurons without including every detail we know about their behaviour. We may also find some common principles within biological networks disguised beneath their evolutionary specializations.

2.2 Making a model network oscillate

I want to move on now to describe some attempts to develop self-organizing model networks that display oscillatory outputs. The objective was to mimic the rhythmic behaviour of motor pattern generating networks in a homogeneous network of simple model 'neurons'. As is clear from earlier discussion and from Chapters 11 - 14 (by Selverston & Mazzoni, Roberts, Burrows & Laurent, and Robertson, respectively), starting with a homogeneous network may seem odd. However, a further aim of this work will be to use learning rules similar to those used in more conventional networks to modify the connection strengths in the network to achieve these behaviours. The work therefore falls somewhere between the complexity and temporal nature of the biological networks described in other chapters and the mathematically tractable nature of network models used principally to mimic cortical functions. This work is in a preliminary stage but I hope will show the potential of the approach.

2.2.1 The model neuron

Neurons found in biological oscillatory networks display a wide range of physiological properties. As a starting point I modelled a simplified 'neuron' giving realistic time-dependent behaviour, and with the exception of the distribution of connections allowed between layers of the network, all units were identical.

Each unit was modelled with the following properties:

1) The unit was considered to be a single isopotential node. It had a resting potential of –70 mV, and a threshold for spiking of –55 mV. The unit fired if this spiking threshold was exceeded (Figure 2.1A). Unlike real neurons, the rate of approach towards the threshold had no effect on the moment at which it spiked.

2) Upon spiking, a unit could affect other units. Non-spiking interactions were not modelled. Positive connections (via a positive synaptic weight) resulted in a depolarizing excitatory post-synaptic potential (an EPSP), negative connections in an inhibitory PSP (an IPSP). The magnitude of the PSP was dependent on the synaptic weight of the connection, and on the immediate post-synaptic membrane potential (Figure 2.1B).

3) Synapses could take on any value between fixed limits so that the maximal depolarization from the resting potential reached by an EPSP was about 24 mV, or –24 mV for the maximal inhibitory input.

4) The membrane potential was repolarized after each spike (Figure 2.1A), introducing some refractory behaviour into the unit's responses.

5) The networks received one of two types of external input or drive to maintain some spiking activity. First, pacemaking activity was simulated in some units by introducing ramping excitatory inputs. The membrane potential would be gradually driven to the spiking threshold, the unit would spike, and the ramp input for just that unit would be reset. Alternatively, units could receive continuous tonic input sufficient to hold the membrane potential of the isolated unit just below threshold. In a network of interconnected units, this usually allowed some spiking activity to be maintained.

6) No other electrophysiological properties were modelled although post-inhibitory rebound and adaptation to spiking are features that might be sufficiently common in biological networks to consider including.

The computer model was of course digital with an iteration rate that was equivalent to 1 msec of simulation time. The choice and simulation of neuronal properties was dictated by two constraints. The first was to mimic as closely as possible the real nature of neurons. This is best done by implementing Hodgkin-Huxley equations or similar procedures but is computationally expensive. The second constraint was to abstract just sufficient temporal behaviour while keeping the computational steps as small as possible.

This is important for simulating networks of 'neurons' with limited computer power in a practical time, and is the approach I have favoured. The 12-unit networks described later ran on a IBM-compatible PC at a rate of roughly 1 second of simulation time (and synapse updating) per minute.

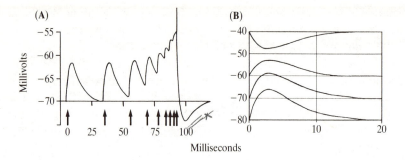

Figure 2.1 Responses of the model neuron to excitatory inputs. In **A** a barrage of inputs drives the membrane potential to the threshold for spiking. In **B** the membrane potential is held at levels around the resting potential, demonstrating attenuation and reversal of excitatory PSPs.

At each iteration all excitatory and inhibitory inputs from other units were multiplied by the respective synaptic weights and summed. The total input was then scaled according to the current membrane potential of the unit. This was necessary to limit the potential within +/–20 mV of the resting potential, and crudely mimics the effects of reversal potentials for ionic currents (Figure 2.1B). The lower reversal potential was set at –90 mV, so that if the membrane potential was close to that point inhibitory inputs would be greatly attenuated, and excitatory inputs maximized. The upper reversal potential was set at –50 mV and had complementary effects, attenuating excitatory inputs and maximizing inhibitory inputs. If the membrane potential was driven beyond either reversal potential by an intense barrage of inputs (and this was rarely seen in the small networks considered here), the effect of the input was reversed and would bring the unit back towards its normal operating potential. After this adjustment, the input pulse was added to the membrane potential and passed through a second order low-pass filter. This mimics the temporal properties of real neurons, producing an EPSP or IPSP with a time course of about 20 iterations (Figure 2.1B).

When a unit reached its spiking threshold a flag was set to indicate the fact. For only the next iteration of the computer model this unit could then provide input to others via a table of synaptic weights. It also generated a self-inhibitory input (of constant magnitude) that acted at the next iteration as an after-hyperpolarization, repolarizing the membrane potential after each spike (Figure 2.1A). The flag for the unit was then reset. These spikes were not actually present in the membrane potentials of the units, and only the time of their occurrence and their post-synaptic effect was modelled. To visualize them on the computer screen a line representing a 'spike' was drawn rising from the trace of the membrane potential (Figure 2.1A).

2.2.2 A simple network

A network of these model 'neurons' can easily be made to show rhythmic behaviour if one or more units is given pacemaking properties. This was shown by

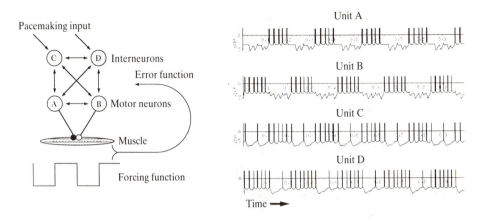

Figure 2.2 A small network. Cells A and B are motoneurons, C and D are pacemaking interneurons. The four traces on the right show an example of the membrane potential and spiking activity in the network. After testing the range of output patterns found in this net a square-wave forcing function was defined, and the error function used to alter synapse weights.

providing ramping excitatory inputs to two units of a 4 unit network (Figure 2.2). The ramps were set to random starting values for each simulation. Synaptic strengths between the units were chosen by a search through all possible weights, in steps of 10% of the maximum values allowed.

What became immediately clear was that many different configurations of this network could display rhythmic behaviour, the waveforms could be complex, and the period of the output was not readily matched to the period of the ramp function. This is because the ramps could be reset not only when they reached the spiking threshold but also by spikes induced by excitatory input from the other units. The period of spiking in interconnected units could therefore be different from the period in an isolated unit. However, the networks were extremely sensitive to the phase of the input ramps, and the same network could show radically different patterns of activity if the two pacemaking units were started at different phases of their natural period.

Attempts to teach these networks a particular pattern of behaviour were generally unsuccessful. The output of the network was monitored by its effects on a 'muscle'. The spike trains of the two 'motoneurons' (Units A & B, Figure 2.2) were linearly subtracted and filtered heavily. This mimics the effect expected on a muscle or limb by two antagonistic motoneurons.* The synapses between 'motoneurons' and 'muscle' were therefore of fixed signs and magnitudes. A desired output or forcing function was then defined as a square wave signal (Figures 2.2 and 2.3). The difference (error) between the desired and observed muscle position - or length or tension, it makes little difference what the output is considered to represent - was used to increase or decrease each synaptic weight so

* * like as for knee reflex.

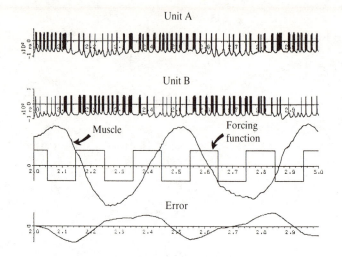

Figure 2.3 An attempt to teach the small network. The upper two traces indicate spiking activity of the motoneurons, the third trace the muscle output and forcing function, the bottom trace the heavily filtered error signal used to alter synapse weights.

as to minimize the current error. Despite the very strong learning rule these attempts invoked, where the desired direction of change of each synapse weight could be defined, few simulations showed any systematic changes in their output pattern. Instead, they would shift from one state to another or get stuck in patterns that were often quite unrelated to the desired pattern (Figure 2.3). The pacemaking units were acting like coupled non-linear oscillators and the range of output patterns that they could adopt, while large (Kauffman, 1969), could not match the arbitrary patterns I had chosen as a target.

Similar neural models have been developed that rely on post-inhibitory rebound, plateau potentials or pacemaking activity to maintain activity (e.g. Roberts, Chapter 12; Friesen & Stent, 1977; Perkel & Mulloney, 1974; Satterlie, 1985; Segundo *et al.*, 1987) but the results suggest that the type of output patterns that can be formed depend on what cellular properties are included in the model (Getting, 1983; Matsuoka, 1985). This is no bad thing if one aims to mimic a known biological system. My aim was slightly different. I wanted the networks to learn an output pattern chosen without any clear idea of the possible patterns they could form. So a network was required that had the potential to produce a wide a range of patterns.

2.2.3 A bigger network

The next stage was then to remove all pacemaking units and demonstrate that groups of simple non-pacemaking units could still be made to oscillate without having to invoke more complex electrophysiological properties.

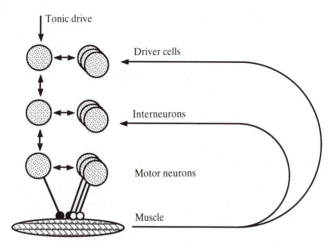

Figure 2.4 A bigger network. There are four cells in each layer; each cell connects with the other three, and with all cells in the neighbouring layers. There is no connection between motoneuron and driver cell layers. Feedback of muscle position is available only to the upper two layers, and external sub-threshold inputs only to the driver cells.

The network used is shown in Figure 2.4. Each unit is identical to the units described previously. They are arranged in three layers, informally representing driver neurons, interneurons and motoneurons. Each unit in a layer is connected to all others in the layer, including itself. The connections between layers were asymmetric: each 'driver' output onto all four 'interneurons'; each of these in turn output back to all drivers as well as onto all four 'motoneurons'. The motoneurons projected back to the interneurons, and to the muscle. The same filter as used in the 4-cell network was used to represent a muscle excited (or shortened) by the spikes of two of the motoneurons and inhibited (or lengthened) by the other two. Finally the 'muscle position' signal was fed back onto all drivers and interneurons. Connections from the muscle back to the motoneurons were avoided, as they usually resulted in saturation due to positive feedback.

The synaptic strengths were initially set randomly and a random number of units started with their membrane potential just above the spiking threshold. The driver cells received tonic sub-threshold excitation. The behaviour of the network was assessed by calculating the auto-correlation function (ACF) of the muscle output signal every 1000 iterations. Peaks in the ACF indicated periodicity and were therefore used as a measure of the merit of each configuration. A single random change in the synaptic table was then made and the ACF recalculated after a further 1000 time steps. 'Evolutionary' selection of the better of each pair of networks was used to progress towards configurations that were highly periodic. About 30% of runs ended with the network falling into inactivity. Once this happened, it could not

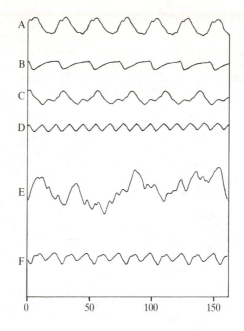

Figure 2.5 Examples of the output of the 12-cell network after 'evolution' towards oscillatory behaviour. Traces **A-D** were produced in the deterministic model. Trace **E** is an example evolved with stochastic thresholds; trace **F** shows the behaviour of the same network when the threshold was made deterministic.

spontaneously restart as the only external input was sub-threshold. In this case all synaptic weights were randomized and evolution started again.

An encouraging diversity of behaviours was found (e.g. Figure 2.5A-D), suggesting that the larger number of units in the network provided sufficient complexity and range to be able to match particular desired patterns.

2.2.4   *Stochasticity in the network*

Learning requires that different responses to a given stimulus be tested against some desired response. Alternatively, different stimuli can be presented and the response to each assessed. For my network there is no external stimulus: the network must spontaneously produce oscillations. So in order to implement a learning rule there must be some way for the network to vary its behaviour, in a 'trial and error' or 'generate and test' fashion (see Barto, Chapter 5). There are several methods to choose from. The evolutionary approach just described is one but is obviously not appropriate for learning *during* the behaviour - during the 'lifetime' of the model. To allow continuous variation of the network, I have allowed the threshold for spiking in each unit to vary randomly by a small amount at each iteration. (Noise with a Gaussian distribution, zero mean and 0.8 mV standard deviation was added to the –55 mV spiking threshold.) It should be stressed that while this may not be biologically realistic, neurons are certainly stochastic devices (Holden, 1976) and one can expect fluctuations in release of transmitter and in post-synaptic responses that would have very similar outcomes to a variation in spike threshold. This randomness also serves to weaken any effect of the regularity of the iterations of the simulation on its behaviour. Before going on to include a learning algorithm in the model, it was important to test the effects of this randomness. The same evolutionary procedure as described above was therefore repeated.

Introducing this noise into the network severely reduced the periodicity of the output, and very few configurations were now found that showed strong rhythm in the presence of the noise. However, most of these unpromising configurations (Figure 2.5E) showed some periodic behaviour if the noise was removed whilst keeping the synaptic weights unchanged (Figure 2.5F). In other words, the evolutionary selection procedure could produce, in the presence of noise, networks that were essentially oscillatory but that could not express their oscillations fully because of the randomness of the spike threshold.

2.2.5 Learning in the network

The last step in this story is to describe attempts to get self-organization in the above network from a random starting point. It is clear that many biological networks, and especially the pattern generating systems discussed in other chapters, are not developed during the lifetime of the organism through synaptic changes in a randomly pre-connected network. In other words the networks have not learnt to oscillate but have been developed through evolutionary changes over many, many generations. However, it would be interesting to compare structures of networks that have arrived at oscillatory behaviour from both avenues. It is also possible that rules may be found that can find 'optimum' configurations of a given network, in much the same way as some connectionist learning rules can optimize performance at a task.

Each unit in the network contributes only a small part to the output of the system. Their behaviour must be taken in context of the activity of other units in the network. By default, periodicity in the output can only be assessed over some finite time interval. Units should not be rewarded or punished on the basis of present responses and the effect of each can only truly be assessed over some time, perhaps even over a cycle period of the oscillation. There is therefore a difficult credit-assignment problem. It seems likely that rules needed to learn to oscillate will be similar to those discussed by Barto (Chapter 5). Therefore the rule will probably need an 'eligibility trace' through which current behaviour of a unit can be assessed at a future moment when appropriate assessment is available. To keep things simple, I have tried not to introduce any new 'neural' property to the units which might be required to maintain a trace of activity in each synapse. Instead I used the following simple rule, applied each time a unit spiked:

$$\Delta w_{ij} = k\, w_{ij}\, a_i\, R \quad \text{if } y_j \neq z_j \tag{2.1}$$

where w_{ij} is the synaptic weight from unit i to j, k is a constant, a_i is the activity of unit i (0 or 1), R is the reward signal (positive or negative), and y_j is the output of unit j ($y_j = 1$ because the rule is only applied when j spikes). z_j is the expected action of j (0 or 1) at each moment, given by its membrane threshold with respect to the average spike threshold of -55 mV.

In other words, if randomness in the spike threshold causes unit j to spike when the membrane potential is below the true threshold of -55 mV, then the synaptic weights from all active input units will be changed. Those exciting unit j during positive reward or those inhibiting j during negative reward will be enhanced; those inhibiting j during positive reward or exciting j during negative reward will be reduced. The reward/punishment signal was again based on the auto-correlation of the muscle, but because of the processing time involved in calculating an auto-correlation function (ACF) each time any unit spiked, a recursive function was applied that approximates the ACF but does not give an accurate estimate of signal power. (Instead of performing the complete ACF at each time step, a new 'entering' value of the signal was cross-multiplied across the portion of the signal under consideration and added, while the 'leaving' value was similarly cross-multiplied but subtracted.) The presence of peaks in this function was taken as a positive reward, the absence as negative. The reward function was also scaled by the inverse of the peak height so that changes in synaptic weights would be greatest when the peak signal 'power' was low or absent, and would reduce as 'peak power' increased. It was hoped that this would allow the network to settle in configurations evoking strong periodic behaviour.

This rule does indeed produce periodic behaviours in most instances, with some periodicity evident in 16 out of 22 trials. However, as found in the 'evolutionary' approach, random activity in the net masked the true nature of the output. In only 2 of the 22 trials, running for between 100 000 and 1 million iterations (100 - 1000 s of simulated time), was powerful periodic behaviour seen in the presence of the stochastic spiking threshold (Figure 2.6A). In 14 cases (Figure 2.6B) periodicity was only clearly seen when the randomness of the spike threshold was removed (Figure 2.6D). In the remaining 6, running for between 300 000 and 900 000 iterations, there was little evidence of oscillatory output either before or after the randomness was removed. Plots of the peak of the ACF function during learning showed considerable scatter: some rapidly increased to a peak with few reversals whereas others showed little evidence of a consistent increase in ACF value.

2.2.6 Summarizing the 'hybrid' network

These preliminary experiments have shown that the approach taken here is feasible. Homogeneous networks of simple model neurons can indeed be found that can produce oscillatory behaviour. There are however difficulties in using the ACF function to assess behaviour. One is that all periodic waveforms have strong ACF

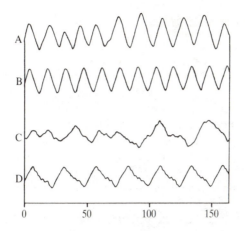

Figure 2.6 Two examples of the output of the network after learning to oscillate. Traces **A** and **C** are those shown at the end of the learning process, with random thresholds; **B** and **D** show the same networks when the randomness was removed.

peaks so there are many possible 'solutions'. The network may well get trapped in these local solutions without reaching the more powerful periodic states. Furthermore, it seems likely that rules better than mine could be produced to control learning in these networks. In particular rules seem to be needed that can gradually reduce the stochastic process as a solution is reached. Also, the rule used (Equation 2.1) does not incorporate the sort of memory trace used by Sutton & Barto (1981). This may improve performance since there is a delay between the network behaviour and accurate assessment of its periodicity. It would be interesting to develop a comparative assessment scheme whereby the output could be compared to a *known* biological pattern. If successful this approach could be used in reverse, not to generate rhythm but to recognize it. With sufficiently large networks it might be possible to recognize complex waveforms, perhaps even patterns of speech (Tank & Hopfield, 1987).

There are several ways in which the functions of units in these networks need to be assessed. Analysis of the connections within the networks is difficult because of the relatively large number of units used (with 108 modifiable synapses): as yet I cannot see any clear pattern emerging when comparing networks with their output patterns. One way forward may be to selectively eliminate single units in the network, or even single synapses, to determine if some units are more necessary than others or if there is redundancy in the network. The number of units in the network could also be varied, and the effect on its behaviour studied.

Finally, it is worth pointing out the ease with which the random search procedure generated periodic behaviours. This may be a useful interim strategy to produce network 'hypotheses' to compare with biological systems until more efficient learning rules are developed.

2.3 Concluding remarks

A few more general comments could also be made. A point made earlier, and clearly shown in other chapters of this book, was that most biological networks consist of highly different individuals. My model has a rather simple model neuron and only changes in synaptic strengths in the networks were made. As mentioned earlier, there is no reason to limit changes to the synapses, and it would be equally possible to alter dynamic properties of individual units. Another approach, perhaps more suited to the volumes of data on pattern generating networks, would be to model the different types of units in the correct numbers and to use learning rules to set the connection strengths. In other words, the synapses could be set at random and the network trained against the pattern of behaviour known to be produced in the animal.

The second point is about the 'eligibility trace' that provides such strength to Sutton & Barto's (1981) algorithms. In their systems a separate trace is provided for each synapse, providing a record of the previous action taken for a particular input. EPSPs and IPSPs in a neuron's membrane potential also indicate the synapse's 'response' to inputs. Over time, the membrane potential will be correlated with the output of the neuron. This could therefore be used as a brief, natural 'eligibility trace' in each dendrite reflecting the recent activity across its synapses. Changes in synaptic strength would then need to be made dependent on the post-synaptic potential at the moment of reward, which does not seem impossible. Of course most PSPs may be too brief to act as effective traces but Stratford *et al.* (Chapter 16) suggest that the membrane potential of pyramidal cells may not return to the resting level for up to 200 milliseconds, providing a more useful time scale. In order to 'generate and test', however, the synapses need to exhibit some fluctuation in responses, equivalent to the random threshold used here or to a random decision function (Sutton & Barto, 1981). We cannot expect there to be neurons that would respond to an input sometimes with EPSPs and at other times with IPSPs but it is probable that some pre-synaptic terminals fail to release sufficient transmitter to produce a post-synaptic response. It may therefore be possible to site the 'unexpectedness' function (Equation 2.1) at the synapse itself rather than in the post-synaptic spiking mechanism.

Third, the networks modelled here are very susceptible to small changes in spike threshold (Figures 2.5 and 2.6) or to the phases of pacemaker cells (Figure 2.3). They are unrealistically dependent on accurate real numbers (see Mitchison, Chapter 3, and Laughlin, Chapter 17). Biological pattern generating networks are much more robust, and even tolerate attack by neurobiologists with considerable success. So biological networks may have fail-safe properties ensuring that the correct pattern is produced despite fluctuations in the responses of their constituent units. It is tempting to speculate that some of the diversity found amongst the neurons in these systems may be involved in this overdesign. If this is so, we may in future be able to separate those features fundamental to pattern generation from those added in the course of evolution just to keep the pattern robust. The networks also seem to need some way to reduce the stochasticity in their units as they develop to allow full expression of their oscillatory behaviour. This may be analogous to developing nervous systems, where competition and death of supernumerary connections gradually reinforces the effect of some pathways over others, and so increases the 'signal-to-noise' ratio in the mature network.

The last point, really a summary of the arguments raised in Sections 2.1.1 - 2.1.4, is that we should look to connectionist models as a way of testing identified biological systems, perhaps as a way of learning to recognize the functions of cells embedded in networks, and as a way of generating alternative configurations of networks to study both their range and their specificity.

Acknowledgements

This work was supported by King's College Research Centre and by the SERC. I am grateful to Graeme Mitchison, Richard Durbin and Gilles Laurent for their comments.

References

Andersen P. & Andersson S.A. (1968) **Physiological basis of the alpha rhythm.** Appleton-Century-Crofts, NY.

Buhmann J. & Schulten K. (1986) Associative recognition and storage in a model network of physiological neurons. **Biol. Cybern. 54**, pp. 319-335

Bullock T.H. (1976) In search of principles in neural integration. In: **Simpler Networks and behaviour.** J. Fentress (ed.) Sinauer Assoc., Sunderland, Mass., pp. 52-60

Crick F.H.C. & Asanuma C. (1986) Certain aspects of the anatomy and physiology of the cerebral cortex. In: **Parallel Distributed Processing: Explorations in the Microstructure of Cognition.** Vol. II. pp. 333-371, J.L. McClelland & D.E. Rumelhart (eds.) MIT Press, Cambridge Mass. & London.

Delcomyn F. (1980) Neural basis of rhythmic behaviour in animals. **Science 210**, pp. 492-498

Dowling J.E. (1987) **The retina.** Belknap Press, Cambridge, Mass. & London.

Dumont J.P.C. & Robertson R.M. (1986) Neuronal circuits: An evolutionary perspective. **Science 233**, pp. 849-851

Friesen W.O. & Stent G.S. (1977) Generation of a locomotory rhythm by a neural network with recurrent cyclic inhibition. **Biol. Cybern. 28**, pp. 27-40

Frohn H., Geiger H. & Singer W. (1987) A self-organizing neural network sharing features of the mammalian visual system. **Biol. Cybern. 55**, pp. 333-344

Fukushima K. (1988) Neocognitron: A hierarchical neural network capable of visual pattern recognition. **Neural Networks 1**, pp. 119-130

Getting P. (1983) Mechanisms of pattern generation underlying swimming in *Tritonia*. II. Network reconstruction. **J. Neurophysiol. 83**, pp. 1017-1035

Gilbert C.D. (1983) Microcircuitry of the visual cortex. **Ann. Rev. Neurosci. 6**, pp. 217-248

Gray C.M., König P., Engel A.K. & Singer W. (1989) Oscillatory responses in cat visual cortex exhibit inter-columnar synchronization which reflects global stimulus properties. **Nature 338**, pp. 334-337

Gray C.M. & Singer W. (1989) Neuronal oscillation in orientation columns of cat visual cortex. **Proc. Nat. Acad. Sci. USA 86**, pp. 1698-1702

Harris-Warrick M. & Flamm R.E. (1986) Chemical modulation of a small central pattern generator circuit. **TINS 9**, pp. 432-436

Hillis W.D. (1988) Intelligence as an emergent behaviour; or, The songs of Eden. **Proc. Am. Acad. Arts & Sci. 117**, pp. 175-189

Holden A.V. (1976) **Models of stochastic activity of neurons.** Springer, Berlin.

Hopfield J.J. & Tank D.W. (1986) Computing with neural circuits: a model. **Science 233**, pp. 625-633

Ito M. (1984) **The cerebellum and neural control.** Raven Press, NY.

Kandel E.R. (1976) **Cellular basis of behavior.** W.H. Freeman, San Francisco.

Kauffman S.A. (1969) Metabolic stability and epigenesis in randomly constructed genetic nets. **J. Theor. Biol. 22**, pp. 437-467

Kawato M., Furukawa K. & Susuki R. (1987) A hierarchical neural network model for control and learning of voluntary movement. **Biol. Cybern. 57**, pp. 169-186

Kurogi S. (1987) A model of neural network for spatiotemporal pattern recognition. **Biol. Cybern. 57**, pp. 103-114

Lapedes A. & Faber R. (1986) A self-optimizing non-symmetrical neural net for content addressable memory and pattern recognition. **Physica D 22**, pp. 247-250

Laurent G.L. & Burrows M. (1989) Intersegmental interneurones control the gain of reflexes in adjacent segments by their action on non-spiking local interneurones. **J. Neurophysiol.** in press.

Lehky S.R. & Sejnowski T.J. (1988) Network model of shape-from-shading: neural function arises from both receptive and projective fields. **Nature 333**, pp. 452-454

Linsker R. (1986) From basic network principles to neural architecture: Emergence of spatial-opponent cells. **Proc. Nat. Acad. Sci. USA 81**, pp. 3088-3092

Lorente de Nó R. (1933) Studies on the structure of the cerebral cortex. **J. Psychol. Neurol. 45**, pp. 382-438

McCrohan C.R. (1988) Modification of central pattern generation in invertebrates. **Comp. Biochem. Physiol. 90A**, pp. 17-22

MacGregor R.J. & Tajchman G. (1988) Theory of dynamic stability in neuronal systems. **J. Neurophysiol. 60**, pp. 751-768

Matsuoka K. (1985) Sustained oscillations generated by mutually inhibiting neurons with adaptation. **Biol. Cybern. 52**, pp. 367-376

Miall R.C. (1989) The storage of time intervals using oscillating neurons. **Neural Computation**, in press.

Mobbs P.G. (1982) The brain of the honeybee *Apis mellifera*. I. The connections and spatial organization of the mushroom bodies. **Phil. Trans. R. Soc. Lond. B 298**, pp.309-354

Perkel D.M. & Mulloney B. (1974) Motor pattern production in reciprocally inhibitory neurons exhibiting post-inhibitory rebound. **Science 185**, pp. 181-183

Poulton E.C. (1974) **Tracking skill and manual control.** Academic Press, London.

Reichert H., Rowell C.H.F. & Griss C. (1985) Course correction circuitry translates feature detection into behavioural action in locusts. **Nature 315**, pp. 142-144

Satterlie R.A. (1985) Reciprocal inhibition and post-inhibitory rebound produce reverberation in a locomotor pattern generator. **Science 229**, pp. 402-404

Segundo J.P., Diez Martinez O. & Quijano H. (1987) Testing a model of excitatory interaction between oscillators. **Biol. Cybern. 55**, pp. 355-365

Selverston A.I. (1980) Are central pattern generators understandable? **Behav. Brain Sci. 3**, pp. 535-571

Selverston A.I. (1988) A consideration of invertebrate central pattern generators as computational data bases. **Neural Networks 1**, pp. 109-117

Selverston A.I. & Moulins M. (1985) Oscillatory neural networks. **Ann. Rev. Physiol. 47**, pp. 29-48

Shepherd G.M. (1978) Microcircuits in the nervous system. **Sci. Am. 238**, pp. 92-103

Shepherd G.M. (1979) **The synaptic organization of the brain.** Oxford University Press, Oxford

Sompolinski H. & Kanter I. (1986) Temporal association in asymmetric neural networks. **Phys. Rev. Lett. 57**, pp. 2861-2864

Sutton R.S. & Barto A.G. (1981) Toward a modern theory of adaptive networks: Expectation and prediction. **Psychol. Rev. 88**, pp. 135-171

Tank D.W. & Hopfield J.J. (1987) Neural computation by concentrating information in time. **Proc. Nat. Acad. Sci. USA 84**, pp. 1896 -1900

Torras C.i.G. (1986) Neural network model with rhythm-assimilation capacity. **IEEE Sys. Man Cybern. 16**, pp. 680-693

Zipser D. & Andersen R.A. (1988) A back-propagation programmed network that simulates response properties of a subset of posterior parietal neurons. **Nature 331**, pp. 679 - 684

3

Learning Algorithms and Networks of Neurons

Graeme Mitchison

3.1 Introduction

It is not difficult to see why neural networks have such a power to fascinate. They possess all the charm of self-programming automata, they often produce elegant or unexpected solutions to problems, and they even hold out a promise of solving problems which have resisted the onslaught of more conventional AI techniques. Neurobiologists might reasonably feel that this should have some bearing upon the objects of their own study. After all, these artificial networks are built out of neuron-like elements, and the brain is often mentioned - albeit with a touch of defocus - as the ultimate source of inspiration for such structures. Yet it is by no means clear what relationship these networks have to real nervous systems.

There is one direction in which this recent work can reasonably be expected to benefit neurobiologists. The learning algorithms can be used to generate networks which perform a certain task, and one can then ask whether units so created resemble those in real nervous systems. Examples of this approach are the applications of back propagation by Kristan *et al.* (Chapter 10), Lehky & Sejnowski (1988), and Zipser & Andersen (1988). The last of these is particularly instructive because the task which the network performs - effectively the subtraction of eye position from retinotopic position - is trivially easy for a digital computer but requires a considerable apparatus of neurons. The message here is that some of the complexity of neuronal machinery may be a consequence of the limited computational repertoire of neurons.

Another use for connectionist theory is more speculative, but it is this which will be pursued in this chapter. To what extent can the learning rules for artificial networks give insight into learning in nervous systems? One problem is that many of the learning rules seem very contrived and biologically implausible. For instance, back propagation requires the evaluation of complex analytic expressions and also requires a knowledge of synaptic weights further on in the processing stream from a given cell. Another problem is that the algorithms often take a long time to arrive at their solutions, sometimes requiring millions of cycles through the entire data set. Furthermore, the number of cycles needed may escalate rapidly as the number of units is increased, and, since the current models use only small numbers of units, this poses a severe problem of scaling. What hope is there of producing realistic models?

I argue that one should not be too discouraged by such considerations, but should look into the general features of algorithms and ask what seems to be essential to the nature of the task being performed. This may suggest characteristic structures or circuitry which can be used to diagnose the type of operation being carried out by neurons.

3.2   An overview of learning algorithms

In this section I give a brief résumé of the properties of some learning algorithms which are discussed in other chapters in this book. There is a loose order here: first, single layer learning nets, then many-layered nets, both in the context of supervised learning, and finally unsupervised learning algorithms. I follow Miall's usage in calling the components of theoretical networks 'units' and reserving the term 'neuron' for the real thing. A net receives a number of inputs in the form of axons which synapse onto its units; the state of activity of such an axon will also be termed an input (e.g. 'the ith input is 1'); an 'input pattern' is the pattern of activity over all the inputs. An analogous usage will be followed for outputs and output patterns. An 'event' is an instance of an input pattern and its corresponding output pattern, and the 'event set' is the set of all events which a network should ideally learn.

I consider first nets where the units are of a very simplified kind: linear threshold devices which fire (produce an output of 1) when the sum of their inputs, weighted by the strengths of the synapses, exceeds some threshold value. It is natural to assume that the inputs take the same values as the output, namely 0 or 1. The associative net (Longuet-Higgins *et al.*, 1970) makes the further assumption that the weights of the synapses are either 0 or 1, initially all 0. In the original version of the net there was a set of output units, but it is helpful to restrict attention to a single unit. Such a unit is trained as follows: when the desired output is 0 we do nothing; when it is 1 we set all the synapses whose inputs are 1 to the value 1 (and leave them unchanged if they are already 1). The threshold is set equal to the number of 1's in the input, an operation which could be performed by an inhibitory neuron which subtracted a measure of the total input activity.

It can be shown that the trained unit can give correct responses to a number of events. How many events can be learnt depends on the extent to which they are uncorrelated and on how sparse they are - the fewer 1's in each input pattern and in the output the more events can be learnt. A rule of thumb is that errors begin to occur when about half the synapses have been set to 1.

In some ways the associative net is neurobiologically attractive. The learning phase could be implemented by supposing that there is a second input to the dendrites of a neuron which has a strong depolarizing influence whenever the desired output is 1. Thereafter this training input can be absent, and the appropriate input pattern will fire the cell. Learning is achieved in one trial, which, as we shall see, is far from being the case with other algorithms. Performance is greatly improved when the input and output patterns are sparse, and in fact an extreme degree of sparseness is generally required for the algorithm to function efficiently. For instance, if the probability of an input or output being active is 0.1, then only about 70 random events can be stored. This follows because after 70 events the probability of a synapse being set to 1 is 1/2, as the probability of both input and output being 1 in any one event is $(0.1)^2 = 0.01$ and $(1 - 0.01)^{70} = 1/2$, approximately. If we consider a neuron to be 'active' when its firing rate is more than half of its maximal response rate, then the coding by neurons responsive to faces, described by Rolls in Chapter 8, appears to be less sparse than this (see Figure 8.2c), and one would have to conclude that there could be only limited learning within the category of faces using the mechanism of the associative net. But if there were a subpopulation of very infrequently firing cells, many more events could be stored using that subpopulation; for instance, if there were neurons which fired strongly with a probability of 10^{-3} or less, then more than 7×10^5 events can be stored. This would make the associative net a much more attractive proposition. Note that a subpopulation of cells with such a low firing probability (and hence high stimulus specificity) might easily escape detection.

The perceptron learning algorithm (Rosenblatt, 1962; Minsky & Pappert, 1987), which is an error correction algorithm, avoids this severe limitation, though at a certain price as we shall see. The principle of the algorithm is very simple. The event set is cycled through repeatedly; when the output is correct, nothing is done; when a 1 is wrongly generated the inputs are subtracted from the present synaptic weights; when a 0 is wrongly generated the inputs are added. The synaptic weights are no longer 0 or 1 but take integer values, (assuming the inputs are 0 and 1, or other integers). This gives greater flexibility and allows many more events to be stored. For instance, if a cell has 10^4 synapses (Cragg, 1975) and if the probability of the neuron firing is 0.1, then about 4×10^4 events can be stored instead of the 70 for the associative net. Furthermore, this result does not depend crucially upon low probability firing of neurons. If the probability is 0.5 the number falls to 2×10^4 (see Gardner, 1988, and Mitchison, 1987, for the basis of such calculations).

Even if the task is not simple association, it is clear that the perceptron learning algorithm is more powerful than the switching of binary synapses underlying the associative net. The price to be paid is that the algorithm can be slow, in the sense that many cycles through the data set are required, and can also generate very large synaptic weights. These evils can be minimized by using the algorithm below its optimal performance, as discussed later.

Closely related to perceptron learning is error minimization by gradient descent. Here the synaptic weights are adjusted so as to minimize the square of the difference between the desired output and that generated by the network, summed over the event set. This algorithm requires the output of the unit to be a continuous function of its summed inputs, so some smooth threshold function is used in place of the discrete switch of the linear threshold unit. As with perceptron learning, the event set is cycled through repeatedly, making changes to synaptic weights, until, if possible, some tolerably small error is attained. This algorithm allows the outputs to be set, approximately at least, to any number between 0 and 1, which can be regarded as a firing rate. Again, there is a price to be paid for achieving the more exacting goal; the synaptic weights must be more accurately specified and convergence will generally be slower even than perceptron learning.

Back propagation (Rumelhart *et al.*, 1986) uses exactly the same principle of minimizing the error by steepest descent, though in the context of more general multi-layer networks. It is the algorithm with the best record for finding solutions to a wide range of problems (e.g. Chapter 10). There are two reasons why it is not immediately attractive as a neuronal model. One is the requirement for a rather elaborate calculation involving the post-synaptic weights of a unit. The other is the large number of iterations through the event set which are often needed to obtain solutions.

It is possible to imagine circuitry which would allow the direct calculation of something resembling the error term in back propagation; I consider this in the next section. An alternative approach was taken by Barto & Jordan (1989). If noise is introduced within units, this causes variations in the output of the network and thereby allows each unit to form an estimate of the role it plays in producing the output. For example, if the noise causes a unit to fire when the summed input is subthreshold, and if this leads to a correct output for the whole network, then the unit should increase the synaptic weights associated with that input so that it is more likely to fire in future when given that input. This strategy requires a more elaborate kind of unit which keeps track of both the summed input and its firing record. The idea that neurons might resemble 'intelligent' units of this kind, and that ensembles of such units might have great computational power, is discussed by Barto in Chapter 5. Barto & Jordan's noise-based version of back propagation is certainly elegant and economical in its demands on circuitry; the main drawback is that it is even slower than conventional back propagation.

An algorithm which is much faster than back propagation is that used in the committee machine (Nilsson, 1965). This only applies to a very specific class of networks made of linear threshold units, and it works by adjusting synaptic weights only in those hidden units which are closest to threshold. A modification and slight generalization of the committee machine was investigated by Richard Durbin and myself (Mitchison & Durbin, 1989). In the event of a wrong output, our algorithm selected only one hidden unit, this being the unit closest to threshold, and added or subtracted the inputs from its synaptic weights, as in perceptron learning. Because this rule effectively requires the smallest amount of change to achieve a given goal we called this algorithm 'least action'. It could be implemented neuronally by switching off those neurons which have just been active in an event, lowering the threshold of all other neurons, and choosing that cell which fires most strongly when the input pattern is presented again. This procedure is appropriate when the goal is to generate a '1'. When a '0' is required, the procedure of choosing the *least* active neuron seems highly implausible; but the most active inhibitory neuron could play the same role.

We have found that, within the limits of those tasks which require only a single output, least action is dramatically faster than back propagation. Richard

Durbin has pointed out that Kohonen's algorithm for activity-dependent mapping (Kohonen, 1984), which shares the feature of selecting a single unit in each cycle of operation, is also much faster than the continuous mapping algorithm developed by Durbin & Willshaw (1987). This suggests that discrete algorithms which incorporate an element of selection or competition may be far superior to their continuous, perhaps more mathematically natural, counterparts. Since competition is a process which has many precedents in biological systems, and could presumably be implemented neuronally by inhibitory mechanisms, algorithms of this kind should be further explored.

Competitive learning (Rosenblatt, 1959; Grossberg, 1980; Rumelhart & Zipser, 1986), in which only that unit which responds most strongly to an input is reinforced, is perhaps the most straightforward example of such a mechanism. The effect of competitive learning is, roughly speaking, to cause the units to share out the input space in such a way that each unit comes to respond to a set of input patterns which lie close together; if the inputs fall into groupings, the units may come to represent individual groupings. Although competitive learning is essentially an unsupervised process, it can sometimes be used to generate appropriate outputs by extending the input space to include both the input patterns and their associated output patterns; in other words, the outputs are presented at the 'input end' of the net. This encourages the selection of groupings of inputs which are associated with the same output. If the output from this layer is fed to a second layer, where competitive learning also occurs, these groupings may come to be signalled by the firing of a particular neuron in the second layer (Rumelhart & Zipser, 1986). Once the groupings have been learnt, presenting the inputs alone can generate the appropriate response in this layer.

Rolls (Chapter 8) conjectures that such a mechanism may be used for cortical processing. Back projections from the hippocampus carry multi-modal information back to earlier cortical areas; competitive learning in these areas will generate representations which incorporate some of this higher knowledge, even when the input from the back projections is subsequently removed (see his Figure 8.9). In broad outline, this is an attractive idea which deserves to be pursued further both biologically and computationally.

Barlow & Földiák's decorrelation model (Chapter 4) also generates codings, and could be used in a multi-layer system in precisely the same fashion that Rolls proposes for competitive learning. How do the codings it produces compare with those generated by competitive learning? Decorrelation yields codings with certain theoretically desirable properties. For instance, if a set of outputs is to be associated to the inputs by least squares minimization, then the eigenvalues of the distribution of inputs recoded by Barlow & Földiáks's model are of equal length, giving an optimal rate for learning by steepest descent (Luenberger 1984). By contrast, competitive learning may make the eigenvalues more unequal, and hence decrease the learning rate. A simple example is given by three input patterns $(1,1,0)$, $(1,0,1)$ and $(0,1,1)$, presented with equal frequencies; here the ratio r of largest to smallest eigenvalues is 4. Competitive learning transforms these into $(1,1/2,1/2)$, $(1/2,1,1/2)$ and $(1/2,1/2,1)$, for which $r = 16$.

Note that one could obtain a decorrelated coding in this example by applying the competitive rule not only to the learning stage but also to the responses of the coding units (as implicitly assumed in Rumelhart & Zipser 1986), so that the recoded patterns would become (1,0,0), (0,1,0) and (0,0,1), respectively. However, this would imply that events were represented by single units, which rapidly becomes impracticable as the size of the input set increases. An interesting compromise is offered by the rule used by Rolls (Chapter 8), which selects the most prominent responses in such a way as to achieve the desired degree of sparseness.

Although decorrelation may give an optimal learning rate there is no guarantee that a given set of outputs will actually be learnable, in the sense that synaptic weights can be found which generate these outputs. In some circumstances, competitive learning may produce codings which are better from this point of view than decorrelated inputs. To show why this might be, we can interpret decorrelation as a second order approximation to a coding by units whose firing patterns are statistically independent. In such a coding, a unit comes to represent a component of a set of input patterns; for example, some set of visual features which occur commonly together. In competitive learning, a unit represents an average of some subset of input patterns which are similar; for example, some particular kind of visual scene. In the case of a learning task like object recognition, a component coding may be appropriate. But if the outputs are related more to particular classes of input, competitive learning may provide the better coding. This highlights the fact that the type of coding required depends not only on the inputs but also on the relation that these have to the outputs.

The neural requirement for decorrelation is a set of connections which can either enhance or suppress the joint firing of neurons. This does not violate the rule that a neuron cannot deliver both excitatory and inhibitory outputs, for, as pointed out by Barlow & Földiák (Chapter 4), the connections could be entirely excitatory but added to an inhibitory baseline. This inhibitory baseline might, for instance, be proportional to the average activity in a neighbourhood of cortex. It is important to note that a switch from positive to negative correlation between two units does not require a change of sign in the firing of one of the units: correlation should be measured relative to the mean firing rate (formally $\langle(o_i - \langle o_i\rangle)(o_j - \langle o_j\rangle)\rangle$ in the notation of Barlow & Földiák), so that a negative correlation can be produced by the suppression of the firing rate of one unit below its mean rate.

The simplest neuronal model for competitive learning would use mutual inhibitory interactions between neurons to select the most strongly firing unit (Grossberg 1976). However, in view of the noisiness of neuronal responses (see Laughlin, Chapter 17), it is unlikely that a single unit can be reliably selected, and in fact a more robust representation, in which several units are selected, may be preferable. A natural way to achieve this is to replace pure inhibition by a centre-surround operation of local excitation and wider-ranging inhibition. Then a localized set of neurons will be selected, giving rise to a spatially continuous representation. The resulting algorithm is closely related to Kohonen's activity-dependent mapping algorithm (Kohonen, 1984) which selects the unit that is most active in response to an input and causes not only that unit but also its neighbouring units to strengthen their response to the input. The effect of local excitation, or of Kohonen's neighbourhood interactions, is to produce a mapping of event space on a neural substrate such as the cortex.

A variant of this type of model has been proposed by Pearson *et al.* (1987). Here a mapping onto the somatosensory cortex is generated while allowing the connection strengths of neurons to vary in a Hebbian fashion. More precisely, a wide-ranging inhibition of fixed strength is combined with a pseudo-Hebbian rule for local excitatory connections. Under these conditions, groups of strongly interconnected units are formed. This simulation is presented as an example of the process of group selection (Edelman, 1987), though the groups actually emerge by a process of synaptic competition rather than by selection from a pre-existing repertoire (see Crick, 1989). It is not clear what functional purpose such groups would serve. It is possible to obtain a good simulation of the broad features of the somatosensory map without generating groups (Ritter & Schulten, 1986), by using Kohonen's algorithm, so the groups are not needed for making a plausible map. Moreover, their presence introduces a redundancy since all the receptive fields in a group are similar (because of their strong mutual excitatory connections). The resulting representation is therefore far from the type of coding produced by decorrelation. While it would certainly be interesting if such groups were found in any cortical area, there seems little evidence for them as yet. Similarity of receptive fields of neighbouring neurons is not in itself evidence; the hallmark would be clusters of very similar receptive fields separated by abrupt shifts. A recent detailed mapping study of somatosensory cortex (Favorov & Whitsel, 1988), despite reporting a certain systematic pattern of receptive field overlap, does not give much support for a group-like structure.

3.3 Biological plausibility of error correction

As remarked by McLaren (Chapter 9), the psychology literature gives support to the notion of error correction in learning. For some tasks there may be an ideal behaviour from which an explicit error measure can be derived. But other tasks, such as the pole balancing problem discussed by Barto *et al.* (1983), require the building up of an internal measure of error, and it may be that this is in fact the commonest kind of learning. Despite this, I consider here explicit error correction, where a target value for the output of a network is given.

The simplest kind of error correction rule updates the ith synaptic weight w_i by $\Delta w_i \approx I_i(T - R)$, where I_i is the input to the ith synapse, R is the unit's output and T is the target value of this output for the given input (see McLaren, Chapter 9, who uses E and A_{sj} for my T and I_i, respectively). Note that, owing to the reversal of sign, this is like an *anti-Hebbian* law $\Delta w_i \approx - (\text{Input})_i \cdot (\text{Output})$, a type of learning rule which has been proposed by Uttley (1979). In fact error correction could be implemented by subtracting the target value T from R by inhibition, (see Figure 3.1a), and then applying the anti-Hebbian rule $\Delta w_i \approx - I_i(R - T)$.

One difficulty with this is that the inhibition will alter the output of the unit, and may therefore prevent a correct computation of error further up in the processing stream. Moreover, with the particular rule given here we are led to the absurd situation that the perfectly trained unit will generate a zero response to all inputs. One way round this would be to deliver the inhibition *after* the unit has signalled, so that there would be a second phase of error correction after all the processing steps are complete. In other words, a memory of the recent activity R of the unit is retained at the synaptic site and the weight change only takes place when subsequent inhibition by T occurs.

The idea of an error correcting phase for learning in neuronal systems is not so unrealistic, and in fact there would seem to be considerable advantages in having several different phases of computation, since many of the structures required for the primary processing task could also be used for learning without incurring unwanted interactions between these operations. My proposal can therefore be regarded as an alternative to the kind of scheme proposed by McLaren, though of course Nature may well have inclined towards neither approach.

Despite its appealing simplicity, a Hebbian (or anti-Hebbian) rule is not necessarily easy for a neuron to implement since some measure of the output R has to be made available to all input synapses. This might be achieved by a regenerative mechanism which propagates information from the cell body back up the dendrites (Pellionisz & Llinas, 1977). Alternatively, the output might be registered by some further neural elements and fed back to the neuron. This leads us to consider a more general class of error-correcting mechanisms. Indeed, as soon as one goes to a multi-layer system one can no longer expect there to be a target value T for each unit as in the model considered above. In the case of back propagation, for instance, where the error is measured in the final output layer, the update rule for synaptic weights takes the form $\Delta w_i \approx (\text{input})_i \cdot (\text{error term})$, where the error term is a product of the output error (in the final layer), of synaptic weights of connections made by the unit further on in the processing stream, and of various other terms derived from threshold functions (Rumelhart *et al.*, 1986). Although complicated, the error term depends on the firing rate and connections of the whole unit and not on any property of the particular synapse. In a neuron, therefore, the change in synaptic weight could be computed from the local input at that synapse together with a global error signal which might, for instance, be generated by an appropriately distributed set of synaptic inputs.

How difficult would it be for neurons to compute the error term in back propagation? Some components of the term (e.g. certain derivatives of the threshold function) may be inessential, but computation of the post-synaptic weights of connections made by the cell is important since these define how the effect of the neuron's activity is distributed, and hence allow the contribution of the neuron to the error to be estimated. This is known as the credit assignment problem (Minsky, 1961; Barto *et al.*, 1983), and is likely to play an essential part in any multi-layer learning system. How might these synaptic weights be read?

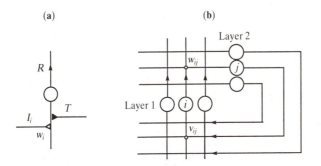

Figure 3.1 Some error-correction circuits. (a) shows an arrangement which allows a unit to perform error correction by means of an anti-Hebbian rule for adjusting the weight of synapses. The output of the neuron is R; in a simple linear unit we can assume R is the depolarization inside the unit. There is an inhibitory input (filled triangle) of strength T, where T is the target value. The total depolarization is then $(R - T)$, so the anti-Hebbian rule becomes:

$$\Delta w_i = -(R - T) .$$

(b) illustrates the arrangement which allows synapses v_{ij} on a feedback path (from layer 2 to layer 1) to be set proportional to the synapses w_{ij} from layer 1 to layer 2. Suppose the cell labelled i in layer 1 fires at some fixed rate, 1 say. The input to cell j in layer 2 will be w_{ij}, and we assume it fires at a rate proportional to w_{ij}, say kw_{ij}. The product of pre- and post-synaptic activities at the synapse labelled v_{ij} is then kw_{ij} and it is assumed that v_{ij} is set to this value.

Parker (1985) has proposed a scheme for doing this that relies upon creating reverse connections which learn at the same time as the forward connections. I suggest here an alternative mechanism, more in the spirit of my proposal that different aspects of learning are carried out at different times. Two layers are connected by forward synapses of weight w_{ij} and backward synapses of weight v_{ij} (Figure 3.1b), and the aim is to arrange that $v_{ij} = kw_{ij}$, for some constant k. This can be done by having one unit at a time in layer 1 fire. Suppose unit i fires at some fixed rate and excites unit j in layer 2 in proportion to the weight w_{ij}. The weight v_{ij} can then be learnt by setting it equal to the product of the input activity (i.e. the activity of unit j in layer 2), which is proportional to w_{ij}, and that of unit i in layer 1, which we take to be some constant. Note that this is not the usual Hebb rule, for it is not the rate of change of the weight but its actual value which is dictated by the product of pre- and post-synaptic activities. Note also that it is not actually necessary for only one neuron at a time to be active; the same result can be achieved if the activities of units in the first layer are uncorrelated. If these activities are denoted by A_i, then the weight v_{1j}, say, will be specified by $A_1(\Sigma A_i w_{ij})$, and this is proportional to w_{1j}, provided that $A_1 A_i = 0$, $i \neq 1$ and $A_1^2 > 0$.

The point of this somewhat artificial scheme is that it shows that there is nothing neuronally unlawful about setting up a reverse pathway devoted to credit assignment. This pathway would allow each neuron to form an estimate of the influence it has upstream in the processing flow. This can be compared to the extensive averaging which is necessary in the gradient following algorithm of Barto & Jordan (1989), where each unit has to single out the contribution to the output error that is due to its own intrinsic noise as opposed to that due to the noise of other units. If the reverse pathways in the cortex were tuned by the kind of mechanism I am proposing, one would expect to see a period of distinctive activity, perhaps of widespread sparse firing. This would not need to be carried out at every learning trial but only after many changes had accumulated. One possibility is that this kind of operation could be performed off-line, during sleep.

This brings us back to the point mentioned above, that an error correcting system may have several phases of operation. We have been led to consider three such phases: the transmission of the signal, the subsequent correction via feedback from the output stages, and the tuning of the feedback system. The second of these would have to happen soon after the first, so as to make the correction to the appropriate set of synapses. This phase might be triggered by a non-specific learning signal; in the cortex it might originate from a diffuse system.

All the models considered here require error-correcting signals to be generated during learning. There are certain anatomical requirements for a neuronal system transmitting such signals. They should be able to reach all parts of a neuron's dendrites, or at any rate those parts where modifiable synapses occur. As pointed out by Marr (1969), the climbing fibres in the cerebellum are well placed to perform such a task for Purkinje cells, but there seems to be no comparable structure in the cortex. The signal presumably comes from areas which lie ahead in the processing stream, which would suggest that the reverse cortico-cortical pathways are used. These are thought to terminate in the superficial or deep layers (Crick & Asanuma, 1986), and may therefore contact the more distal regions of dendritic fields, such as the upper part of the apical dendrites. In fact, what is most important for the error message is not that it should be constant over the cell body (since synapses can adjust their responses to the overall size of the signal), but that the different components of it, received from different cells in the next cortical area, should be thoroughly mixed, so that each synapse makes the correct credit assignment. One might guess, therefore, that the appropriate arrangement would be one where the error inputs were clustered together and lay some distance from other inputs. It is possible that the extremal distribution of the back projections achieves this pattern, but it would be interesting to examine a compartment model (Stratford *et al.*, Chapter 16) to see whether this was electrically plausible.

3.4 Scaling of learning algorithms

As we have seen, algorithms of the error correction type require a number of cycles through the data set. It is not clear how much rehearsal occurs in the learning of skills by humans or other animals, but one might be happy to contemplate, say, 10 or even 100 cycles through a data set, while a requirement for 10^4 cycles would engender some disbelief. In general, as one scales up a learning task there is an increase in the number of cycles taken to achieve the goal. Given our inability to simulate networks of biological dimensions, it is important to have some basis for extrapolation. Similar comments apply to the range of synaptic weights needed for the task; one can simulate the noisiness of synaptic transmission (see Laughlin, Chapter 17) by allowing a synapse only a limited number of distinguishable weight values.

Perceptron learning is a conveniently simple algorithm on which to study the effects of scaling. A suitable question to ask here is how many cycles are necessary to learn a set of random input vectors with random outputs. The probability of being able to learn the data set (irrespective of the number of cycles) decreases with the number of events to be learnt. If n is the number of inputs, then the probability of successful learning is 1/2 when there are $2n$ vectors and decreases rapidly close to this value (Cover 1965). The task of learning $2n$ events therefore lies close to the limit and can be regarded as a difficult task, whereas learning n events, say, is an easy task and can be achieved with probability close to 1. As Figures 3.2a & b show, not only are more cycles required for the harder task, which is unsurprising, but the scaling is different, being very approximately quadratic (over the range considered) for the learning of $2n$ events and linear for learning n events. Even in the case of the easier task, however, the number of cycles required to reach 90% success rate increases undesirably fast, its extrapolated value for $n = 10^4$ being about 1000 cycles.

Richard Durbin has suggested that one should relax the task so that one no longer attempts to learn the whole training set correctly but allows a proportion of wrong responses to members of the training set. Figure 3.2c shows the effect of allowing 12.5% errors in learning $2n$ events. Note that what is plotted here is the probability of success - i.e. of learning the training set with at most 12.5% errors - in the number of cycles shown on the horizontal axis. The scaling has been improved from approximately quadratic to almost linear dependence on n. The effect of error tolerance is therefore somewhat similar to that of learning a smaller event set.

A conspicuously different result is obtained when 12.5% errors are allowed with the easier task of learning n events. As Figure 3.2d shows, scaling effects have almost disappeared; beyond an initial rise, there is little evidence of a further increase in time requirements with larger n. If one can extrapolate from this set of data, the implication is that between 10 and 20 cycles is enough to ensure more than 90% success, regardless of the number of input patterns.

Turning now to the question of the range of synaptic weights required, one can crudely limit their size by truncating them so that they lie within the range $-\beta \leq \text{weight} \leq \beta$. If the inputs are integers the weights will also be integers, so there will be $2\beta + 1$ values possible between $-\beta$ and β. Consider the task of learning a set with a tolerance of 12.5% error. Bounding the weights between $-\beta$ and β will reduce the success rate if β is too small; let us take, as our criterion of an acceptable bound, that it should permit a 90% success rate within 20 cycles (in other words, that 90% of data sets should be learnt, with a tolerance of 12.5% errors, in 20 cycles). Suppose that the inputs are binary, so that the value for the input at each

(a)

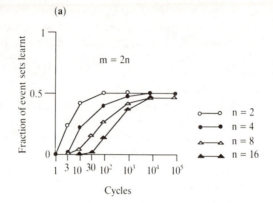

(b)

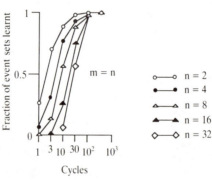

Figure 3.2 (a) The success rate of perceptron learning in the task of learning random patterns as a function of the number of cycles through the event set. The number of input patterns, m, was twice the number, n, of inputs to the unit. Each point indicates the fraction of event sets learnt in 500 trials. In each trial a set of random inputs and outputs was generated. Each output was either 0 or 1; the inputs were sets of n integers in the range 0 to 1000 (similar results were obtained if the individual inputs were 0 or 1). The fraction of successes eventually reaches the theoretical optimum of 0.5. If the horizontal spacing of the individual graphs is compared in the region where the fraction is about 0.25 then it is found that each doubling of n gives rise to a displacement equivalent to a ratio of very roughly 4 in the number of cycles, indicating a quadratic dependence of cycles on n. (b) The same as (a), but for $m = n$. The fraction of successes now reaches a value of (almost) 1. Measuring the displacement between graphs in the region where the fraction of successes is 0.5 indicates an approximately linear dependence of cycles on n. (c) The same as (a) but now a learning trial is counted a success if there are not more than 12.5% of false responses in each event set. Also the individual inputs are binary (0 or 1). The eventual success rate is actually a little larger than 0.5 because of the more lenient learning criterion. The dependence of cycles on n is more like (b) than (a), though a little above linear. (d) This shows the dramatic improvement in scaling behaviour obtained when $m = n$ and 12.5% of errors is allowed in each event set. There is an increase in cycles in going from $n = 8$ to $n = 32$, but thereafter there is only the **(Cont.)**

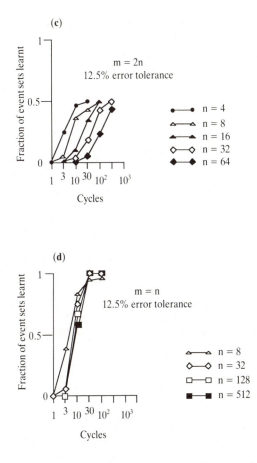

(Fig. 3.2 cont.) smallest increase which may be interpreted as a steepening rather than a shift of the learning curve. Note that the values of *n* increase by factors of 4 here, rather than 2 as in (a) to (c).

synapse is either 0 or 1. At each cycle there are *n* events and therefore at most *n* subtractions or additions of 0 or 1 from a given synaptic weight. The largest amount which could be added to a weight in 20 cycles is therefore 20*n*. As Table 3.1 shows, the acceptable bound varies not as *n* but as $\sqrt{n}$, suggesting that the additions and subtractions are noise-like. A good approximation to the acceptable bound is empirically found to be $1.31\sqrt{n}$, which extrapolates to a range of ±131 when $n = 10^4$, equivalent to about 8 bits per synapse (or 7 bits if negative weights are carried by inhibitory cells).

This result can be translated into a measure of the use made of synaptic information. If there are *n* input lines and hence *n* synapses, there is a total of 8*n* bits available in all of the synaptic weights. As each correct output carries one bit of information and as *n* events are being learnt, the correct performance delivers *n* bits.

Since 12.5% errors are allowed, this is reduced to $0.5n$ bits (that is, $p\log_2 p+(1-p)\log_2(1-p)$ bits, with $p = 0.125$), which implies that about 6% of the information in the synapses has been used. Compared to this, the associative net performs poorly when the firing probability is 0.1, for then there are 10^4 bits per unit (viz. 10^4 synapses each worth one bit) and only 70 stored events, each worth 0.4 bits (viz. $p\log_2 p+(1-p)\log_2(1-p)$ bits, with $p = 0.1$), so only 0.3% of the information in the synapses is used. For units with 10^4 synapses, the associative net comes into its own only when the firing frequency is approximately 10^{-3}, when about 70% of the information in the synapses is used.

Table 3.1 This table shows how the range of synaptic weights needed for perceptron learning to reach a specified level of performance at a task scales with n, the number of inputs. The task is that of learning a set of n random, binary vectors, allowing 12.5% of errors in the set. The acceptable range of synaptic weights is that which allows a 90% success rate at this task within 20 cycles. The synaptic weights are allowed to take positive or negative integer values; ß defines the permitted upper and lower bounds, ß and $-$ß, respectively, so the total range of values is 2ß$ + 1$. Also shown in the table are the values of $1.31\sqrt{n}$, which give a good approximation to ß for all but the lowest value of n.

n	ß	$1.31\sqrt{n}$
8	4-5	3.7
16	5	5.2
32	7-8	7.4
64	11	10.5
128	15	14.8
256	21	21.0

3.5   Temporal patterns

In Chapter 2, Miall suggests that more attention should be paid in network modelling to temporal patterns of neuronal events. One aspect of this is considered by Longuet-Higgins (Chapter 6), who asks how temporal sequences (i.e. sequences of pulses separated by specified time intervals) can be learnt. More precisely, he asks what kind of neuronal machinery can generate a specific temporal sequence in response to an input (also a temporal sequence). Such a device might be used to memorize particular time sequences of action, as in the case of musical rhythms. But it could also be used to extend the range of neuronal coding so that the signals between groups of neurons took account of timing and not just firing rate.

Longuet-Higgins proposes that the temporal patterns should be translated into spatial patterns by means of delay lines. The first pattern is sent along a slow delay line, the second pattern along a fast line; whenever two pulses coincide (in position and time) a synapse between the two lines is activated. As one possible biological realization of this, he proposes that the slow delay line might be an axon making

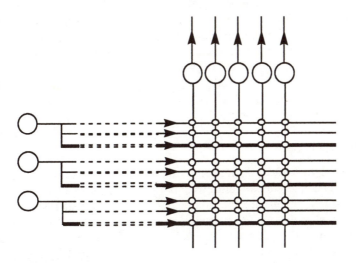

Figure 3.3 A network for learning spatio-temporal patterns. The axons of the input units have a number of branches with different conduction velocities (shown as horizontal lines of different thicknesses) which intersect the dendrites of the output neurons at synapses (small circles). There is a substantial stretch of the input axons (dotted lines) before the input dendrites are reached; because of this the input pulses arrive with different delays at the input dendrites. (The time taken to travel between different output dendrites within the network is assumed to be insignificant.) It is important that the differences in the delays should not be too large, for then an output pulse might occur during a gap between the arrival of two delayed versions of the same input pulse. To avoid this, the differences in delay should be approximately the width of a pulse, probably a few milliseconds. The synaptic learning rule could be any of the single layer rules discussed in Section 3.2, with the additional requirement, of course, that learning operates only on pre- and post-synaptic pulses which arrive within a specified time window.

multiple synapses onto the body of a neuron or one of its principal dendrites. One difficulty with this proposal is that even a thin axon conducts pulses at about 10 cm/s, so the time taken for a spike to travel a millimetre - the length of a sizeable apical dendrite of a cortical pyramidal cell - is about 10 ms, which is not long compared with the time for passive conduction, even within a thick dendrite. One can ask whether there might be structures capable of generating longer time delays. One possibility would be to have a set of axons with different conduction velocities branching from the same input neuron (Figure 3.3); other possibilities include axons which take zig-zag excursions between their synaptic contacts, delays in the form of multiple synaptic pathways, and so on.

The network in Figure 3.3 is shown with several inputs and outputs, to emphasize the point that such a network can function as a spatio-temporal version of the original associative net (Longuet-Higgins *et al.*, 1970). There is a slight difference between this and a network which uses 'time delay' synapses of the kind proposed by Longuet-Higgins in Chapter 6. In the former there is, in effect, a synapse for each time delay, rather than a single synapse which becomes committed to a given time difference. The result is that several different time delays can be encoded between the same input and output lines. This network can be trained in a manner similar to the original associative net. Alternatively, it can be trained by the perceptron learning algorithm, in which case patterns with a richer temporal structure can be stored at the cost of allowing each synapse a small number of distinct weight values.

Conclusions

This brief survey of learning algorithms has shown that, while many of them may not immediately lend themselves to a neuronal incarnation in conventional elements, they can usually be adapted in some way that makes them more biologically plausible while preserving an important aspect of their function. An algorithm may also suggest some novel biological component. A good example of this is Longuet-Higgins' suggestion that delay lines could be used for storing temporal sequences. This invites a search for extra-slow-conducting axons, or for structures that perform an equivalent function (Figure 3.3). One could also look for the synapse he proposes that learns a time-delay; this would certainly be a spectacular find.

The key element in Barlow & Földiák's decorrelating model is an anti-Hebbian synapse. Those who go in search of Hebbian synapses would do well to bear in mind that, if their experiments do worse than draw a blank, they may have discovered something of considerable interest. The theoretical arguments given by Barlow & Földiák in favour of a decorrelated coding are compelling, and an anti-Hebbian synapse is the natural device for generating it.

Error correction is the basis of some of the most powerful algorithms. McLaren (Chapter 9) has suggested specific circuits for accomplishing error correction, the more elaborate versions of which do not violate any of our current notions of neuronal plausibility. I have taken a different tack in this chapter and proposed that simpler circuitry may be possible if there are a number of distinct phases to error correction. This allows the anti-Hebbian synapse to appear in a new guise, as an element which adjusts its strength so as to minimize error in the output of a neuron. There is a hidden assumption here, which is that it should be possible to select a given period - a short time interval immediately following an error message - during which the synaptic weight can be changed, the synapse being unmodifiable at other times. A requirement of this kind is probably concealed in many other algorithms, and is perhaps not biologically unreasonable.

Algorithms which incorporate competition or selection seem computationally very powerful and superior in speed to more mathematically tractable or conventional processes such as minimization by gradient descent. The committee machine, competitive learning and Kohonen's activity-dependent mapping algorithm all embody such a selective process. This is an encouraging state of affairs since the machinery needed to accomplish competition or selection, namely some kind of lateral inhibition, has the highest biological credentials. However, what is required is probably more like recursive or iterative lateral inhibition, which is needed to select the most active neuron (or set of neurons). As Barlow & Földiák point out, there is little evidence for mutual inhibition between two neurons, but the same effect could be accomplished by mutual excitation, which has better experimental support, against a background of inhibition.

Finally, I turn to the question which, in one form or another, preoccupies those who make network models. How much computation is required by a given algorithm, and how does this scale with problem dimension? I have taken the example of perceptron learning of random binary vectors and showed that, when the algorithm is used below capacity and with some tolerance for error, rather few cycles are required. Furthermore, there seems to be little increase in cycle time with increasing numbers of inputs. The range of synaptic weights required does not show quite such good behaviour, increasing approximately as the square root of the size of the input set, and reaching a value of over 100 states when there are 10^4 inputs (roughly the number of synapses on an average cortical neuron). It might be possible to learn sparse inputs with a much more limited range of weights.

Though the scaling behaviour in this task is quite promising, not all problems can be learnt so easily. For instance, the standard solution to the symmetry problem ('signal 1 when a binary string is symmetrical about its midpoint') requires hidden units with components which grow exponentially with input dimension (Rumelhart *et al.*, 1986). However, this is not the kind of problem which human beings can readily solve, for it must be born in mind that the geometrical context of the problem is not available to the network - it can as easily solve the problem if the inputs are randomly scrambled. This serves to remind us that current algorithms are in many ways unrealistic. Sometimes (as with symmetry) they can do too much, and at other times (as with almost all tasks handled effortlessly by humans) they can do too little. The attempt to discover biological counterparts for them might therefore seem a little premature, and indeed if carried out too literally this would be so (Chapter 1). But the way forward lies not in perfecting in isolation a theory of networks, nor in carrying out a vast exercise in pure neuroanatomy and physiology, but in an interplay between the two subjects.

Acknowledgements

I thank both my fellow editors for their comments; particular thanks are due to Richard Durbin for his insightful criticisms.

References

Barto A.G. & Jordan M.I. (1989) Gradient following without back-propagation in layered networks. **Proc. IEEE First Ann. Conf. on Neural Networks**, San Diego, CA.

Barto A.G., Sutton R.S. & Anderson C.W. (1983) Neuronlike adaptive elements that can solve difficult learning control problems. **IEEE Trans. Sys., Man & Cybern. SMC-13**, pp. 835-846

Cover T. (1965) Geometrical and statistical properties of systems of linear inequalities with applications in pattern recognition. **IEEE Trans. Elect. Comp. 14**, pp. 326-334

Cragg B.G. (1975) The density of synapses and neurons in normal, mentally defective and ageing human brains. **Brain 98**, pp. 81-90

Crick F.H.C. (1989) Neural Edelmanism. **TINS**, in press.

Crick F.H.C. & Asanuma C. (1986) Certain aspects of the anatomy and physiology of the cerebral cortex. In: **Parallel Distributed Processing**. Vol. 2, pp. 333-371, D.E. Rumelhart & J. McClelland (eds.) MIT Press, Cambridge, Mass. & London.

Durbin R. & Willshaw D. (1987) An analogue approach to the travelling salesman problem using an elastic net method. **Nature 326**, pp. 689-691

Edelman G.M. (1987) **Neural Darwinism**. Basic Books, New York.

Favorov O. & Whitsel B.L. (1988) Spatial organization of the peripheral input to area 1 cell columns. I. The detection of 'segregates'. **Brain Res. Rev. 13**, pp. 25-42

Gardner E. (1988) The space of interactions in neural network models. **J. Phys. A: Math. Gen. 21**, pp. 257-270

Grossberg S. (1976) Adaptive pattern classification and universal recoding. Part I Parallel development and coding of neural fieature detectors. **Biol. Cybern. 23**, pp. 121-134

Grossberg S. (1980) How does the brain build a cognitive code? **Psych. Rev. 87**, pp. 1-51

Kohonen T. (1984) **Self-organization and associative memory**. Springer Verlag, Berlin

Lehky S.R. & Sejnowski T.J. (1988) Network model of shape-from-shading: Neural function arises from both receptive and projective fields. **Nature 333**, pp. 452-454

Longuet-Higgins H.C., Willshaw D.J. & Buneman O.P. (1970) Theories of associative recall. **Quart. Rev. Biophys. 3**, pp. 223-244

Luenberger D.G. (1984) **Linear and nonlinear programming**. Addison-Wesley, Reading, Mass.

Marr D. (1969) A theory of cerebellar cortex. **J. Physiol. 202**, pp. 437-470

Minsky M.L. (1961) Steps towards artificial intelligence. **Proc. IRE 49**, pp. 8-30

Minsky M.L. & Pappert S. (1987) **Perceptrons**. MIT Press. Cambridge, Mass., & London.

Mitchison G.J. (1987) The organization of sequential memory: sparse representations and the targetting problem. To appear in **Proc. Bad Homburg Conf. on Brain Theory** 1987; also King's College Research Centre Memo, BIP 2

Mitchison G.J. & Durbin R.M. (1989) Bounds on the learning capacity of some multi-layer networks. **Biol. Cybern 60**, pp. 345-356

Nilsson N.J. (1965) **Learning Machines**. McGraw-Hill, New York.

Parker D.B. (1985) Learning-Logic. **TR-47**, Center for Computational Research in Economics and Management Science, MIT

Pearson J.C., Finkel L.H. & Edelman G.M. (1987) Plasticity in the organization of adult cerebral cortical maps: a computer simulation based on neuronal group selection. **J. Neurosci. 7**, pp. 4209-4223

Pellionisz A. & Llinas R. (1977) A computer model of the cerebellar Purkinje cell. **Neurosci. 2**, pp. 37-48

Ritter H. & Schulten K. (1986) On the stationary state of Kohonen's self-organizing sensory mapping. **Biol. Cybern. 54**, pp. 99-106

Rosenblatt F. (1959) Two theorems of statistical separability in the perceptron. In: **Mechanisation of Thought Processes**: Proceedings of a symposium held at the National Physical Laboratory, November 1958. Vol 1, pp 421-456, HMSO, London.

Rosenblatt F. (1962) **Principles of Neurodynamics**. Spartan, NY.

Rumelhart D.E. & Zipser D. (1986) Feature discovery by competitive learning. In: **Parallel Distributed Processing**. Vol. 1 pp. 151-193, D.E. Rumelhart & J. McClelland (eds.) MIT Press, Cambridge Mass. & London.

Rumelhart D.E., Hinton G.E. & Williams R.J. (1986) Learning internal representations by error propagation. In: **Parallel Distributed Processing** Vol. 1 pp 318-362, D.E. Rumelhart & J. McClelland (eds.) MIT Press, Cambridge Mass. & London.

Uttley A.M. (1979) **Information transmission in the nervous system**. Academic Press, London.

Zipser D. & Andersen R.A. (1988) A back-propagation programmed network that simulates response properties of a subset of posterior parietal neurons. **Nature 331**, pp. 679-684

4
Adaptation and Decorrelation in the Cortex
Horace Barlow & Peter Földiák

Summary

Any small region of the cortex receives input through a large number of afferent fibres, and transmits efferent output to other regions of the brain. If the units interact according to an anti-Hebbian rule, the outputs define a coordinate system in which there are no correlations even when the input fibres show strong correlations. The idea that cortex performs such decorrelation has several theoretical merits and fits some prominent facts about the cortex:

1) It would be advantageous in making effective use of the narrow dynamic range that is characteristic of cortical neurons.

2) The absence of correlations would make it easier to detect newly appearing associations resulting from new causal factors in the environment.

3) It provides a role for recurrent collaterals, which are a conspicuous feature of cortical neurons, especially in striate areas.

4) It may account for the after-effects of adapting to patterned stimuli.

5) It could account for part, at least, of the effects of experience during cortical development.

6) It can improve the performance of Hebbian learning rules in associative networks.

4.1 How is the cortical image interpreted?

Many readers will be familiar with the picture of neural activity in the primary visual cortex that has been revealed by the work of Hubel (1988), Wiesel and many others over the past two or three decades, but most will probably agree that nobody knows quite what will happen next.

Let us put the problem this way: what can these signals for lines, edges, textures, movements, disparities and colours mean without any background

54

knowledge of the world? Are they not like single letters without a language? And without knowing what effects they produce, the occurrence of activity in a nerve cell does not mean any more than the production of silver grains means to the camera. You have to know something about the interpretive system before you can understand what the nerve impulses mean.

In this paper we are concerned with one particular aspect of this system, namely the way it acquires, stores, and uses background knowledge of the sensory environment. Probably everyone will agree that visual perception uses knowledge of images and their ways to reach a valid interpretation of the current scene; to illustrate this, ask yourself when you last tripped, or avoided tripping, over a shadow. According to current knowledge a shadow will stimulate an 'edge-detector' in V1 as effectively as the image of a doorstep, so why is it that you do not treat shadows as if they were doorsteps all the time? Possibly current knowledge is incomplete and it is certainly worth asking how our interpretive system distinguishes them.

There are two groups of people who are acutely aware of the major task facing the interpretive system in going from the 2-D images our eyes provide, to the world of 3-D objects that we can usually construct with astonishing reliability. The first are the perceptual psychologists, and few have appreciated the problem from this point of view better, or more deeply, than did Helmholtz nearly a century and a half ago (Helmholtz, 1925); that fact perhaps indicates how slow and difficult progress has been using classical psychological methods. Much more recently, those concerned with robot vision and computer image interpretation have tried to mimic our everyday perceptual performance - and having so far failed, they are very impressed by what our brains do so effortlessly.

One of the basic problems, understood since Helmholtz's time and formalized by Poggio, Torre & Koch (1985), is that 2-D images do not provide all the information that is needed for the reconstructions that our minds perform. Assumptions are necessary to make this possible, and if these assumptions are to work they must be based on valid expectations about the nature of the world we inhabit. How are these expectations formed? What are they based upon? How are they stored? How are they accessed when needed? We think that well-known adaptation phenomena provide strong clues to the solution of this puzzle.

4.2 Adaptation to patterns

Aristotle described the waterfall phenomenon, now known as the motion after-effect: you gaze at a waterfall for about a minute, then when you transfer your gaze to the rocks or foliage at the side they appear to be moving upwards. The idea that this may be something to do with entraining eye movements can be ruled out by using a rotating spiral. The effect is easily visible, though the after-movement is not very fast or vigorous - a sort of drift. It is confined to the region of the visual field exposed to the adapting movement.

The explanation usually given, and actually dating back to Sigmund Exner (1894), is that the period of adaptation fatigues elements responding selectively to motion in a particular direction, and it has been shown that something of this sort does happen with directional and other types of pattern selective cells (Barlow & Hill,1963; Maffei, Fiorentini & Bisti, 1973; Vautin & Berkeley, 1977; Ohzawa, Sclar & Freeman, 1985). When you continue stimulating such a cell the response declines; then when you stop, the maintained discharge is suppressed and its responsiveness is impaired. There is usually no adapting effect from stimuli to which the cell does not respond. Thus the explanation offered, for instance for the motion after-effect, is that continued motion in one direction imbalances the responses from units signalling opposite directions, so that a stationary, non-moving, object appears to move in the reverse direction.

Similar adaptation effects can be obtained with many patterned stimuli. Gibson (1933, 1937) noted after-effects from viewing curved lines, and Gilinsky (1968), Pantle & Sekuler (1968) and Blakemore & Campbell (1969) independently discovered that a plain grating causes decreased sensitivity to gratings of similar frequency and orientation. As shown in Figure 4.1, adapting to coarsely spaced lines makes lines appear more finely spaced, and vice versa (Blakemore & Sutton, 1969), and tilted lines cause lines to appear tilted the other way.

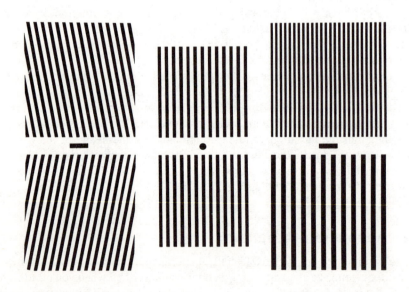

Figure 4.1 The visual system changes its characteristics when it adapts to grating patterns. Look at the black bar between the pair of tilted gratings for about 30 seconds, then shift your gaze to the round dot between the central pair of vertical gratings: they will appear tilted in the opposite direction to that to which the corresponding region of the visual field has just been adapted. Similarly the apparent spacing of the gratings can be changed by adapting to the pair of gratings on the right (from Blakemore, 1973).

Finally there is the mysterious McCollough (1965) effect. Adaptation consists of looking at a red, horizontal, grating for about 5 s, then shifting your gaze to a green, vertical, grating for another 5 s, then back to the red and so on for a few minutes. When you then look at a test pattern consisting partly of horizontal, partly of vertical, colourless gratings, you will see the horizontal parts tinted green, the vertical parts red. If you think the test pattern itself is tinted, tilt your head through 90°, and observe that the tints reverse.

The important point about the McCollough effect is that it persuaded people to realize that one is adapting to *contingencies* (red if horizontal, green if vertical), rather than to a primary sensory quality (for a review, see Stromeyer 1978). The issue is blurred by the fact that there probably are neurons selectively sensitive to these contingencies (Michael, 1978), so that the 'fatigue of pattern selective neurons' explanation still holds water. But there are at least three reasons to think there is more to adaptation than this.

We first warn against the assumption that, because a stimulus is effective in activating a single neuron, it is that activation alone that causes change in the neuron's responsiveness. The adapting stimuli will generally excite large numbers of neurons having the same type of pattern specificity, and we think it is this joint excitation that is the important contingency for causing adaptation. Thus for the loss of sensitivity that follows viewing a plain grating the contingency would be the joint excitation of many neurons all tuned to the same orientation and spatial frequency; likewise for the disturbances in perception illustrated in Figure 4.1. Though the grating would certainly be an effective stimulus for many individual neurons, we think it is the joint excitation of a group of them, and the resulting changes in their interactions, that causes changes in their responsiveness. A mechanism that might bring about such group effects will be proposed shortly.

The second point is that images are full of non-accidental associations; although we make the phenomenon observable by introducing *abnormal* contingencies, the *normal* patterns of contingent excitation must continually produce their effects on the mechanism. If adaptation to these naturally occurring contingencies is a mechanism producing positive functional effects, it should not be called fatigue.

The third point follows from this: the naturally occurring contingencies are precisely what the interpretive mechanism needs to know about to provide valid expectations upon which reliable interpretations of 2-D images depend. This is so because these natural contingencies result from the properties of real objects in the real three dimensional world, and this is what provides the eye with its normal diet of images. We therefore think the adaptation mechanism is fundamentally important for acquiring, storing and accessing valid knowledge about the normal environment, and hence 'fatigue' is a thoroughly inappropriate term for it.

One can look at this from many different points of view, and we shall first present it as a necessary mechanism, given the poor dynamic range of cortical neurons. Next we shall suggest a physiological process that might bring it about and an idealized model of this process. Finally, we shall return to a discussion at the perceptual level.

4.3 The need for contingent adaptation

Most people are familiar with the idea that normal light adaptation adjusts the response range of neurons to the range of luminances actually present in the image. Figure 4.2 shows at the top a hypothetical distribution of luminances over an image at a low light level, and another at high. Below are shown hypothetical response curves of 'on' and 'off' signalling neurons, and how they shift with mean luminance of the image.

Something of this sort really does happen; Figure 4.3 shows responses of two retinal ganglion cells in the cat. The intersections of the pairs of curves with the abscissa show the levels to which the retina was adapted; the ordinates show how many extra impulses were elicited when the luminance at the centre of the receptive field was briefly stepped up or down to other neighbouring values on the abscissa. Clearly the response range shifts with adapting luminance, and this is necessary because the range of possible input luminances is very large, while the range of possible outputs is strictly limited.

Now the available response range of neurons can be wasted in a different way. Suppose that, for whatever reason, two neurons very nearly always respond together; the available response space spanned by the two neurons will not be properly utilized, and Figure 4.4 shows what can be done about it. The top left shows a hypothetical plot of the response Ψ_A of one neuron to physical variable A against the response Ψ_B of another neuron to physical variable B. For simplicity, we have assumed uniform, rectangular distributions for each of them. If they are uncorrelated, the scatter diagram fills the whole plane uniformly. If each neuron can discriminate 4 levels of activity, all 16 possible states occur with approximately equal probabilities, and the limited representational possibilities of these two neurons would be fully utilized. The results in Barlow *et al.* (1987) suggest that four reliably distinguishable levels may be an optimistic estimate of the dynamic range of cortical neurons.

Next suppose the physical variables A and B are positively correlated, so the scatter diagram would then look like the one at top right. Clearly it would be inefficient for the two neurons to respond simply to physical variables A and B as before, because their responses would then be strongly correlated and the representational space would not be filled. An oblique coordinate system should be adopted so that the response Ψ_A is given by the projection on Ψ_A parallel to the Ψ_B axis, and vice versa. The diamond-shaped response pattern would now match the scatter of the points, and all representational possibilities would again be utilized.

At bottom right the distribution is plotted with the responses Ψ_A, Ψ_B as the orthogonal axes, and the dotted vectors show the directions of the original physical stimuli A and B in this plot. The vector for A slopes backwards, and this means physical stimulus A has a negative or inhibitory effect on Ψ_B, the neuron that originally responded only to B. Similarly B has an inhibitory effect on Ψ_A.

To summarize the argument of this section, when two physical variables are strongly correlated one might expect two neurons, each of which responds predominantly to one of them, to develop mutual *repulsion* so that if a physical

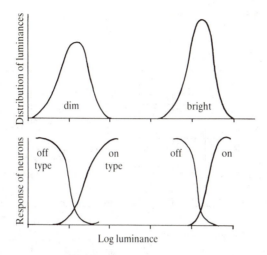

Figure 4.2 This illustrates the way retinal ganglion cell response characteristics change when the mean luminance of a scene changes. The top pair shows hypothetical distributions of luminance in a dim and a bright scene. Below are shown the hypothetical responses of retinal neurons to the luminances in the scenes; on-type neurons respond to increases and off-type to decreases, but without a shift in their characteristics when the mean luminance changes, the signals would not cover the appropriate luminance ranges.

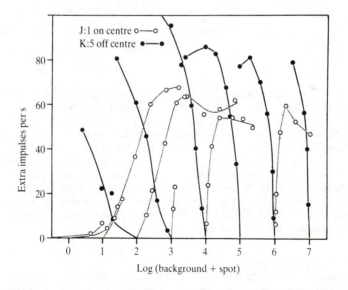

Figure 4.3 Actual retinal neurons behave as illustrated diagrammatically in Figure 4.2. The retina was adapted to the 7 different luminances at the points on the abscissa intersected by the curves. The luminance at the centre of the receptive field was then transiently shifted upwards for the on-centre unit (solid lines), or downwards for the off-centre unit (dashed lines), and their responses for such shifts of luminance are plotted as ordinates (from Barlow, 1969).

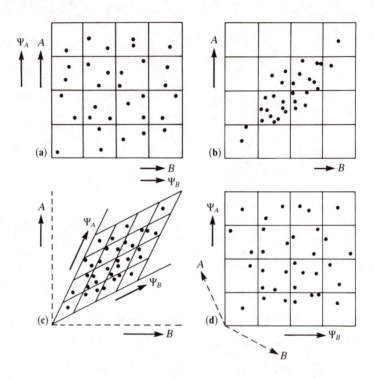

Figure 4.4 The limited dynamic range of neurons would be better used if their responses were uncorrelated. Such a state is shown in (**a**), where two uncorrelated physical stimuli A and B cause responses Ψ_A and Ψ_B in two neurons: all the distinguishable responses occur, as indicated by the presence of dots in all the squares. In (**b**) the physical stimuli are strongly correlated, and many of the distinguishable response states do not occur, indicated by empty squares. The solution is to make the response axes oblique, as in (**c**), where the response Ψ_A is given by the projection of a point on the oblique axis Ψ_A in the direction given by Ψ_B ; the lozenge shaped region now fits the pattern of correlated signals and all possible signals are generated. In (**d**) the orthogonal axes are the responses of the two neurons, and the dashed lines show the directions of the physical stimuli A and B; it will be seen that A slopes backwards, signifying that physical stimulus A has an inhibitory effect on the response Ψ_B, and similarly B inhibits Ψ_A.

variable excites the one it will inhibit the other, and vice versa. Such mutual inhibition is of course a well known feature of sensory ganglia, and the only new suggestion here is that its strength should be variable and adjusted according to the strength of the correlation between the activities of the two neurons under consideration. This argument stems simply from the desirability of utilizing fully the representational space offered by elements of limited dynamic range.

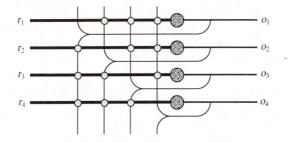

Figure 4.5 The idealized linear network with outputs o_i feeding back to the inputs r_i through modifiable connections; the strength of mutual inhibition increases when outputs are positively correlated. In matrix notation $\mathbf{o} = \mathbf{r} + \mathbf{Wo}$, so after an initial transient, $\mathbf{o} = (\mathbf{I} - \mathbf{W})^{-1}\,\mathbf{r} = \mathbf{T}\,\mathbf{r}$, where $\mathbf{T} = (\mathbf{I} - \mathbf{W})^{-1}$ is the overall transfer matrix of the network.

4.4   An idealized model

We are suggesting that there can be two kinds of adaptation: each single unit adapts to the mean values of its own input, while an inter-unit mechanism stores and discounts expected relationships between input variables. To demonstrate the effect of this mechanism we considered a simple model similar to Kohonen's novelty filter (1984). It consists of a number of linear units with inputs r_i, outputs o_i, and modifiable feedback connections between them (Figure 4.5).

The output of each of the N units is determined by the external input to that unit plus the feedback it receives from the other units, i.e. the outputs of the other units weighted by the synaptic strengths.

$$o_i = r_i + \sum_{j=1}^{N} w_{ij} o_j \tag{4.1}$$

Initially the synapses are not effective, $w_{ij} = 0$. The network is trained by repeatedly taking patterns out of a predetermined, large set and presenting them on the input lines. The outputs will satisfy the above equation after an initial transient has occurred, which is not simulated.

For the definition of the learning rule it seemed convenient (but may not be necessary) to use a scaled version of the output variables, O_i, defined to have unit variance ($\langle O_i^2 \rangle = 1$), and calculated as $O_i = o_i / \sqrt{\langle o_i^2 \rangle}$, where $\langle \rangle$ denotes averaging over the set of patterns. After reaching a stable output for each input pattern, the strengths of the synapses change very slightly according to the following symmetric, anti-Hebbian rule:

$$\begin{aligned} \Delta w_{ij} &= -\alpha\, O_i\, O_j \quad &&\text{if } i \ne j; \\ \Delta w_{ii} &= 0 \quad &&\text{otherwise} \end{aligned} \tag{4.2}$$

where α is a small positive constant determining the rate of adaptation. If α is small enough, the synaptic weights between two units will change in (negative) proportion to the correlation between the output activities of the units taken over the whole input set. This means that if two output variables are initially positively correlated, then inhibition between them will gradually get stronger, making them less correlated, and the network can only reach a stable state ($\langle\ \Delta w_{ij}\ \rangle = 0$) when the outputs of all pairs of units are uncorrelated: $\langle\ O_i O_j\ \rangle = 0$ if $i \neq j$, and as $\langle\ O_i^2\ \rangle = 1$, the correlation matrix tends to the identity matrix. The modification rule is unsupervised and local, the information about the activity of the pre- and post-synaptic units being available at synapse w_{ij}.

Figure 4.6 shows a correlated input distribution (each dot representing an input vector) and the output of a network consisting of two units after a few cycles of training.

The speed of convergence decreases with the number of units, but as Figure 4.7 shows, the covariance matrix of the outputs approaches the identity matrix at a nearly exponential rate.

4.5   Relation to Kohonen's novelty filter

The network and modification rules are the same as the novelty filter described by Kohonen & Oja (1976), with one minor difference; our output variables do not feed back on themselves, but are gain-controlled to have unit variance. As a result the output does not go to zero for a 'familiar' input. We also look upon the filter as performing a somewhat different task. Instead of learning a specific set of inputs (the number of which is smaller than the number of units) and signalling the projection of the current input on the complementary subspace of the set of learned vectors, we regard our network as learning the average relations between a large ensemble of inputs - its covariance matrix - and using this knowledge to generate uncorrelated signals. The number of pattern vectors can be arbitrarily large ($\gg N$), or the input can be thought of as a continuous function of time.

4.6   Decorrelating taste signals

It is known that the information about the four basic tastes (sweet, sour, bitter, salty) is not carried by separate fibres; instead each fibre carries a mixed signal with different relative sensitivities to the four substances (Pfaffman, 1941; Sato, 1980). This lack of segregation has always been puzzling, partly because it contrasts with other sensory pathways, but also because the task of separating the mixed-up taste qualities does not appear a simple one. The puzzle would be lessened if neural networks can easily decorrelate sensory signals along the lines we have described, so we have tried out our algorithm on a simulated taste system.

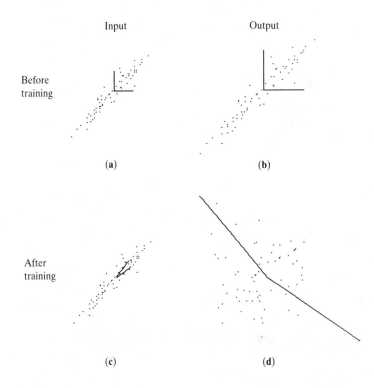

Figure 4.6 The dots represent a correlated set of vectors on (a) the inputs and (b) the outputs of a network consisting of two units before training. After training these are transformed to (c) and (d). Axes in the output space indicate the projections of the base vectors of the input space and vice versa.

If we assume independent distributions for the concentrations of the four taste substances to which the animal is exposed, the inputs to the units will be correlated because of the overlap in the relative sensitivities between any two units. During simulated training the outputs of the network become uncorrelated, but this does not mean that we get our original variables back. For instance, if the external signals S (sour) and B (bitter) are originally uncorrelated with normal distributions of equal variance, then $S+B$ and $S-B$ are also uncorrelated, as is any other rotation of the coordinates. Depending on the way the signals are mixed on the inputs the network will implement the transformation that can be achieved by a symmetric feedback matrix. If one wants to get not only an uncorrelated combination of variables but the original variables themselves, one has to assume a special property of the original signals. For instance, the concentrations of the four basic taste substances can only take positive values and in this case the only transformations that will keep all the output values positive (and uncorrelated) will be the ones that restore the original variables. Any other transformation will cause negative components in the outputs for some vectors.

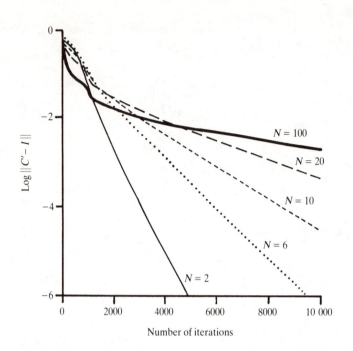

Figure 4.7 The rate of adaptation of the decorrelating network. For the purpose of estimating the speed of the convergence of the network, the input is assumed to have a Gaussian distribution, so it is not necessary to represent the input distribution as a set of patterns and its covariance matrix **V** uniquely defines it. For each input distribution the time of convergence will be different, so it can be estimated by averaging over a large number of randomly chosen input distributions. The covariance matrix of the outputs, **C**, can be calculated from each input covariance matrix, **V**, as: $\mathbf{C} = \mathbf{T} \, \mathbf{V} \, \mathbf{T}^T$, which converges to the unit matrix during training. Single-unit adaptation is modelled by its effect on the covariance of the scaled output, $C'_{ii} = 1$, so $\mathbf{C}' = c_{ij} \, / \sqrt{c_{ii} \, c_{jj}}$. Initially the connections are ineffective, $w_{ij}(0) = 0$, and they change as:

$$w_{ij}^{(k+1)} = w_{ij}^{(k)} - \alpha \, C'_{ij}^{(k)} \text{ if } i \neq j$$

after k cycles of training. Let's denote the expression $\frac{1}{N} \sqrt{\sum_{ij} (a_{ij} - b_{ij})^2}$ by $\| \mathbf{A} - \mathbf{B} \|$ for matrices **A** and **B**. To measure the precision of the convergence we can use the quantity $\| \mathbf{C}' - \mathbf{I} \|$ to indicate how close the covariance matrix of the output is to the unit matrix. The diagram shows these values averaged over 100 runs for $N = 2, 6, 10, 20$ and averaged over two runs for $N = 100$. The random input covariance matrices were generated as: $\mathbf{V} = \mathbf{M} \mathbf{M}^T$ where the elements of **M** were taken from an even distribution on the interval [0,1]. α was 0.001 for this simulation, and for this value 1 out of 100 runs oscillated and only converged with a smaller α. This one was replaced by an additional run. For higher values of α the convergence gets significantly faster, but a higher proportion of runs will oscillate.

A modified version of the model uses this assumption that the variables cannot take negative values in order to restore the original variables. Here the concentrations are taken from exponential distributions, chosen because these are simple distributions limited to positive values, and the synaptic modification rule is slightly modified:

$$\Delta w_{ij} = -\alpha \left(g(O_i)\, O_j - 1 \right) \quad \text{if } i \neq j \qquad (4.3)$$

where

$$g(x) = \begin{cases} x & \text{if } x \geq 0 \\ d \cdot x & \text{if } x < 0 \end{cases} \qquad (4.4)$$

and $d > 1$. Note that here O_i denotes the output scaled so that $\langle O_i \rangle = 1$ (rather than $\langle O_i^2 \rangle = 1$).

The zero point of our model variables (O_i) is assumed to correspond to the spontaneous firing rate of real neurones, and small negative values to firing below spontaneous rate. This rule behaves like the previous one as long as all outputs stay positive, but as soon as one of the O_i's goes slightly negative (meaning 'no firing') for one of the input patterns the negative value of that unit gets multiplied by d, a large positive constant, making Δw_{ij} positive. This results in a decrease of inhibition on the unit that went negative until all the patterns occupy the positive region of the output space only, restoring the original variables sweet, sour, bitter and salty.

It is known that in higher stages of the taste system some individual cells become more selective to only one of the basic tastes (Yamamoto *et al.*, 1985; Scott *et al.*, 1986), and our model shows how this might be achieved. When decorrelating many different groups of fibres in parallel, it would be advantageous to have the same coordinate system for each group, and having units selective for the primary qualities might, for instance, enable a salt-hungry animal to recognize what it lacks. Of course there is more to taste than correcting the confusion caused by the initial failure of the system to segregate the qualities on to separate pathways.

4.7 Local decorrelation in images

A decorrelating network can easily handle more than the four inputs shown in the model, but it cannot handle anything like the number that are involved in the images coming from the eyes. Furthermore the local connections in the striate cortex, which would be involved in the mutually inhibitory or excitatory connections between neurons, only extend for distances of the order of millimetres. Hence one must consider what decorrelation performed on local patches of the image could achieve, and first we need to clarify the nature of the information stored.

Note that simple automatic gain controls on each of the input lines might be said to store the mean values of each input, for the settings of the gains tell one how to derive a standard output level from each input. What is the information about the input that is stored in the model's matrix of inhibitory coefficients?

Without inhibition the outputs would be correlated in the same way as the inputs, while with the appropriate inhibitory coefficients the outputs are uncorrelated. Since the matrix of inhibitory coefficients compensates for the input correlations, it can be said that they store knowledge of the covariance matrix of the input in the normal environment. The pattern of saccadic eye-movements over a scene will cause the covariances to be averaged for different positions, but the values for different separations and orientations will be preserved and effectively yield the auto-correlation function. From this one can obtain the complete local power spectrum of the input images by Fourier transformation. Hence a decorrelating network stores knowledge of the power spectrum of its input and will be expected to show adaptive changes when exposed to images that have mean local power spectra or auto-correlation functions that differ from those to which they have previously been adapted.

Since decorrelation depends upon the local power spectrum, it is easy to see that many of the adaptation effects we have described are exactly what would be expected. What is interesting, however, is that this explanation does *not* at first sight seem to entail elements that are specifically tuned to different spatial frequencies, as in the usual 'channels' explanation (Braddick *et al.*, 1978). A decorrelating network would, it seems, necessarily adapt to stimuli that cause peaks in the local power spectrum, and would proceed to flatten them, simply because, with the moving eye, it is the power spectrum that drives the decorrelation process. On this view adaptation does not depend on the selectivity of the output neurons in the way that is often assumed, so one should be very cautious in accepting the existence of selective adaptation as evidence for neurons with specific selectivity for the adapting stimulus.

Notice that a network decorrelating N inputs uses of the order of N^2 synapses to store the power spectrum, which only requires N coefficients for its specification. As Kohonen (1984) points out, a sparse pattern of feedback connections should be sufficient to do this, or alternatively one might devise a means of storing more about the input in a completely connected network: for instance the different synapses might use different updating coefficients to produce different adaptation rates, or the feedback paths might be delayed by varying times in order to decorrelate temporal as well as spatial associations.

4.8 Temporal aspects

The normal environment is presumed to be whatever has happened in the recent past, and something needs to be said about how fast these normal expectations are formed. The evidence about this from experiments on pattern adaptation is curious. Fifteen seconds adaptation produces quite easily detectable after-effects, which usually persist for only a short time. Very thorough adaptation, on the other hand, can produce after-effects that are said to last many days, and long persistence is aided by the absence of other sensory experiences, as during sleep (MacKay & MacKay, 1974). Probably the decay is not a single exponential, but has a long tail, and perhaps one should not assume that there is only a single stage process. It seems premature to go into detailed discussion of the possibilities offered by hierarchies of decorrelators until the simplest mechanism has been better defined.

To summarize, we think that modifiable mutual inhibition provides a plausible explanation for pattern adaptation, and that it is a mechanism for acquiring, storing and using information about the normal pattern of contingent excitation of a group of inputs. Access to this store of knowledge occurs automatically whenever the system is used, and its effect is to make the representational elements independent in the normal environment.

4.9 Anatomical plausibility

Modern methods have enormously improved our knowledge of the neuro-anatomy of the cortex, but in spite of this it is still insufficient to exclude the vast majority of models. We may, however, have succeeded in picking one of these rare ones, for we suggest (see Figure 4.5) that there are direct inhibitory connections between the cortical output neurons (mainly pyramidal cells), and such connections are not thought to exist. We have two possible answers to this. First, the inhibition may be relayed through one of the classes of neuron that are thought to mediate intra-cortical inhibition; since there is unlikely to be one such neuron for every output neuron, this would necessitate decorrelating groups of neurons rather than individual ones, which weakens some of our arguments. Another possibility is that the modifiable connections are in fact excitatory, but with the strength of the feedback modified in the anti-Hebbian direction, and perhaps superimposed on a background level of inhibition from a wider range of other cortical neurons. This is an attractive possibility since the anatomical evidence suggests that the majority of the excitatory input synapses on cortical neurons derive from the recurrent collaterals of other cortical neurons in the vicinity. At first such positive feedback sounds explosively unstable, but of course the anti-Hebbian feature would tend to stabilize it, for it would strongly discourage joint firing of many neurons. It requires more modelling to see if any such scheme might work.

Another unrealistic feature of the present model is the assumption of high accuracy real variables for input and output in place of low accuracy pulse trains. There are also problems if the number of outputs exceeds the number of degrees of freedom, or dimensionality, of the inputs. It is clearly very much an idealized version of what may actually be going on, and the attempt to make it anatomically realistic has hardly begun.

4.10 Significance for early steps in image analysis

The model works on the principle of a null instrument such as a Wheatstone bridge, where the variable element in one arm is adjusted to balance the potential drop caused by the unknown element in the other; the ease of detecting very small deviations from zero makes the method extremely sensitive and accurate. The light adaptation mechanism illustrated in Figures 4.2 & 4.3 does something of the same sort, for when the mean luminance changes, the neurons respond initially, but this is then reduced to a low level, so the neurons are again sensitive to small deviations from the new mean luminance. But in the neural network proposed here, the null principle is applied to something more interesting than a voltage or a luminance, for it is part of the associative structure of the images that is balanced out.

Now, a null instrument is particularly sensitive to whatever measure of its input is nulled; are we particularly sensitive to the local properties of images that the network adapts to and compensates for? That's too big a question to try to answer here, but it is striking how many of the primary types of visual analysis do depend upon pairwise relationships between constituent elements - what is sometimes referred to as 'second order structure'. Examples in static images are texture, orientation, and disparity, and motion can be added if one considers the analysis of successive images. The moiré effects described by Leon Glass (1969) are particularly impressive from this point of view; the method of making them produces a peak in the local auto-correlation function, and their visibility is strongly resistant to dilution by noise in the form of unpaired dots (Maloney *et al.*, 1987). Thus the detection of associative structure may be a very important part of early, local, image analysis in perception, but decorrelation may also explain certain higher level effects.

4.11 Helmholtz's unconscious inference

Helmholtz knew that the system that interprets messages from the eye has expert knowledge of the sorts of things that do and do not happen in images, and that this knowledge is applied whenever we perceive anything. The mechanism we have suggested, based upon the adaptation phenomena we described, is perhaps involved in such an interpretive system, but before showing how it might do this, some examples of inference or induction in perception will be described.

Some of the best evidence that knowledge derived from experience of the real world is used by the interpretive system comes from experiments and observations on stereoscopic vision, though of course this does not mean experience is not required in monocular vision. We shall have to describe the phenomena rather than demonstrate them, but it is much more convincing if you can see the effects for yourself; this requires a stereo-viewing system in which you can reverse the images to the two eyes, and move your head while viewing a fixed stereo-pair.

Consider first a simple pair consisting of three vertical lines seen by each eye, with the central line displaced slightly to the right in the left eye's image; the result is of course that it is seen lying slightly in front of the two flanking lines. That is normal stereoscopic vision; it is remarkable that it wasn't discovered until 1838, by Wheatstone, and its late discovery shows how unaware one is of the subtlety of perceptual mechanisms.

If you now consider interchanging left and right eye images it is easy to see that rightward displacement of the centre line in what is now the right eye's image should cause it to be seen behind the flanking pair, and that is precisely what happens. Now repeat the experiment with a stereo photograph of a complex scene such as one views in the Victorian drawing room stereoscope. (This would probably involve separating and remounting the pair.) The result is not what one would expect. At isolated points the scene with the reversed stereo-pair shows evidence of reversed apparent depth, and the whole scene creates a sense of unease, or something being wrong. Although it lacks convincing depth, the overall scene looks surprisingly normal, so that most of the evidence provided by the binocular disparities of matched features in the two images must have been rejected or ignored.

Upon reflection one sees that making use of these cues would often lead to paradoxes in perception. For instance if the scene included a table top seen from above, near and far edges would be reversed and it would not look horizontal, so the objects on it would have to be glued to it. Furthermore the occlusion of the (originally) far edge by an object would be paradoxical - the edge ought to occlude the object. It is clear that something interferes with the utilization of disparity cues that do not 'fit-in', though it is an open question at this point whether it is high-level, possibly cognitive, knowledge of facts such as the way objects rest on table tops, or local, low-level, experience of the slant implied by perspective cues and the relationships between occlusions and disparities; we would prefer the latter.

There are many perceptual phenomena that seem to imply that the brain has much stored knowledge of images and their ways, and applies this knowledge instantly and automatically. One example is the 'toytown effect', which occurs when a stereo-pair of a scene is taken with the camera positions separated by a distance greater than the separation of the two eyes. This enhances the stereo depth effect, but it also gives the impression that the scene is not real, but a reduced scale model. Other examples are the diminutions in apparent size (*micropsia*) that result from placing a prism in front of one eye that requires increased convergence, or a lens that requires additional accommodation.

Describing the perceptions resulting from unusual forms of visual stimulation Helmholtz (1925) said 'such objects are always imagined as being present in the field of vision as would have to be there in order to produce the same impression on the nervous mechanism under conditions of normal use'. A particularly striking demonstration of this rule can be obtained when looking at a projected stereo-pair. If you move your head sideways (translating, not rotating) while looking at such a scene it appears to move, following your head as you move to the left and following it back as you move to the right. If you close one eye this impression of movement instantly ceases. At one level an explanation of this effect is that stereo-disparity tells you there are objects at different distances; but if there were, and the objects were fixed, then they would be displaced relative to each other when you move your head. This doesn't happen, and the only geometrical solution is that the objects themselves moved; this is what would be happening under 'conditions of normal use', so that is what you see. Again, our perceptual mechanism seems to have expert knowledge of what happens to images in the real world; perhaps all this knowledge comes in our genes, but we think a very natural explanation follows from our model.

Normally when you move through a scene there is a predictable relation between the stereo depth information and motion parallax - the relative motions of the images of objects at different distances. Wherever in the brain motion and stereo messages come together, the pattern of covariation of the neurons sensitive to stereo and motion parallax will be such that mutual inhibition builds up between certain sets of them. Because of the special nature of paired stereo images projected on a flat surface, when you move your head you continue to get stereo depth information, but the motion parallax cue is missing; inhibition on the covariant motion parallax neurons from the stereo neurons is unopposed by the 'expected' stimulation from motion cues, and the resulting imbalance of the motion signalling neurons causes the perception of motion in the direction contrary to that expected if the scene had been real.

Of course one needs to record from neurons that behave in this way before being fully convinced, but we think it may be possible to explain many instances of perceptual inference along these lines.

Conclusions

We started by saying that, although a lot has been discovered about the patterns of impulses that occur in the visual cortex, one cannot really understand how the world is represented in our heads without knowing about the system that interprets these patterns of impulses. We think it is a promising idea that decorrelation by anti-Hebbian mutual interaction is part of this interpretive system: it would acquire, store and make allowances for the pairwise associations in past sensory experience, thereby helping us to detect the new associations that indicate new causal factors in the world around us. Obviously we should attempt to identify the components of our network with those of the anatomical network in the cortex, and we hope to find if pattern adaptation of cortical neurons follows the expectations of the theory. We also think decorrelation may play a role in determining the susceptibility of early cortical development to modified visual experience, and we hope to explore its importance in preparing a representation of sensory information that can be used efficiently by associative networks with positive Hebbian rules.

References

Barlow H.B. (1969) Pattern recognition and the responses of sensory neurones. **Ann. New York Acad. Sci. 156,** pp. 872-881

Barlow H.B., Hawken M., Kaushal T.P. & Parker A.J. (1987) Human contrast discrimination and the contrast discrimination of cortical neurons. **J. Optical Soc. America A 4,** pp. 2366-2371

Barlow H.B. & Hill R.M. (1963) Evidence for a physiological explanation of the waterfall phenomenon and figural after-effects. **Nature 200,** pp. 1345-1347

Blakemore C. (1973) The baffled brain. In: **Illusion in Nature and Art.** R.L.Gregory & E.H.Gombrich (eds.) pp. 8-47, Duckworth, London.

Blakemore C. & Campbell F.W. (1969) On the existence of neurons in the human visual system selectively sensitive to the orientation and size of retinal images. **J. Physiol. 203,** pp. 237-260

Blakemore C. & Sutton P. (1969) Size adaptation: a new aftereffect. **Science 166,** pp. 245-247

Braddick O.J., Campbell F.W. & Atkinson J. (1978) Channels in vision: Basic aspects. In: **Handbook of Sensory Physiology Vol VIII; Perception.** R. Held, H.W. Leibowicz & H.L. Teuber (eds.) pp. 1-38, Springer, New York.

Exner S. (1894) **Entwurf zu einer physiologischen erklärung der psychischen erscheinungen.** I Theil, Franz Deuticke, Leipzig und Wien.

Gibson J.J. (1933) Adaptation, after-effect and contrast in the perception of curved lines. **J. Exp. Psychol. 16,** pp. 1-31

Gibson J.J. (1937) Adaptation with negative after-effect. **Psychol. Rev. 44,** pp. 222-244

Gilinsky A. S. (1968) Orientation-specific effects of patterns of adapting light on visual acuity. **J. Optical Soc. America 58,** pp. 13-18

Glass L. (1969) Moiré effect from random dots. **Nature 223,** pp. 578-580

Helmholtz H. von (1925) **Physiological Optics.** Translated from 3rd German Edition (1910) Volume III. The theory of the perceptions of visions. Optical Society of America, Washington.

Hubel D. H. (1988) **Eye, Brain, and Vision.** Scientific American Library, New York.

Kohonen T. (1984) **Self-organization and Associative Memory.** Springer, Berlin.

Kohonen T. & Oja E. (1976) Fast adaptive formation of orthogonalizing filters and associative memory in recurrent networks of neuron-like elements. **Biol. Cybern. 21,** pp. 85-95

MacKay D.M., & MacKay V. (1974) The time course of the McCollough effect and its physiological implications. **J. Physiol. 237,** 38-39P

Maffei L., Fiorentini A. & Bisti S. (1973) Neural correlate of perceptual adaptation to gratings. **Science 182,** pp. 1036-1038

Maloney R.K., Mitchison G.J. & Barlow H.B. (1987) The limit to the detection of Glass patterns in the presence of noise. **J. Optical Soc. America A 4,** pp. 2336-2341

McCollough C. (1965) Color adaptation of edge-detectors in the human visual system. **Science 149,** pp. 1115-1116

Michael C.R. (1978) Color vision mechanisms in monkey striate cortex: simple cells with dual opponent color receptive fields. **J. Neurophysiol. 41,** pp. 1233-1249

Ohzawa I., Sclar G. & Freeman R.D. (1985) Contrast gain control in the cat's visual system. **J. Neurophysiol. 54,** pp. 651-667

Pantle A.S. & Sekuler R.W. (1968) Size detecting mechanisms in human vision. **Science 162,** pp. 1146-1148

Pfaffman C. (1941) Gustatory afferent impulses. **J. Cell. Comp. Physiol. 17,** pp. 243-258

Poggio T., Torre V. & Koch C. (1985) Computational vision and regularisation theory. **Nature 317,** pp. 314-319

Sato T. (1980) Recent advances in the physiology of taste cells. **Progress in Neurobiology 14,** pp. 25-67

Scott T.R., Yaxley S., Sienkiewicz Z.J. & Rolls E.T. (1986) Gustatory responses in the frontal opercular cortex of the alert Cynomolgous monkey. **J. Neurophysiol. 56,** pp. 876-890

Stromeyer C.F. III, (1978) Form-color after-effects in human vision. In: **Handbook of Sensory Physiology,** Vol 8. R. Held, H.W. Leibowicz & H.L. Teuber, (eds.) pp. 97-142, Springer, New York.

Vautin R.G. & Berkeley M.A. (1977) Responses of single cells in cat visual cortex to prolonged stimulus movement: neural correlates of visual after-effects. **J. Neurophysiol. 40,** pp. 1051-1065

Yamamoto T., Yugama N., Kato T. & Kawamura Y. (1985) Gustatory responses of cortical neurons in rats. II. Information processing of taste quality. **J. Neurophysiol. 53,** pp. 1356-1369

5

From Chemotaxis to Cooperativity: Abstract Exercises in Neuronal Learning Strategies

Andrew Barto

Summary

In this chapter I draw on parallels that have been made between neurons and free-living unicellular organisms, to explore the idea that basic neural learning mechanisms have an abstract structure similar to that of the chemotactic behavior of certain free-living unicellular animals. The major line of support that I bring to bear on this hypothesis consists of theoretical and computational results relating to the collective behavior of neuron-like units that implement the suggested learning mechanism. These results show that such neuron-like units are capable of learning how to behave as effective decision makers in distributed systems and are able to learn how to cooperate with one another to solve problems that the individual units are not able to solve. The considerable range of collective behavior that emerges from a few simple principles, suitably refined, suggests that behavior patterns seen in unicellular organisms might serve as models for aspects of the learning capabilities of mature neurons.

5.1 Introduction

A large part of contemporary computer science is devoted to the study of parallel and distributed processing. Although parallel processing and distributed processing are often not distinguished, computer scientists do make a distinction between them that, while not being completely sharp, nicely encompasses the perspective I take in this chapter. When multiple processors cooperate closely to perform a task that somehow has been divided among them, the term parallel processing applies. The term distributed processing, on the other hand, applies when multiple processors cooperate more loosely in performing separate tasks (Kleinrock, 1985). In the first case, a problem's potential for concurrency is exploited to achieve a faster solution; whereas in the second, distribution is forced on the system by natural circumstances. Distributed processing systems come about, for example, when the data do not arise from a localized source and decisions, which may not act through a central authority, have to depend on remotely generated data and have outcomes dependent on decisions made at other sites.

Neural networks and neurally-inspired connectionist systems are generally seen as exemplifying principles of parallel processing. Indeed, these are examples *par excellence* of systems using closely coupled processors to carry out complex computations with remarkable speed. I can hardly disagree with this categorization, but having pointed out that the distinction described above is not sharp, in this chapter I emphasize aspects of neural networks that are more closely akin to those emphasized in distributed processing. In order to do this, it is necessary to shift from viewing a neural network as a massively parallel computational system to viewing a network as a confederation of units that face special difficulties in achieving their local goals because of their spatial distribution, limited means of communication, and lack of access to centralized control information. This shift in perspective requires some idea of what a unit's local task is so that it makes sense to think of a network as a distributed processing system. We have to modify the assumptions often made in studies of theoretical neural networks, that the processing units are *simple* and that nearly everything of interest in a network is the result of the interaction of many units.

In this chapter I draw on parallels that have been made between neurons and unicellular organisms to explore the idea that basic neural learning mechanisms have an abstract structure similar to that of the adaptive strategies possessed by certain free-living unicellular animals. One of the motivations for studying unicellular organisms, such as *Paramecium* and certain kinds of bacteria, is that, while being relatively easy to study, there are similarities between the cellular mechanisms of these organisms and those of excitable cells such as neurons (Koshland, 1980; Hinrichsen & Schultz, 1988). One factor making these organisms useful models is that because they are free-living, correspondences between cellular mechanisms and cellular behavior can be particularly clear, as when, for example, depolarization causes *Paramecium* to swim backwards (Hinrichsen & Schultz, 1988). Most important for my purposes, however, is the apparent clarity with which one can attribute functional significance to cellular behavior and thereby establish correspondences, albeit speculative ones, between mechanisms and the adaptive utility of behavior. The backward swimming of *Paramecium*, for example, plays a role in an avoidance response, and the swimming of the bacterium *Escherichia coli* can be understood in terms of chemotactic behavior that causes the bacterium to approach and remain in the vicinity of nutrients (Koshland, 1980).

Not only do behavioral patterns such as these remind us that single cells can exhibit subtle and complex behavior, these patterns can be abstracted and elaborated to serve as the basis for a neuronal model of learning. According to this model, instead of modulating swimming behavior, neurons adjust their firing tendencies under the influence of changing levels of substances analogous to the attractants and repellents that modulate bacterial movement. Hence, the suggestion is that chemotactic-like mechanisms operate in neurons, not just during development where neurotrophic factors synthesized in target fields influence neuron growth and survival, but in mature neurons where they manifest themselves not as movement strategies, but as mechanisms underlying learning.

The major line of support that I can bring to bear on this hypothesis consists of theoretical and computational results relating to the *collective* behavior of neuron-like units that implement the proposed learning mechanism, and much of what follows is devoted to describing these results and their place within the relevant theoretical traditions. These results show that neuron-like units, implementing learning rules of the type suggested by chemotactic behavior, are capable of learning how to behave as effective decision makers in distributed systems. They are able to make progress toward achieving local goals in spite of the uncertainty produced by their limited local views and their limited ability to control important system variables. Most important is the fact that distributed systems composed of this type of unit are able to learn how to solve problems that the individual units are not able to solve. A form of cooperativity emerges from the collective behavior of these units that may be of significance in helping to understand aspects of the adaptive behavior of aggregates of cells.

Despite my emphasis on the collective behavior of relatively complex neuron-like units with capabilities motivated by the study of unicellular organisms, it is not my intention to argue that nervous systems are colonies of loosely interacting, autonomous cells, or that neurons and chemotactic unicellular organisms are particularly closely related in an evolutionary sense. Aspects of the behavior of neural networks might be more understandable if our view shifted a bit toward the view that individual neurons have their own agendas, but no adequate account of real neural networks can ignore the specialized nature of neurons or the high degree of network structure present in nervous systems.

The perspective presented here has developed over a number of years, beginning with the hypothesis of Klopf (1972, 1982) that many aspects of memory, learning, and intelligence can be understood by viewing neurons as self-interested agents, and continuing with my research in collaboration with a number of colleagues (e.g. Barto, 1985; Barto *et al.*, 1986; Barto & Anderson, 1985; Barto, 1986; Barto & Jordan, 1987). I also draw heavily on the research of M.L. Tsetlin, the Soviet cybernetician whose studies of learning automata and their collective behavior conducted in the 1960s appeared in English in 1973 (Tsetlin, 1973). Some of the examples I use were presented by Tsetlin in a 1965 address to a section of the Physiological Society (appears in English in Tsetlin, 1973). I use these examples to draw attention to Tsetlin's work, which is not widely enough known, and because I know of no better examples. This line of research has continued as the theory of stochastic learning automata, reviewed by Narendra & Thathachar (1974). I also draw heavily of the research of D.E. Koshland on bacterial chemotaxis and its relation to neurobiology (Koshland, 1980) and of Yu-Chi Ho (1980) on decentralized decision making. I omit technical details as much as possible in this presentation, leaving the interested reader to consult the references.

5.2 Neurons and unicellular organisms

Providing biological motivation for the learning methods to be considered are the capacities of free-living unicellular organisms for goal-directed motility and similarities that have been noted between these organisms and neurons. Much of the study of single-cell movement is based on its potential relevance to cell motility in multicellular organisms, for example, to the migration of embryonic cells in morphogenesis and epithelial cells in wound healing. Other studies, however, are motivated by the relevance of unicellular organisms as models of the membrane mechanisms and behavior of excitable cells. For example, one reason the ciliated protozoan *Paramecium* is being studied is because it responds to sensory stimulation by Ca^{2+}-mediated depolarization which causes backward swimming by reversing the ciliary beat. With repolarization, the cells swim forward again but in a new direction. Overall, the behavioral response seems to be regulated by eight different ionic conductances together with the participation of cAMP and cGMP (Hinrichsen & Schultz, 1988).

Bacteria such as *Escherichia coli*, *Bacillus subtilis*, and *Salmonella typhimurium* are also studied for their potential relevance to neurobiology. The work of Koshland (Koshland, 1980) most clearly explores the possible relationship between bacterial chemotaxis and neuronal function. Even though they are not eukaryotes, bacteria share many of the properties of neurons. Like neurons, they have chemical receptors for sensing their environments, they contain a signal processing system of moderate complexity, and they produce a response: release of neurotransmitter in the neuron's case and the reversal of flagellar rotation in that of the bacteria. Bacteria also show adaptation, memory, and sensory integration that may resemble those processes in neurons (Koshland, 1980). Lackie (1986) provides additional information on bacterial chemotaxis and other movement strategies of single cells.

Most relevant to the neuronal learning method I describe below is the chemotactic behavior of bacteria such as those studied by Koshland. Such a bacterium propels itself along a relatively straight path by rotating its flagella, which form a bundle. Upon reversing the direction of flagellar rotation, the bundle becomes disorganized, which causes the bacterium to stop and tumble in place. As the flagella continue to rotate in this new direction, they reorganize and cause the bacterium to again be propelled on a straight path but in a new, randomly determined, direction. A kind of chemotaxis, which is the directed response to a chemical substance in the environment, results because the frequency of flagellar reversal is modulated by movement with respect to levels of attractant and repellent chemicals. Reversal frequency decreases if movement is toward higher attractant concentrations and increases if movement is toward lower concentrations. Repellents have the opposite effect. This modulation of flagellar reversal biases locomotion so that the bacterium finds, and remains near, places of maximal attractant concentration or minimal repellent concentration. It is an effective strategy, particularly when the gradient information is very noisy.

This behavior pattern has been called the 'Run-and-Twiddle Strategy': if things are getting better, keep doing what you are doing; if things are getting worse, do something else (Selfridge, in press). It is called klinokinesis with adaptation when played out over space by bacteria. Klinokinesis refers to the alteration of the direction of travel, and adaptation refers to the fact that the sensory system responds to changes in concentration rather than to absolute concentrations. We may also recognize in 'Run-and-Twiddle' a variant of the 'Win-Stay / Lose-Shift' strategy that has been studied by psychologists. In this case, winning and losing respectively correspond to swimming towards higher and lower attractant concentrations (or lower and higher repellent concentrations). An important distinction between the 'Run-and-Twiddle' behavior of bacteria and the usual form of 'Win-Stay / Lose-Shift' is that the latter behavior pattern is deterministic whereas the former is probabilistic. It is the *probability* of changing swimming direction (i.e. of twiddling or shifting) that is increased by losing, and it is the *probability* of swimming in the same direction (i.e. of running or staying) that is increased by winning. As I discuss below, the probabilistic nature of this behavior pattern is important because it has advantages when uncertainty is present in the task.

Koshland (1980) proposed a model for the regulation of bacterial tumbling that is relevant here because it suggests how aspects of the neuronal learning rule I describe below could be produced by neurons. That is, one can postulate a mechanism for altering neuronal firing rate in response to afferent signals that is analogous to how a bacterium's sensory signals may alter the frequency of flagellar reversal. Although the details of how a model of tumble regulation might apply to neurons has to await the description of the neuronal learning rule given below, it is appropriate to describe Koshland's model of tumble regulation here. According to this model, flagellar reversal is controlled by the concentration of a chemical response regulator, X, that ordinarily varies randomly about a background level X_{crit}. When the concentration of X is above X_{crit}, tumbling is suppressed; when below X_{crit}, tumbling frequency is enhanced (Figure 5.1). The response regulator, X, is formed from a substrate, W, with a rate V_f, and decomposed with rate V_d to product Y. Ordinarily, V_f approximately equals V_d, so that the concentration of X shows a small variation about a fixed level. This shared value of V_f and V_d is, in turn, regulated by the rate at which attractant and repellent molecules bind to receptors. This is hypothesized to occur by means of alterations in the reactions that produce the enzymes required for the formation and decomposition of X. Swimming through higher attractant concentrations results in higher, but still equal, values for V_f and V_d. Higher repellent concentrations result in lower values for V_f and V_d. Thus, the absolute levels of attractant and repellent concentrations do not influence the background concentration of X and hence do not alter tumble frequency, as is appropriate to describe the behavior of bacteria sensing uniform levels of attractants and repellents over time.

However, in the model it is assumed that the *rates* at which V_f and V_d change in response to *changes* in attractant and repellent concentrations differ, with V_f changing more quickly than V_d . Thus, upon sensing an increase in attractant

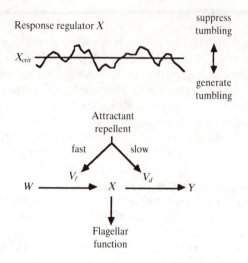

Figure 5.1 A model for bacterial chemotaxis from Koshland (1980).

concentration, the concentration of X undergoes a transient increase due to V_f being temporarily larger than V_d. This transiently suppresses tumbling. Similarly, decreases in attractant concentration, or increases in repellent concentrations, cause transient decreases in the concentration of X and increases in tumble frequency. As long as attractant concentrations are increasing, as when the bacterium is swimming up an attractant hill, tumbling remains suppressed as V_d lags behind V_f. Similarly, tumbling is enhanced upon swimming down an attractant hill. According to this model, then, both the adaptation to constant levels of attractant and repellent concentrations and the short-term memory required to provide the information needed to determine attractant and repellent gradients are produced by the dynamics of the cellular biochemistry and not (of course) by networks of cells.

5.3 Control and uncertainty

The first step in translating and extending chemotactic-like behavior patterns into specific hypothetical neuronal learning rules is to place these behavior patterns within a theoretical context that can help us extract their fundamental features. In trying to place the bacterium's klinokinesis with adaptation within a theoretical context, one first regards it as a simple hillclimbing method, as indeed it is, but to stop there obscures some of the issues involved in understanding the nature of this behavior. The hillclimbing consequences of the bacterium's behavior pattern are part of a global view that goes beyond the local task faced by the organism from moment to moment. Probabilistic 'Win-Stay / Lose-Shift' is an appropriately microscopic characterization of the *strategy*, but what kind of *task* is faced locally by the organism? It is not the usual hillclimbing task.

I think this local task is best characterized as a *control task* under conditions of uncertainty. The bacterium interacts in a closed-loop fashion with an environment on which its actions exert only modulatory control. It does not have the ability to place itself instantaneously anywhere in space (as is often assumed in framing more abstract optimization tasks); it does not even have the ability to choose a specific direction of travel. Moreover, it has neither a sufficiently rich sensory repertoire nor a sufficiently elaborate internal representation of its local environment, we may safely assume, to allow it to determine which of its two actions (reversing or not reversing flagellar rotation) is the best at any instant. Probabilistic 'Win-Stay / Lose-Shift' (where winning, staying, losing and shifting are all suitably defined in terms of spatial movement) is a control rule that produces effective hillclimbing behavior, given the kinds of attractant distributions encountered, despite the bacterium's restricted capabilities in directly controlling and sensing its environment.

A free-living cell faces uncertainty due to the complexity of the medium in which it lives and its limited local view. A cell in a multicellular organism faces uncertainty for the same reasons, but in this case, these factors arise in part from the decentralization implied by the distributed nature of the system. Remote components can have only limited information about each other and the overall system of which they are parts. Following Wheeler (1985) we distinguish between two types of uncertainty: *endogenous* uncertainty is uncertainty due to unknown aspects of the behavior of other components in the same system; *exogenous* uncertainty is uncertainty due to unknown aspects of the system's external environment and chance external events. In the examples described below, both kinds of uncertainty are factors, but let us first examine a deceptively simple decision problem involving uncertainty.

5.4 A decision problem under uncertainty

Suppose you are given two coins, which are distinguishable as Coin 1 and Coin 2, and you are to conduct a series of trials, or experiments, in each of which you select one of the coins, flip it, and note the outcome (head or tail). Nothing is known about the coins except that they may not be fair. The object of your task is to select a coin at each step, based on knowledge of the history of previous selections and observations, so as to maximize the expected number of heads over some finite or infinite time interval. Clearly, you would like always to select the coin with the larger probability of turning up heads, but you do not know, in fact, you can never know with certainty, which coin this is. Two factors influence each selection: (1) the desire to use what you already know about the coins to obtain immediate payoff, and (2) the desire to acquire more knowledge about the coins in order to make better selections in the future. More generally, the first factor is the desire to *control* the environment based on the current level of knowledge in order to improve performance, whereas the second factor is the necessity to *identify* the environment in order to make better control decisions in the future. These two factors - the need to control and to identify - ordinarily conflict: the best decision according to one is not best according to the other. Identification requires performing experiments designed to probe the environment for new information, something that by its very nature requires abandoning short-term performance goals. We can see the control/identify conflict in the task faced by the chemotactic bacterium. The bacterium's movement must not only bring it toward higher attractant concentrations but must also serve to detect the gradient of the attractant through the comparison of successively sensed attractant levels.

The decision problem just described in terms of two coins is probably the simplest example showing the control/identify conflict. It is known as the 'two-armed bandit' problem, studied first by Thompson (1933). It is a problem involving the sequential allocation of experiments and has both theoretical and practical importance (the coins, for example, may be replaced by two clinical treatments and the trials by patients). Berry & Fristedt (1985) provide a comprehensive treatment of this subject and a useful annotated bibliography. This class of decision problem is of interest here because the hypothetical neuronal learning rule we explore is a direct extension of one type of strategy that has been applied to these tasks.

5.5   Stochastic learning automata

Of the several theoretical traditions that have developed around the problem of the sequential allocation of experiments, I focus on the theory of learning automata, which originated in the work of the Soviet cybernetician M.L. Tsetlin (1973) and is currently being pursued by engineers (Narendra & Thathachar, 1974), where stochastic learning automaton algorithms are the primary subjects of study. Similar algorithms were independently developed by mathematical psychologists (e.g. Estes, 1950, Bush & Mosteller, 1955). Figure 5.2 shows a stochastic learning automaton interacting with a random environment. At each time step in the processing, the automaton randomly selects an action from a set of possible actions $\{a_1, \ldots, a_n\}$, where a_i is chosen with probability p_i. The environment then evaluates the action and transmits a payoff back to the automaton. For simplicity, we consider only the case in which the payoff is either 'success' or 'failure', but the theory extends to the case of a range of payoff values. The environment determines the payoff according to a set of probabilities $\{d_1, \ldots, d_n)\}$, where d_i is the probability of delivering success given that action a_i was selected. Upon receiving the payoff, the automaton updates its action probabilities depending on the action chosen, its current action probabilities, and the payoff received.

Rules for updating action probabilities increase the probability of the action chosen if the payoff indicates success, and decrease it if the payoff indicates failure. The other action probabilities are adjusted so that the new probabilities still sum to one. The magnitudes of these probability changes as functions of the current probabilities are critical in determining the performance of the update rule. Beginning with no knowledge of the success probabilities, the objective of the

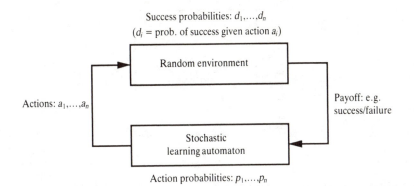

Success probabilities: $d_1,\dots,d_n$
(d_i = prob. of success given action a_i)

Random environment

Actions: $a_1,\dots,a_n$

Payoff: e.g.
success/failure

Stochastic
learning automaton

Action probabilities: $p_1,\dots,p_n$

Figure 5.2 Stochastic learning automaton interacting with a random environment.

automaton is to improve its expectation of success over time. Ideally, it should eventually choose, with probability 1.0, the action corresponding to the largest success probability. Many different algorithms have been studied under a number of different performance measures, and many convergence results have been proven (Narendra & Thathacher, 1974).

It is important to note that although the action probabilities, p_i, $i = 1,\dots,n$, must sum to one, the success probabilities, d_i, do not have to because they are the probabilities of success conditional on the action selected. For example, consider the case of two actions - the case corresponding to the 'two-armed bandit' problem where d_i is the probabability of Coin i coming up heads. Each point in the unit square 'contingency space' shown in Figure 5.3 represents a pair of head probabilities, (d_1, d_2), for two possible coins. Assuming that $d_1 > d_2$, so that Coin 1 is the best, we can restrict attention to the lower triangle. If we knew, *a priori,* that the point corresponding to the task being faced falls within a restricted region of contingency space, we could take advantage of this knowledge in devising an algorithm.

For example, the point (.6, .4) corresponds to a task in which the probabilities happen to sum to one. This task is relatively easy because the best action (select Coin 1) tends to yield success more than half the time, whereas the other action tends to yield success less than half the time. If we knew that the success probabilities summed to one, we could devise a simple algorithm that would do well; in fact, we could determine (in the limit) the best action without ever performing one of the actions. The difficulty is that we would like an algorithm that converges to the best action for tasks falling anywhere within contingency space. It turns out that this is not so easy, and in general it is necessary to continue to perform *both* actions with non-zero probability in order to counter the control/identification dilemma.

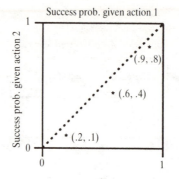

Figure 5.3 Contingency space for the two-action case.

Consider, for example, the tasks corresponding to the points (.9, .8) and (.2, .1) in the contingency space of Figure 5.3. In the first task, both actions yield success with a high probability, making it difficult to decide which is the best. Unsophisticated algorithms often converge to the inferior (but still good) action. In the second task, failure usually results no matter what action is chosen. Unsophisticated algorithms tend to oscillate under these conditions. Fortunately, there are fairly simple stochastic learning automaton algorithms that are able to approach optimal performance for arbitrary contingencies. Here I omit details, which involve subtle issues of stochastic convergence, and simply call such learning automata *competent*. That such learning automata choose their actions probabilistically contributes importantly to their competency. The hypothetical neuronal learning rule we have studied uses a probabilistic firing mechanism because it is an elaboration of a competent stochastic learning automaton.

I would like to make two additional observations about learning automata before turning to their collective behavior. First, the 'Win-Stay / Lose-Shift' strategy in its deterministic form is the first learning automaton studied (Robbins, 1952; Tsetlin, 1973). It is an example of a learning automaton and has been shown to perform better than a totally random strategy for selecting actions, but is far from optimal in these types of decision tasks. Note that the deterministic 'Win-Stay / Lose-Shift' strategy is similar in some respects to an error-correction neuronal learning rule, such as the perceptron rule, in that such a rule only changes weights upon error. In contrast, the rules we consider here change weights more upon success than they do upon failure, a feature essential for their performance in uncertain environments.

A final observation about the learning automaton formalism concerns the meaning of the 'environment.' This is an abstract formalism designed to allow certain kinds of theoretical questions to be framed precisely, and one should not underestimate the degree of its abstraction when relating the formalism to biological systems. In particular, Figure 5.2 shows the environment directly computing the payoff and the learning automaton having a specialized input for receiving it.

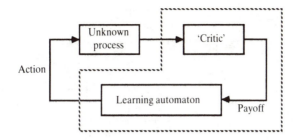

Figure 5.4 An alternative way to view the interaction between a learning automaton and its environment.

However, this is an abstraction that can be implemented in many ways, including that shown in Figure 5.4 in which a learning automaton and a 'critic' (which may itself be adaptive as described by Barto *et al.*, 1983), comprise a learning system (within the dotted lines) that does not receive specialized payoff signals from its environment. In the description of the neuron-like unit given below, the unit has a specialized input pathway for receiving payoff because this seems to be the simplest way to implement the learning rule. However, one can consider units to which payoff is effectively delivered via many pathways, which may also carry other kinds of information, by regarding the unit as preferring some input patterns over others. This kind of implicit payoff may be a more appropriate model for some purposes.

5.6 Collective behavior of learning automata

The random environment shown in Figure 5.2 is an extremely general model of an environment that behaves unpredictably. The ability of a competent learning automaton to improve performance in any such environment serves that automaton well when it has to interact with an environment containing other learning automata. This is the basis for understanding the behavior of collections of learning automata. Figure 5.5 shows a collection of N learning automata interacting with a common environment. The payoff to each automaton depends on the actions of the other automata in addition to its own action. Two different cases are usually studied. In the simplest, each automaton receives the same payoff. This is known as the team problem, or more technically, the 'decentralized team problem with incomplete information' (Narendra & Thathachar, 1974). In a game problem, on the other hand, each automaton receives a different payoff. In this case there may be conflicts of interest among the automata, and the question of what constitutes optimal collective behavior involves the difficult questions studied by game theorists.

A variety of theoretical results exist about the performance of learning automata in team and game problems. In team problems, competent learning

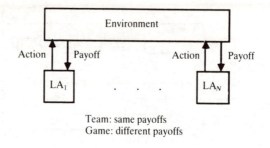

Team: same payoffs
Game: different payoffs

Figure 5.5 A collection of N learning automata interacting with a common environment.

automata have been shown to monotonically improve their performance (Narendra & Wheeler, 1983). In the case of zero-sum games (games of pure conflict), competent learning automata converge to the game's solution in an appropriate probabilistic sense (Narendra & Thathachar, 1974). To illustrate team and game tasks, I briefly describe two examples that Tsetlin presented in a 1965 lecture to physiologists (Tsetlin, 1973).

The first example is the so-called Goore game (although it is a team problem) which I describe as Tsetlin did in terms of human players. Suppose there is a referee and a number of players. The referee can see the players but the players cannot see one another. At the sound of a buzzer, each player is to raise one or two hands. The referee determines what percentage of players raised one hand, then pays each player a fixed amount with a probability that depends on this percentage (for example, according to the functional relationship shown in Figure 5.6). The process repeats each time the buzzer sounds. It can be shown that for any number of players implementing a competent learning automaton strategy, the process converges so that eventually the payoff probability is maximized. The result requires a payoff probability function that has a single maximum, such as that shown in Figure 5.6. Using this particular function, eventually 20% of the players will raise one hand at the sound of the buzzer.

In a Goore game, then, each learning automaton (player) receives the same payoff which is determined by the total number of learning automata that performed the designated action. This is a special case of a team problem where, more generally, the payoff to all the automata can depend on the *pattern* of automaton actions and not just their count. From the perspective of any individual learning automaton, the task is to try to maximize individual payoff in the face of the exogenous uncertainty produced by the probabilistic payoff procedure (Figure 5.6) and the endogenous uncertainty produced by the activity of the other automata - activity that is not directly observed. As far as any of the players is concerned, there are no other players, only a noisy, and non-stationary, environment.

One of the reasons Tsetlin was interested in the Goore game was its potential relevance to the process by which motor units are recruited. If the collection of players is thought of as a motor neuron pool, then the learning process is capable of

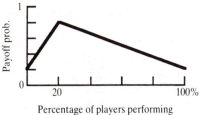

Figure 5.6 Payoff probability as a function of collective action in the Goore game (after Tsetlin, 1973).

adjusting the number of motor neurons that fire. What is perhaps most interesting about this is that, as Tsetlin points out, the payoff does not have to be determined based on the count of the number of neurons firing; it can depend on, say, the total force generated by the motor units, or perhaps on more distal consequences of motor unit activity. The learning process would still produce the required number of active motor neurons (assuming the team does not get stuck in a local optimum). Thus, the collection of learning automata can discover how to achieve some target configuration without requiring an agent in its environment that already knows how the target can be achieved, as would be required if only supervised learning were at work.

Let us look briefly at another example of collective behavior, again following Tsetlin (1973), by considering what he called the distribution game, which, unlike the Goore game, involves players that receive different payoffs. Imagine a collection of animals, each of which feeds from one of a set of feeding troughs. Each trough contains a certain amount of food. At a signal, each animal selects a feeding trough without any form of communication with the other animals. The amount of food each animal receives at each trial depends on the number of animals that have also chosen that trough at that trial. We assume the total amount of food in a trough is divided equally among the animals that approach it. The troughs are then refilled with the same amount of food as before, the signal occurs again, and the process repeats for a sequence of trials. Unlike the team situation, here the players receive different amounts of payoff and can have conflicts of interest. However, to the players, the situation appears identical to that of the Goore game, and competent learning automata learn to distribute themselves in a way that is 'just as reasonable as for people who would know the contents of each trough' (see Tsetlin, 1973, pp. 115-118).

Why do learning automata have to be competent in order to operate effectively as team or game players? Recall that a competent learning automaton is one that can learn which of its actions is best in the absence of *a priori* restrictions on the contingencies it faces. When a learning automaton's environment in part consists of other learning automata, then it faces contingencies that are constantly changing as the other automata are learning (a non-stationary environment). There is no guarantee, therefore, that the contingencies faced by any of the automata in the collection will remain in any pre-designated region of contingency space. If an automaton happens to be confronted with particularly easy contingencies, it will learn quickly; confronted with difficult contingencies, it will learn more slowly but will not prematurely settle on the wrong action. Learning automata that are not sufficiently competent, such as deterministic learning automata, will sometimes learn to participate in appropriate collective behavior and sometimes not.

In order to apply learning automata to the tasks just described - the Goore game and the distribution game - it had to be assumed that the players were not able to communicate directly with one another. This is because the learning automaton formalism (Figure 5.2) does not have provision for input to the automaton other than the payoff signal. Tsetlin made the following comment:

> 'We have discussed very simple forms of behavior, and for this reason we limited ourselves to the simplest types of automata. The exchanges of information among these automata takes place in the language of penalties and rewards. Although this language seems universal enough, it would, however, be interesting to also look at more complicated automata that possess some specialized language to communicate with other automata. Such automata are needed to describe more complex forms of behavior. These more complex behavioral forms necessitate the use of much more diverse information.' (Tsetlin, 1973, p. 125.)

Our research has focussed on extending the theory of learning automata in the direction Tsetlin suggested in this quoted passage. We now consider more elaborate learning automata that are more like neurons because they make decisions conditionally on input signals which provide information about the state of their environments.

5.7   Associative learning automata

Figure 5.7 shows a learning automaton receiving information, which we call context input, in addition to the payoff signal from its environment (cf. Figure 5.4). The bold arrows in Figure 5.7 are intended to suggest that those pathways potentially transmit massive amounts of data; that is, they represent vector rather than scalar signals. The associative learning automaton must learn how to act conditionally on the context input in order to maximize its expected payoff. Whereas the learning automata described above have to learn a *single* optimal action (or perhaps a single optimal probability for each action), an associative learning automaton tries to learn a *rule*, or mapping, associating context input with optimal actions. What action is best depends on the contingencies currently being implemented by the environment, and usually an environment can provide information that can be associated with appropriate actions. One can think of the context input as providing a clue as to the state of the environment. Context input

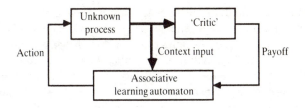

Figure 5.7 A modified version of Figure 5.4 showing an associative learning automaton receiving context input in addition to payoff input.

therefore plays a role similar to that of discriminative stimuli in instrumental conditioning.

Associative learning automata face two kinds of problems. First, they have to learn to classify context input patterns into classes, where all patterns in a given class signal that the same action is best when performed in the presence of any of those patterns. Second, they have to discover what these best actions are. The first problem corresponds to the pattern classification tasks for which a variety of learning rules for neuron-like units have been developed, e.g. the perceptron rule (Rosenblatt, 1961) or Widrow & Hoff's (1960) Least-Mean-Square (LMS) rule. Here, however, there is no teacher able to directly specify desired responses. The learning system has to discover what the best actions are by probing its environment in the manner of a learning automaton.

We have developed numerous algorithms for associative learning automata, but here I focus on the most successful one: the *Associative Reward-Penalty*, or A$_{R-P}$, algorithm, first introduced by Barto & Anandan (1985) and extensively discussed by Barto (1985). It is a hybrid of perceptron/LMS and stochastic learning automaton algorithms that turns out to be closely related to Thorndike's (1911) Law of Effect and to the 'selective bootstrap adaptation' rule of Widrow *et al.* (1973). The A$_{R-P}$ algorithm applies to a neuron-like unit with a number of input pathways for context input and a specialized input pathway for payoff. I describe its behavior informally; details can be found in the references.

The unit has binary output, its two actions being 'firing' and 'not firing'. As is usual, there is a weight for each context input pathway, and the unit's output is determined by the weighted sum of the context input signals. However, the output depends in a random way on the weighted sum: the more positive the sum, the more likely the unit is to fire; the more negative, the less likely it is to fire (this input/output behavior is identical to that of the Boltzmann units of Ackley *et al.*, 1985). Thus, the A$_{R-P}$ unit is like a two-action stochastic learning automaton except that its action probabilities depend on the context input in a manner determined by the synaptic weights. If an action is followed by feedback indicating 'success', the weights are changed so as to make that action more likely in the presence of the context input pattern in which that action was taken (and patterns similar to it). If an action is followed by 'failure', the weights are changed to make that action less likely. The role of the random action-generation process is the same as it is for a stochastic learning automaton: to generate sufficient variety in the unit's behavior so that the identification aspect of the unit's task is accomplished effectively.

Note that it is not the synaptic weights that we vary randomly but the unit's firing activity. It would be quite possible to consider a system in which each synapse were represented by a separate (non-associative) stochastic learning automaton, but then the learning process for a single unit would require solving a team decision problem. Learning in this case would be far less efficient than in the one we are considering, in which knowledge is used about how the individual input signals are combined by the unit. Indeed, it would even be possible, and perhaps interesting, to consider each synapse as containing a team of non-associative learning automata, each representing a neurotransmitter vesicle or receptor engaged in a kind of Goore game. Relying solely on this mechanism would be inefficient in the extreme, but learning automata operating at all these levels and facing locally-defined payoff structures could yield very robust adaptive capabilities.

We see, then, that an AR-P unit in effect just implements the Law of Effect, but the weights have to be updated so that the unit is competent (see Section 5.5) in all of the contexts to which it is exposed, or at least, is competent within the confines of its ability to discriminate contexts. An AR-P unit achieves this (but under the restriction that the context input patterns are linearly independent; see Barto & Anandan, 1985). In addition to its probabilistic action-generation process, a feature of the AR-P unit that is critical for its competency is an asymmetry between the magnitudes of the weight changes that occur in the 'success' and 'failure' cases. A much smaller step size must be used in the case of failure; indeed, as the weight changes made upon failure get smaller, the asymptotic behavior of the unit improves. Competency seems to require updating weights in a manner strikingly different from that of an error-correction rule like the perceptron rule, which changes weights only when its response is incorrect. It may be of more than passing interest that the asymmetry between the success and failure cases, required for an AR-P unit to be competent, exactly corresponds to the change in Thorndike's first symmetrical version of the Law of Effect that he adopted to bring his theory into closer accord with experimental observations (see, for example, Hilgard, 1956).

My colleagues and I have written extensively on the differences between associative learning automata and the more familiar error-correction rules for supervised learning commonly used in artificial neural networks (Barto *et al.*, 1983; Barto, 1985). I limit my remarks here to a few observations about differences between the tasks each is capable of solving. As usually formulated, supervised learning, where a teacher directly specifies the desired responses, does not involve any form of feedback through the environment. The environment simply repeatedly presents input patterns paired with desired responses. This is a form of open-loop learning akin to Pavlovian conditioning. There is feedback involved in error-correction rules, of course, but it is feedback of the unit's own response, which can take place within the unit.

In an alternative formulation of error-correction rules for supervised learning that places the error calculation outside of the unit, there *is* feedback passing through the unit's environment, but it is very different from the evaluative feedback under which associative learning automata operate. According to this formulation, learning occurs under the control of error signals that tell the unit *how* to change its actions, whereas evaluative feedback signals do not do this. In supervised learning, a positive error tells the unit that its response was too high, a negative error tells it that its response was too low, and an error of zero signals the desired state of affairs. On the other hand, in the kind of learning we are considering here, the payoff would be 'failure' for both the cases of positive and negative error, and the learning system would have to make adjustments so as to decrease its tendency to do whatever it did, not just decrease or increase its response as specified by the sign of the error. Moreover, if the environment is noisy, then the adjustments must be made carefully to ensure adequate testing of alternatives. Of course, the payoff signal need not be derived from a signed error in this manner (no error = success, plus and minus error = failure). It can be generated by a critic (Figure 5.7) that knows neither what the actual response was nor what it should have been. A critic can generate a payoff based on knowledge solely of *what* it wants accomplished and not of *how* the learning system can accomplish it.

It should be clear that the kind of learning we are considering can be applied to supervised-learning tasks (Barto & Jordan, 1987), but it applies to more difficult tasks as well. However, the usual error-correction rules for supervised-learning are not competent in the kinds of tasks we are considering here. These tasks involve genuine feedback paths through the learning system's environment as in instrumental conditioning experiments. Describing error-correction as 'trial-and-error' learning, as has often been done, is incorrect and misleading. Trial-and-error really means 'generate-and-test,' which only applies superficially to supervised-learning methods. Learning automata, associative or otherwise, are engaged in learning to *control* their environments, not just to mimic them. Learning to mimic environmental events may be an important process in the construction of mental representations of the environment, but it is not the only process of interest.

Is it plausible that a single neuron could implement a competent associative learning automaton strategy? We can only speculate about possible cellular mechanisms, but Koshland's model of bacterial chemotaxis described in Section 5.2 suggests a starting point. One of the requirements of such a mechanism, if it is to operate in real time, is that it must possess a form of short-term memory to retain a trace of context inputs, and the actions taken in their presence, for sufficient time to allow the return of evaluative feedback. This requires a mechanism more complex than Koshland postulated for bacterial chemotaxis (Figure 5.1), but that model suggests how this short-term memory could be implemented within a cell. We could, for example, replace the tumble regulator X by a randomly varying membrane potential or firing threshold, allowing the firing probability to be conditional on synaptic input. Attractants and repellents would correspond to various neuromodulators delivered via diffuse projections from brain reinforcement centers and from sources that are more local. The detection of changes in the concentrations of these substances could be accomplished as in Koshland's model, and traces of relevant past information could be maintained by similar biochemical means as long as the time interval is not too long (perhaps hundreds of milliseconds to a few seconds). Traces of the recent past history of synaptic activity would have to be maintained in some synaptically-local manner. Sutton & Barto (1981) discuss hypothetical mechanisms for storing these kinds of traces at synapses, and more recent knowledge about cellular mechanisms suggest others (see, for example, Alkon & Rasmussen, 1988). Some of the theoretical issues involving time delays between actions and their consequences have been studied, but this is outside the scope of the present chapter (see Sutton & Barto, 1981; Barto *et al.*, 1983; Sutton, in press).

5.8 Collective behavior of associative learning automata

The behavior of collections of associative learning automata can be more complex than the behavior of the collections of non-associative automata considered above. I present two examples that suggest some of the possibilities. The first example is a team decision problem illustrating some of the important features of decentralized decision making that are absent in the non-associative case, and which I believe may be important in the functioning of the brain. The second example shows how the problem of learning in a layered network can be considered as an extension of the decentralized team decision task, where part of the context input to a unit is determined by the actions of other units.

5.8.1   *Decentralized decision making*

In a tutorial on decentralized statistical decision making, Yu-Chi Ho (1980) used a simple example that emphasizes the 'essentials of team theory by stripping away all unimportant details'. I describe the task just as he did, and then I show how AR-P units learn how to act as effective decision makers in this task. Mr. B, who lives in Boston, and Mr. H, who lives in Hartford (about 100 miles away), need to meet in Worcester, about midway between Boston and Hartford, in order to close a business deal. They decide to meet in Worcester the next day at noon if it doesn't rain, but are unable to communicate further. As Ho says, 'New England weather being what it is, an *uncertainty* has developed about whether or not it is raining in Worcester when H and B are about to depart for their meeting. Of course, each of them has access to his *own* local weather information in his city. This information is in turn correlated with the state of the weather in Worcester as well as with the information received by the other person.' Assuming that both H and B have to be present to conduct their business and that sunshine in Worcester is essential to its successful outcome, Ho postulates the payoff matrices shown in Figure 5.8.

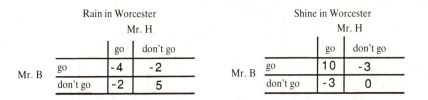

Figure 5.8 Payoff matrices for team decision problem (after Ho, 1980, Figure 1).

Mr. B and Mr. H have to decide whether or not to make the trip to Worcester. More than this, however, we require them to come up with a strategy for deciding when to make the trip depending on their local weather conditions. According to Ho (1980) this problem has the main features of team decision problems (quoting Ho):

1) the presence of *different but correlated* information for each decision maker about some underlying *uncertainty*;

2) the need for *coordinated* actions on the part of all decision makers in order to realize the *payoff*.

If the problem does not have both of these features, then it simplifies. For example, if the cities involved are so far apart that their weather is uncorrelated, then it is does not help to consider local weather conditions; if the tasks to be performed by the decision makers do not require coordination, then the decisions can be made independently.

In the example task, each decision maker can adopt one of four possible decision strategies (different mappings from the two possible local weather conditions to the two possible actions). Thus, there are sixteen possible strategies for the two players, and which one is best depends on the correlations among the weather conditions in the two cities. These correlations arise from the joint probability distribution of the three random variables describing the weather in the three cities. Given such a distribution function, it is possible to determine which of the sixteen strategies yield maximal expected payoff. Figure 5.9 is one such joint distribution given by Ho, and with some computation one can show that the optimal strategy is for both Mr. B and Mr. H to ignore local weather conditions and always travel to Worcester (see Ho, 1980, for details and more complex examples).

This is exactly the kind of problem that associative learning automata, such as AR-P units, should be able to solve. We investigated this by letting two AR-P units play the roles of the decision makers as shown in Figure 5.10. A unit firing means that the decision to make the trip has been made. At each time step, we selected a weather pattern for the three cities according to a given joint probability distribution. The weather selected for Boston was coded as a 0 or a 1 and given as context input to the unit representing the Boston decision maker. Similarly, Hartford's weather provided context input to the other unit. The weather selected for Worcester

Boston	r	r	r	r	s	s	s	s
Hartford	r	r	s	s	r	r	s	s
Worcester	r	s	r	s	r	s	r	s
Prob.	0.25	0.05	0.1	0.1	0.1	0.1	0.05	0.25

Figure 5.9 Joint probability distribution for the weather in Boston, Hartford, and Worcester (r = rain, s = shine; after Ho, 1980, Figure 2).

determined which payoff matrix of Figure 5.8 we used to determine the payoff as a function of the units' actions. We also provided each unit with a variable bias, in the form of a constant input signal multiplied by an adjustable weight, so that it could, if necessary, learn to fire with a high probability when being presented with a context signal of 0. Our simulation experiments suggest that AR-P units are consistently able to find the best strategies for a variety of payoff matrices and weather pattern probabilities, including those shown in Figures 5.8 & 5.9, for which both units learned to stay on.

Despite being able to make decisions conditionally upon context information, the associative learning automata shown in Figure 5.10 have no direct means for communicating with one another. They are therefore unable to agree among themselves upon some course of action *before* they act. This means that this example, as implemented, is a *non-cooperative* problem: no pre-game communication and agreement is possible. The players come to coordinate their actions as a result of the learning process, but no direct coordination is permitted. In contrast, the theory that Ho (1980) discusses is the fully cooperative case in which the players are assumed to be able to communicate with each other when they are designing their strategies, and because he is not studying learning, he does not consider repeated play of the game. He is concerned with the problem of determining what constitutes a good solution to a decentralized decision problem given complete knowledge of the payoff structure and other characteristics of the environment. We have been concerned, on the other hand, with the non-cooperative case and incomplete information, and have focussed on learning. What we can consider within our framework, however, is how decision makers can *learn to cooperate* with one another. I turn now to an example showing how competent associative learning automata can learn how to coordinate their actions for mutual benefit. This takes the form, by now familiar to neural-network researchers, of a layered network.

5.8.2   Layered networks

In previous publications, my colleagues and I described simulation experiments showing how layered networks of AR-P units can learn to solve non-

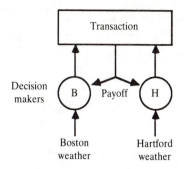

Figure 5.10 Two associative learning automata in a decentralized decision task.

linear associative learning tasks (Barto, 1985; Barto *et al.*, 1986; Barto & Anderson, 1985; Barto, 1986; Barto & Jordan, 1987). Here I describe the simplest of these experiments as an example of a distributed problem solving task in which units learn how to cooperate. Figure 5.11 shows a network of two associative learning automata, labelled A and B, that use the AR-P algorithm. The context input to Unit A provides environmental state information as a stimulus from the environment, and the context input to Unit B tells it which action Unit A has selected (as before, each unit also has a constant input with an adjustable weight so that it can learn to turn on in the presence of a zero as context input). Thus, only Unit A receives input from the environment external to the network, and only the action of Unit B directly influences the payoff. Both units receive the same payoff, making it a team problem.

Suppose we place this network in the following discrimination task. The environment has two states, one of which is selected at random on each trial. When in one state, State 1, the environment responds to Unit B's firing by providing a payoff of 'success' to both units with high probability and 'failure' with low probability; whereas if Unit B does not fire, the State 1 environment responds with 'failure' to both units with high probability and 'success' with low probability. When the environment is in State 0, on the other hand, the contingencies are reversed so that it provides 'success' with the highest probability if Unit B does not fire. The environment signals its state to Unit A by sending a 1 or a 0 to Unit A via its context inputs. Therefore, in order to maximize the expectation of success, the network as a whole should simply construct the identity mapping, producing output 1 in response to input 1, and output 0 otherwise.

If there were no communication link between Unit A and Unit B, only limited success rate could be achieved. Unit B, unable to sense a discriminative stimulus, would solve the task non-associatively by learning always to select the single action that is the best to perform independently of the network input. Unit A, unable to influence the environment at all, would never settle on a consistent action because nothing it could do would matter. The complementary specialities of the two units

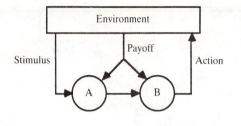

Figure 5.11 A two-layer network of associative learning automata.

have to be combined for the network to achieve an optimal success rate - the units have to cooperate. The interconnecting link from Unit A to Unit B has an adjustable weight that allows Unit A's decision to influence that of Unit B. We set this weight to zero initially in the simulations, and if it is suitably adjusted, then the network can respond correctly to the discriminative stimulus. However, the correct value of the interconnecting weight depends on how Unit A has learned to respond to its input; conversely, the correct behavior of Unit A depends on the value of the interconnecting weight, that is, on how Unit B has learned to respond to its context signal. Thus the two units must adapt simultaneously in a tightly-coupled cooperative fashion. Simulations, more completely discussed in Barto (1985), strongly suggest that the network always converges so as to maximize the expectation of success.

A non-zero value for the weight on the pathway connecting Unit A to Unit B really does mean that the units cooperate, albeit in a limited way. Their activity is no longer statistically independent. To the extent that the weight has large magnitude, there is a *binding agreement* between the units that is acted upon before the network makes an overt action: Unit B responds to what Unit A tells it. Units A and B form a kind of coalition. If the units were reciprocally connected, then the process of agreeing upon an action would take place via an iterative relaxation process, although we have not yet thoroughly studied this case.

Although I have presented this method for learning in multilayer networks in terms of distributed decision making, it has not been my intent to obscure the relationship between this method and other methods for obtaining effective learning in multilayer networks, notably the error back-propagation method (Rumelhart *et al.*, 1986). With a few technical caveats, it appears that layered networks of AR-P units update their interconnection weights in a manner that statistically approximates a gradient of overall network performance as shown by Williams (1986, 1987). Thus, it is not misleading (although not exactly technically correct) to view layered networks of AR-P units, acting as a team, as performing a kind of statistical approximation to the process carried out by error back-propagation.

To gain a better understanding of what happens as layered networks of AR-P units learn, consider a single unit in the interior of a layered network (i.e. a 'hidden unit'). Suppose this unit can vary its output about its current value while the outputs of all the other units remain fixed. By correlating the variation of its output with the consequences of this variation on the overall performance measure for the network, the unit can obtain a good estimate of how its activity influences this measure, that is, it can estimate the derivative of the performance measure with respect to its output at the current point in weight space. From this the unit can easily determine the performance measure's derivative with respect to its weights, and so can alter its weights appropriately. Suppose each unit does this in turn with the other units' outputs fixed. If a unit's new weights are not put into place until all the units have varied their outputs, the result will be a step in weight space according to a good estimate of the gradient of the performance measure. It turns out that it is possible for interacting units to vary their outputs simultaneously to obtain estimates of the appropriate derivatives. This estimation process is made difficult by the endogenous noise produced by the simultaneous variation, but AR-P units are able to sort out the correct information. Note that it would also be possible to vary simultaneously all the network's *weights* to obtain gradient estimates, but this is not done in AR-P networks and it would be considerably slower.

Because the AR-P method estimates gradient information, whereas the error back-propagation method computes it during the backward pass, the AR-P method is considerably *slower* than error back-propagation, which itself is regarded as being too slow for scaling up to large applications. Nevertheless, several things can be said in defense of networks of AR-P units. First, networks of associative learning automata are not restricted to solving supervised-learning tasks; they can be effective for a wide class of decision-making tasks involving uncertainty (which includes supervised learning as a special case) as I have tried to emphasize in this chapter. Second, as I have also emphasized in this chapter, networks of cooperating associative learning automata have a kind of biological plausibility that, in my opinion, algorithms such as error back-propagation lack. The learning of cooperative collective behavior is a very natural consequence of competent associative learning automata interacting under conditions that make it advantageous for the individual units to coordinate their activity. There is no need for a tightly regimented training procedure.

Finally, that competent associative learning automata are robust enough to improve their performance under rather unstructured conditions suggests that this approach may provide new ways of obtaining efficient learning in modularly organized, perhaps hierarchical, adaptive networks. In all the examples I have presented involving associative learning automata, the payoff signal is diffusely broadcast to all the units. Although there are diffuse projections in the brain that could serve this function for large groups of neurons, learning becomes much more rapid as the number of units to which a payoff signal is uniformly broadcast decreases. Sending different and specialized payoff signals to subgroups of units can vastly increase the speed of learning, but requires more knowledge on the part of whatever is serving as a critic, knowledge which may itself be learned with experience. The *global* broadcast of a single payoff signal should be viewed as a *worst case*. Various forms of local reinforcement systems have to exist for large problems to be solvable by this kind of learning. One way of achieving this is suggested by the fact that training can be accomplished by agencies that only know *what* they want accomplished, but not *how* it can be accomplished. Modules can cause things to happen that they cannot do themselves by setting appropriate contingencies for other modules having the necessary expertise and access to the necessary information. Analogies with social and economic systems are obvious, although highly structured regimes that would be unacceptable to organisms like ourselves would have to exist at these microscopic levels. These are issues we are exploring in our current research.

5.9   From chemotaxis to cooperativity

In this chapter I have suggested how adaptive strategies that we know are within the capabilities of single cells can be extended to produce a variety of forms of collective behavior, including the learning of cooperative interactions. To mitigate the degree of speculation unavoidable in hypothesizing that neurons, even just some of them, are competent associative learning automata, I have proceeded in small steps leading from bacterial chemotaxis to cooperative collective behavior, and focussed on theoretical questions that have spawned rich theoretical traditions. That such simple ideas, suitably refined, can underlie a wide range of behavior suggests that the hypothesis is worth serious experimental study.

Acknowledgement

This research was supported by the Air Force Office of Scientific Research, Bolling AFB, through grant AFOSR-87-0030. The author wishes to thank Robert Jacobs for his essential help in preparing some of the material presented here and John Moore for valuable feedback on an early draft.

References

Ackley D.H., Hinton G.E. & Sejnowski T.J. (1985) A learning algorithm for Boltzmann Machines. **Cognitive Sci. 9**, pp. 147-169

Alkon D.L. & Rasmussen H. (1988) A spatial-temporal model of cell activation. **Science 239**, pp. 998-1005

Barto A.G. (1985) Learning by statistical cooperation of self-interested neuron-like adaptive elements. **Human Neurobiol. 4**, pp. 229-256

Barto A.G. (1986) Game-theoretic cooperativity in networks of self-interested units. In: **Neural Networks for Computing.** J.S. Denker (ed.) New York: AIP Conference Proceedings 151, American Institute of Physics, pp. 41-46

Barto A.G. & Anandan P. (1985) Pattern recognizing stochastic learning automata. **IEEE Trans. Sys. Man Cybern. 15**, pp. 360-375

Barto A.G., Anandan P. & Anderson C.W. (1986) Cooperativity in networks of pattern recognizing stochastic learning automata. In: **Adaptive and Learning Systems** K.S. Narendra (ed.) Plenum, New York, pp. 235-246

Barto A.G. & Anderson C.W. (1985) Structural learning in connectionist systems. **Proc. Seventh Ann. Conference Cognitive Science Society**, Irvine, CA.

Barto A.G. & Jordan M.I. (1987) Gradient following without back-propagation in layered networks. **Proc. IEEE First Ann. Int. Conference Neural Networks**, IEEE Catalog #87TH0191-7, vol II, pp. 629-636

Barto A.G., Sutton R.S. & Anderson C.W. (1983) Neuronlike adaptive elements that can solve difficult learning control problems. **IEEE Trans. Sys. Man Cybern. 13**, pp. 834-846

Berry D.A. & Fristedt B. (1985) **Bandit Problems: Sequential Allocation of Experiments.** Chapman & Hall, London.

Bush R.R. & Mosteller F. (1955) **Stochastic Models for Learning.** Wiley, New York.

Estes W.K. (1950) Toward a statistical theory of learning. **Psych. Rev. 57**, pp. 94-107

Hilgard E.R. (1956) **Theories of Learning.** Appleton-Century-Crofts Inc., New York.

Hinrichsen R.D. & Schultz J.E. (1988) *Paramecium*: a model system for the study of excitable cells. **TINS 11**, pp. 27-32

Ho Yu-Chi (1980) Decision theory and information structures. **Proc. IEEE 68**, pp. 644-654

Kleinrock L. (1985) Distributed systems. **Communications of the ACM 28**, pp. 1200-1213

Klopf A.H. (1972) Brain function and adaptive systems - a heterostatic theory. Air Force Cambridge Research Laboratories Research Report, **AFCRL-72-0164**, Bedford, MA.

Klopf A.H. (1982) **The Hedonistic Neuron: A Theory of Memory, Learning and Intelligence.** Hemisphere, Washington, DC.

Koshland D.E. Jr. (1980) Bacterial chemotaxis in relation to neurobiology, **Ann. Rev. Neurosci. 3**, pp. 43-75

Lackie J.M. (1986) **Cell Movement and Cell Behavior.** Allen & Unwin, London.

Narendra K.S. & Thathachar M.A.L. (1974) Learning automata - a survey. **IEEE Sys. Man Cybern. 4**, pp. 323-334

Narendra K.S. & Wheeler R.M. Jr. (1983) An N-player sequential stochastic game with identical payoffs. **IEEE Trans. Sys. Man Cybern. 13**, pp. 1154-1158

Robbins H. (1952) Some aspects of the sequential design of experiments, **Bull. Am. Math. Soc. 58**, pp. 527-532

Rosenblatt F. (1961) **Principles of Neurodynamics: Perceptrons and the Theory of Brain Mechanisms.** Spartan Books, Washington DC.

Rumelhart D.E., Hinton G.E. & Williams R. J. (1986) Learning internal representations by error propagation. In: **Parallel Distributed Processing: Explorations in the Microstructure of Cognition, Vol 1: Foundations.** D.E. Rumelhart & J.L. McClelland (eds.) Bradford Books/MIT Press, Cambridge MA.

Selfridge O. (in press) **Tracking and Trailing.** Bradford Books/MIT Press, Cambridge MA.

Sutton R.S. (in press) Learning to predict by the method of temporal differences. **Machine Learning**

Sutton R.S. & Barto A.G. (1981) Toward a modern theory of adaptive networks: expectation and prediction. **Psych. Rev. 88**, pp. 135-171

Thompson W.R. (1933) On the likelihood that one unknown probability exceeds another in view of the evidence from two samples. **Biometrika 25**, pp. 275-294

Thorndike E.L. (1911) **Animal Intelligence.** Hafner, Darien Conn.

Tsetlin M.L. (1973) **Automaton Theory and Modeling of Biological Systems.** Academic Press, New York.

Wheeler R.M. Jr. (1985) **Decentralized Learning in Games and Finite Markov Chains,** PhD Dissertation, Yale University.

Widrow B., Gupta N.K. & Maitra S. (1973) Punish/reward: Learning with a critic in adaptive threshold systems. **IEEE Trans. Sys. Man Cybern. 5**, pp. 455-465

Widrow B. & Hoff M.E. (1960) Adaptive switching circuits, **1960 WESCON Convention Record Part IV**, pp. 96-104

Williams R.J. (1986) Reinforcement learning in connectionist networks: A mathematical analysis. **Technical Report ICS 8605**, Institute for Cognitive Science, University of California at San Diego, La Jolla, CA.

Williams R.J. (1987) Reinforcement learning in connectionist systems. **Technical Report NU-CCS-87-3**, College of Computer Science, Northeastern University, 360 Huntington Avenue, Boston, MA.

6

A Mechanism for the Storage of Temporal Correlations

H. Christopher Longuet-Higgins

Summary

An important property of associative nets as content-addressable memory models is their capacity to reconstruct the whole of a pattern from part of it; or more generally, when presented with one member of a pair of associated patterns, to recreate the other. A special case is that in which the patterns are pulse sequences, and the first sequence is required to evoke the second. This can be achieved by sending the two sequences, in the correct temporal relation, down two parallel delay lines, one fast and one slow. The earlier sequence is sent along the slow line, and the later along the fast line; wherever one pulse overtakes another, a 'Hebbian synapse' between the two lines becomes activated. Thereafter, when the first sequence is input to the slow line, the second is output on the fast line (together with weaker secondary pulses) in the appropriate temporal relation. It would be of interest to know whether this principle is employed by the central nervous system for the storage and retrieval of temporally structured information.

6.1   Introduction

This note is in the nature of a postscript to an early suggestion (Longuet-Higgins, 1968a), that holographic principles might be employed for the storage and retrieval of temporal information by the central nervous system. For the storage of spatial patterns the hologram (Gabor, 1948, 1949, 1951) has a number of attractive features (van Heerden, 1963; Longuet-Higgins et al., 1970), including content addressability and resistance to damage, and it therefore seemed worthwhile to try and extend the holographic principle into the time dimension. The first model to emerge from this investigation was the 'holophone' - a bank of narrow band-pass filters with individually adjustable gains (Longuet-Higgins, 1968b). The principles underlying its operation were essentially as follows. After the passage of a temporally extended signal, the gain of each filter in the bank was set equal to the amount of energy in the signal at that frequency; thereafter, when the earlier part of

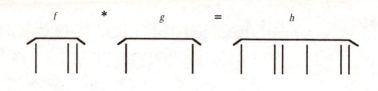

Figure 6.1

the signal was played into the holophone, the later part would emerge automatically, though in slightly garbled form.

It soon became clear, however, that the holophone could hardly be taken literally as a model of temporal memory. Because of a complementary relation (the details of which need not detain us here) between the bandwidths of the filters and the duration of the recorded signal, the memorization of a signal lasting 1 second would require a bank of filters of bandwidth only 1 hertz, and such fine tuning would place quite unrealistic demands on the central nervous system. Gabor (1968) pointed out that this problem would not arise in a system that was based on operations in the time domain rather than the frequency domain; the substance of this important idea will now be outlined briefly.

6.2   Correlations and convolutions

Figure 6.1 illustrates the operation of *convolution*, denoted by an asterisk: a 3-line pattern f is convolved with a 2-line pattern g to yield the 6-line pattern $h = f * g$ called the convolution of f and g. The order of the terms in a convolution makes no difference to the result, but this is not true of *correlation* - a closely related operation. If $f^{\sim}$ is the mirror image of f, then the cross correlation of f with g may be written as $f^{\sim} * g$, whereas the cross correlation of g with f is $g^{\sim} * f$, the mirror image of $f^{\sim} * g$. If f and g are identical the cross correlation of either with the other is simply the auto-correlation function $f^{\sim} * f$, which is left-to-right symmetrical (see Figure 6.2).

Now suppose that f and g are pulse sequences, with f preceding g, and that we want a device that will output g in response to the input f. Then under certain conditions this requirement can be met by a linear filter whose impulse response is $f^{\sim} * g$, the cross correlation of f with g. The reason is to be found in Equation 6.1

$$f * (f^{\sim} * g) = (f * f^{\sim}) * g, \tag{6.1}$$

which asserts that the response of such a filter to the input f equals the convolution of g with the auto-correlation function $(f * f^{\sim})$. If the signal f is sufficiently noise-

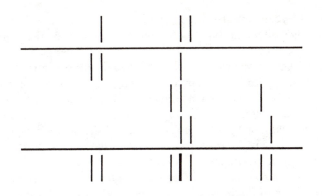

Figure 6.2 The function f (top row) is convolved with its mirror image $f^{\sim}$ (middle rows) to give its auto-correlation function (bottom row), which has a peak in the middle. (No such peak appears in the convolution of f with itself.)

like in character, its auto-correlation function will be sharply peaked at the origin, and the right hand side of Equation 6.1 will then approximate to g itself, as required.

In passing we may note that a signal whose auto-correlation function is small except at zero must have a flat power spectrum (since the power spectrum and the auto-correlation function are Fourier transforms of each other). A single pulse has this property, but a periodic signal does not.

As Dr G.J. Mitchison points out, a slight generalization of Equation 6.1 shows that a mere fragment of the cue f may suffice to evoke the response g. For if f is a sufficiently noise-like signal, and f' is another signal, then the filter's response to f' will be

$$f' * (f^{\sim} * g) = (f' * f^{\sim}) * g \tag{6.2}$$

The term $(f' * f^{\sim})$ on the right hand side of Equation 6.2 is the cross correlation of f with f'; if f' is a sufficiently large fragment of f it will have a peak at the origin like the auto-correlation $(f * f^{\sim})$, and the response of the system to f' will bear a strong resemblance to the desired output g.

6.3 An implementation

In order to implement Equation 6.1, in neural tissue or in hardware, it is necessary to represent time by some physical quantity such as distance, voltage or concentration; a particularly attractive measure is distance along a delay line, where the velocity of propagation links the dimensions of space and time. Braitenberg suggested many years ago (Braitenberg, 1961) that the parallel fibres in the cerebellum might well be fulfilling such a function, but nothing that follows hinges upon this particular hypothesis.

Figure 6.3 shows one way in which the temporal cross correlation between two pulse sequences might be spatially encoded, and subsequently used to reconstruct the later sequence from the earlier one. The horizontal lines at the bottom of the diagram represent a pair of parallel delay lines, one fast and one slow. The earlier sequence f, consisting of two pulses a and b, is input along the slow line; the later sequence g, consisting of pulses c and d, is then input along the fast line. Wherever a fast pulse overtakes a slow one a short circuit is created between the two lines; the pattern of short circuits, resembling the rungs of a ladder, represents the cross correlation of f with g. If, subsequently, the signal f is input to the slow line, a new pulse is generated on the fast line whenever a or b arrives at one of the short circuits. One obtains in this way 8 incipient pulses on the fast line, but of these 8 pulses 2 pairs coalesce to produce signals twice as strong as the others. The resulting pattern of 6 fast pulses is, indeed, the convolution of g with the auto-correlation function of f, and is dominated by the pulses labelled c and d in Figure 6.3.

6.4   Neuronal possibilities

The simplest realization of such a device in neural tissue would be one in which each short circuit from the slow to the fast line was a Hebbian synapse that had been activated by a combination of pre- and post-synaptic activity. The role of the slow line would then be played by the axon of a pre-synaptic neuron, and that of the fast line by another neuron receiving multiple synapses from the first. The anatomical signature of such a system would be a narrow axon making multiple synapses onto the body of the post-synaptic neuron or onto one of its principal dendrites.

Systems of this type suffer, however, from an important limitation: if there are m pulses in the sequence f and n in the sequence g, then the number of synapses needed to encode the cross correlation is m times n, so that for even moderate values of m and n the rungs of the synaptic ladder would have to be impossibly close together. Particular interest therefore attaches to the cases in which f or g consists of a single pulse.

A system that emits a single pulse in response to a specific input sequence constitutes a temporal pattern recognition device; one that emits a specific sequence in response to a single pulse could trigger the performance of a motor routine. A third case is that of a system that learns to respond to a single pulse by waiting for a definite time and then emitting a single pulse. In the style of Figure 6.3 such a system would be represented by a synaptic ladder with only one rung; it would

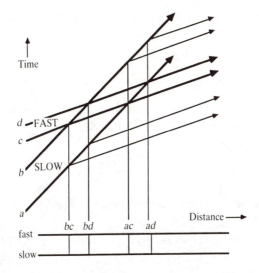

Figure 6.3 Two impulses *a* and *b* along the slow delay line are overtaken by two later impulses *c* and *d* along the fast line, at the places marked *bc*, *bd* etc. Later, the slow impulses *a* and *b* give rise to fast impulses *c* and *d*, and also to weaker secondary impulses.

constitute not merely a Hebbian synapse, but one which reproduced the time delay between the pre- and post-synaptic events in which it participated.

6.5 The association of spatio-temporal patterns

Given a device that learns to respond to an input pulse by emitting an output pulse after a specific time interval, one can build networks that associate pairs of patterns having temporal as well as spatial structure. The simplest possible architecture for such a network is one in which every input line is connected to every output line by a Hebbian-type time-delay synapse - one which learns to associate a pre-synaptic pulse with a post-synaptic pulse at a definite time later. Such a network can readily be taught to associate a sequence of pulses at times t_i along its input lines x_i with a later sequence of pulses at times t_j along its output lines y_j: for every i and j such that $t_i < t_j$ one sets the time delay of the synapse S_{ij} equal to $t_j - t_i$. This recipe for forming spatio-temporal associations is, of course, indifferent to the nature of the synaptic mechanism.

Finally, to propose a mechanism for the storage and retrieval of temporal sequences is not to imply that all sequential information is temporal in character; there are many cognitive skills, such as the memorization of poems or pieces of music, in which timing is of little or no consequence in comparison with sequential order. The manner in which the brain stores such purely ordinal information is, at the present time, an unsolved problem.

Acknowledgements

I am indebted to Dr Graeme J. Mitchison for helpful comments, and to the Royal Society of London for generous research support.

References

Braitenberg V. (1961) Functional interpretation of cerebellar histology. **Nature 190**, p. 539

Gabor D. (1948) A new microscopic principle. **Nature 161,** p. 777

Gabor D. (1949) Microscopy by reconstructed wavefronts. **Proc. Roy. Soc. Lond. A 197**, p. 187

Gabor, D. (1951) Microscopy by reconstructed wavefronts II. **Proc. Phys. Soc. 64**, p. 449

Gabor D. (1968) Improved holographic model of temporal recall. **Nature 217,** p.1288

van Heerden P.J. (1963) A new optical method of storing and retrieving information. **Applied Optics 2,** p. 387

Longuet-Higgins H.C. (1968a) Holographic model of temporal recall. **Nature 217,** p. 104

Longuet-Higgins H.C. (1968b) The non-local storage of temporal information. **Proc. Roy. Soc. Lond. B 171,** p. 327

Longuet-Higgins H.C., Willshaw D.J. & Buneman O.P. (1970) Theories of associative recall. **Quart. Rev. of Biophys. 3**, pp. 223-244. Reprinted in Longuet-Higgins H.C. (1987) **Mental Processes: Studies in Cognitive Science** MIT Press, Cambridge, Mass.

7
Induction of Synaptic Plasticity by Hebbian Covariance in the Hippocampus

Terrence Sejnowski, Sumantra Chattarji & Patric Stanton

7.1 Introduction

Most models of information storage in neural networks rely on changing the synaptic strengths, or weights, between model neurons (Hinton & Anderson, 1989). The weights in these simplifying models are altered by learning rules or algorithms so that the network can later retrieve the stored information, or perform the desired task. A great variety of such learning rules have been postulated, analysed, and simulated (Sejnowski & Tesauro, 1989). Most of these algorithms are based on mechanisms for which there is little or no experimental evidence (Crick, 1989). Indeed, experimental evidence for the long-term alteration of synaptic strengths is very difficult to obtain, and until recently there was no direct evidence for changes of the required duration at any synapse in adult neurons. This situation is rapidly changing as new experimental preparations and techniques are being developed (Alkon, 1987; Kandel *et al.*, 1987; Brown *et al.*, 1989). In this chapter we will explore what is currently known about synaptic plasticity in the mammalian hippocampus and will present experimental data that supports a particular class of learning algorithms.

One of the most popular learning rules is the 'Hebb' rule, which requires the strength of a synapse to increase upon the simultaneous coactivation of pre-synaptic and post-synaptic activity (Hebb, 1949). The defining characteristics of a Hebbian synapse are, first, that it depends only on pre-synaptic and post-synaptic variables, and secondly, that the alteration of the weight depends interactively on these two variables, and not separately (Brown *et al.*, 1989). Thus, a mechanism that depended only on the state of the pre-synaptic neuron, such as post-tetanic potentiation (Katz & Miledi, 1968), would not qualify as Hebbian. This interactive requirement makes the mechanism fundamentally associative. This said, it should be noted that the Hebb rule can nonetheless be implemented by non-associative mechanisms with circuitry of sufficient complexity (Sejnowski & Tesauro, 1989).

Many variations on the Hebb rule have been proposed. For example, some aspects of classical conditioning can be mimicked by a single Hebbian synapse if the temporal sensitivities of the pre-synaptic and post-synaptic elements are suitably

105

arranged (Sutton & Barto, 1981; Tesauro, 1986; Klopf, 1987). There are also good reasons for allowing the sign of the alteration to change, so that selective decreases as well as increases in strength can be made (Sejnowski, 1977b). Thus, it has been proposed that long-term decreases of synaptic strength should occur during conditions when the pre-synaptic and post-synaptic activities are negatively correlated (Sejnowski, 1977a). Similar suggestions have been made for changes in synaptic strengths during development (Bienenstock *et al.*, 1982).

In translating an algorithm like the Hebb rule into testable physiological hypotheses, general terms such as 'activity' must be made explicit. Thus, activity could mean the average level of membrane potential, the stimulation of action potentials, or perhaps the raised level of particular ionic concentrations. Many of these physiological variables are, of course, linked, but one or another of them might be particularly critical to the plasticity. Specific experiments must be designed to determine which variables are the critical ones. In the next section, we will summarize what is currently known about the important variables for the long-term potentiation of synaptic transmission in the hippocampus. Later in the chapter we will present experimental evidence for associative long-term depression as well as associative long-term potentiation of synaptic strength. The conditions under which this plasticity is observed are consistent with a Hebbian covariance model of synaptic plasticity (Sejnowski, 1977a).

7.2 Existing evidence for Hebbian and non-Hebbian synaptic plasticity in the hippocampus

A brief, high frequency activation of excitatory synapses in the hippocampus produces a long-lasting increase in synaptic strength, called long-term potentiation (LTP) (Bliss & Lomo, 1973). Typically, many fibers are synchronously activated for several seconds at frequencies greater than 50 Hz, and the synaptic potentials typically increase by 50-100%. Most of the experiments on LTP have been performed on thin, transverse slices of hippocampal tissue that are maintained *in vitro* in a perfusion chamber. The various regions and layers of cells in the hippocampus can be easily visualized and direct access is possible with recording and stimulating microelectrodes. In addition, pharmacological agents that alter neuronal properties can be easily applied. LTP can be reliably maintained within stimulated slices for the lifetime of the slice, which is around 10 hours. When stimulated *in vitro*, induction of LTP elevates synaptic strengths for weeks or months (Bliss & Gardner-Medwin, 1973).

If LTP depended only on pre-synaptic activation, then it would not be Hebbian, as defined above. The critical test to determine whether LTP also depends on the post-synaptic cell was performed on pyramidal cells in area CA1 by several groups, all of which came to essentially the same conclusion: LTP requires the simultaneous release of neurotransmitter from pre-synaptic terminals coupled with post-synaptic depolarization (Kelso *et al.*, 1986; Malinow & Miller, 1986; Gustafsson & Wigstrom, 1987). However, the plasticity is not critically dependent on action potentials *per se*, since LTP can be induced even when action potentials are selectively blocked in the post-synaptic cell (Kelso *et al.*, 1986; McNaughton *et al.*, 1978). LTP should thus be called pseudo-Hebbian, since the original hypothesis required the post-synaptic cell to be excited or to persistently fire coincidentally with pre-synaptic activity (Hebb, 1949). The consequences of this difference will be taken up in the discussion.

There is a form of long-term plasticity, called associative LTP, that can be produced in some hippocampal neurons when two separate pathways, a test input and a conditioning input that impinge on the same cells, are simultaneously activated (Levy & Steward, 1979, 1983; Barrionuevo & Brown, 1983). In these experiments, a weak test input when stimulated alone does not have a long-lasting effect on synaptic strength; however, when this input is paired with stimulation of a conditioning input sufficient to produce homosynaptic LTP of that pathway, the test pathway is *associatively* potentiated. How is information about the conditioning input transmitted through the dendrites to the synapses from the test inputs? The spread of current from the conditioning input can depolarize the post-synaptic membrane near the synapses of the test input. A voltage-dependent mechanism in the post-synaptic cell could then account for the associative induction of LTP.

The neurotransmitter that mediates the excitatory post-synaptic potentials (EPSPs) in area CA1, and in most long-distance projections in the brain, is likely to be glutamate or a closely related amino acid. There are at least two distinct types of glutamate receptors on the post-synaptic membrane. One of these is responsible for the fast transmission of excitation, the Kainate/Quisqualate, or the K/Q receptor. The other receptor, called the NMDA receptor after the agonist N-methyl-D-aspartate which selectively activates it, has a voltage dependence that permits it to open only when the post-synaptic membrane is strongly depolarized at the same time that glutamate binds to the receptor. The specific NMDA receptor antagonist 2-amino-5-phosphonovaleric acid (AP5) blocks the induction of associative LTP in CA1 pyramidal neurons (Collingridge *et al.*, 1983; Harris *et al.*, 1984; Wigstrom & Gustafsson, 1984). Thus, the NMDA receptor is likely to be an essential component in the Hebbian mechanism underlying LTP in area CA1. Interestingly, AP5 does not block the induction of LTP in another pathway within the hippocampus, that between the mossy fibers and pyramidal cells in area CA3. This observation serves as the starting point for the new experiments that are presented in a later section.

In addition to Hebbian plasticity, non-Hebbian forms of synaptic plasticity have also been found in the hippocampus. Post-tetanic potentiation (PTP) is an elevation of synaptic strengths for many minutes following a high frequency tetanus of the synapse. PTP is a consequence of pre-synaptic mechanisms and does not depend on the post-synaptic cell (Katz & Miledi, 1968; Scharfman & Sarvey, 1985). Another non-Hebbian form of plasticity in the hippocampus is the heterosynaptic depression produced in an unstimulated or weakly-stimulated pathway when another pathway converging on the same neurons is stimulated at a high rate for a prolonged duration (Levy & Steward, 1979, 1983; Lynch *et al.*,

1977). In this case, the depression does not depend on activity of the test input and does not seem to be as long lasting as LTP.

7.3 The covariance model of associative information storage

Probably the most important and most thoroughly explored use of the Hebb rule in neural network models is in the formation of associations between one stimulus or pattern of activity in one neural population and another (Kohonen, 1984). The Hebb rule is appealing for this use, because it provides a way of forming global associations between large-scale patterns of activity in assemblies of neurons using only the local information available at individual synapses. The earliest models of associative memory were based on network models in which the output of a model neuron was assumed to be proportional to a linear sum of its inputs, each weighted by a synaptic strength. Thus,

$$V_B = \sum_{A=1}^{N} W_{BA} V_A \qquad (7.1)$$

where V_B are the firing rates of a group of M output cells, and V_A are the firing rates of a group of N input cells, and W_{BA} is the synaptic strength between input cell A and output cell B.

The transformation between patterns of activity on the input vectors to patterns of activity on the output vectors is determined by the synaptic weight matrix, W_{BA}. This matrix can be constructed from pairs of associated input and output vectors using the simplest version of the Hebb rule (Steinbuch, 1961; Anderson, 1970; Kohonen, 1970; Longuet-Higgins, 1968):

$$\Delta W_{BA} = \varepsilon V_B V_A \qquad (7.2)$$

where the strength of the learning ε can be adjusted to scale the outputs to the desired values.

More than one association can be stored in the same matrix, so long as the input vectors are not too similar to each other. This is accomplished by using Equation 7.2 for each input-output pair. This model of associative storage is simple and has several attractive features: first, the learning occurs in only one trial; second, the information is distributed over many synapses, so that recall is relatively immune to noise or damage; and third, input patterns similar to stored inputs will give output similar to the stored outputs, a form of generalization. This linear model has been generalized to non-linear models of associative memory, which has led to a new class of learning algorithms based on the principle of error-correction (Sejnowski & Tesauro, 1989). In these algorithms, more than one presentation is needed for each input since the storage must be optimized for the entire set of stored patterns.

Numerous variations have been proposed on the conditions for Hebbian plasticity (Sejnowski, 1977a,b; Kohonen, 1984; Levy *et al.*, 1984). One problem with any synaptic modification rule that can only increase the strength of a synapse is that the synaptic strength will eventually saturate at its maximum value. Non-specific decay can reduce the sizes of the weights, but the stored information will also decay and be lost at the same rate. Another approach is to renormalize the total synaptic weight of the entire terminal field from a single neuron to a constant value (von der Malsburg, 1973). One learning algorithm that accomplishes this uses the selective decrease of synaptic strength to accomplish optimal error-correction learning based on storing the covariances between the pre-synaptic and post-synaptic neurons (Sejnowski, 1977a,b). According to this rule, the change in strength of a plastic synapse should be proportional to the covariance between the pre-synaptic firing and post-synaptic firing:

$$\Delta W_{BA} = \varepsilon \left(V_B - \langle V_B \rangle \right) \left(V_A - \langle V_A \rangle \right) \tag{7.3}$$

where $\langle V_B \rangle$ are the average firing rates of the output neurons and $\langle V_A \rangle$ are the average firing rates of the input neurons (see also Chauvet, 1986). Thus, the strength of the synapse should increase if the firing of the pre-synaptic and post-synaptic elements are positively correlated, decrease if they are negatively correlated, and remain unchanged if they are uncorrelated. The covariance rule is an extension of the Hebb rule and it is easy to show that traditional Hebbian synapses can be used to implement it. Taking a time average of the change in synaptic weight in Equation 7.3:

$$\langle \Delta W_{BA} \rangle = \varepsilon \left(\langle V_B V_A \rangle - \langle V_B \rangle \langle V_A \rangle \right) \tag{7.4}$$

The first term on the right hand side has the same form as the simple Hebbian synapse in Equation 7.2. The second term is a learning 'threshold' that varies with the product of the time-averaged pre-synaptic and post-synaptic activity levels. The learning threshold ensures that no change in synaptic strength should occur if the average correlation between the pre-synaptic and post-synaptic activities is at chance level; that is, when there is no net covariance. The time averages in Equations 7.3 & 7.4 should be taken over a time interval that is long compared to the moment-by-moment fluctuations occurring within synapses. In the hippocampus, which has an intrinsic 5-6 Hz theta rhythm, the averaging time should be greater than 200 ms.

The covariance model is based both on information contained in the membrane potentials within populations of neurons and on information transmitted between neurons in the spatio-temporal patterns of spike trains. Recent recordings from pairs of neurons in visual cortex and from local field potentials reflecting pooled activity in hundreds of neurons indicate that oscillatory stimulus-selective correlations are present in cortical networks (Gray & Singer, 1989). Furthermore, experiments with visual stimuli that extend over a wide area of the visual field indicate that these correlations could carry important global information about visual stimuli (Gray *et al.*, 1989). Thus, significant correlations exist between neurons in cerebral cortex that could provide a signal to a covariance storage mechanism.

7.4   Experimental evidence for the Hebbian covariance rule in the hippocampus

7.4.1   *Hebbian synapses in area CA1*

Recently, a new type of synaptic plasticity has been reported in field CA1 of the hippocampus that results in a long-term depression (LTD) of synaptic strengths (Stanton & Sejnowski, 1989). LTD is associative and can be induced in a test input when interacting with a stronger conditioning input on the same dendritic tree, but only if the two inputs are negatively correlated in time. The stimulus paradigm that was used, illustrated in Figure 7.1B, was based on the finding that high-frequency bursts of stimuli spaced 200 ms apart are optimal in eliciting LTP (Larson & Lynch, 1986). The conditioning, or strong stimulus pattern, which was almost always effective in eliciting maximal LTP, consisted of trains of 10 bursts of 5 pulses each at a frequency of 100 Hz, with a 200 ms interburst interval. Each train lasted 2 seconds and had a total of 50 stimuli. The test, or weak stimuli, a train of single shocks at 5 Hz frequency, were given either superimposed on the middle of each burst (positively correlated, or 'in phase'), or symmetrically between the bursts (negatively correlated, or 'out of phase').

The strong stimulus was applied to the Schaffer collaterals and the test stimulus was applied to the subicular input on the opposite side of the recording site, as shown in Figure 7.1A. The weak stimulus train was first applied alone and did not itself induce long-lasting changes. The conditioning site was then stimulated alone, which elicited *homosynaptic* LTP of this pathway but did not significantly alter the amplitude of responses to the test input. When the test and conditioning inputs were activated in phase, the test input synapses were associatively potentiated, as predicted (Figure 7.2A). In contrast, when test and conditioning inputs were applied out of phase, an associative depression of the test input synapses was induced that lasted for hours (Figure 7.2B). The duration of associative LTD was at least 30 minutes (Figure 7.2C) and up to 3 hours following stimulation. The amplitude and duration of associative LTD or LTP could be increased by stimulating input pathways with more trains of shocks. When weak input shocks were applied both superimposed *and* between the bursts, so that the average covariance was zero between test and conditioning inputs, there was no net change in synaptic strength. Thus, the associative LTP and LTD mechanisms appear to be balanced.

A weak stimulus that is out of phase with a strong conditioning stimulus arrives when the post-synaptic neuron is hyperpolarized as a consequence of

(A)

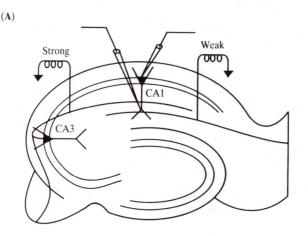

(B)

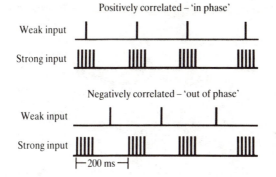

Figure 7.1 Hippocampal slice preparation for area CA1. **A.** Schematic diagram of the *in vitro* hippocampal slice showing recording sites in the CA1 pyramidal cell somatic (stratum pyramidale) and dendritic (stratum radiatum) layers, and conditioning stimulus sites activating Schaffer collateral (Strong) and commissural test afferents (Weak). Hippocampal slices (400 μm thick) were prepared by standard methods and incubated in an interface slice chamber at 34-35°C. Extracellular (1-5 MΩ resistance, 2M NaCl filled) and intracellular (70-120 MΩ, 2M K-acetate filled) recording electrodes, and bipolar glass-insulated platinum wire stimulating electrodes (50 μm tip diameter), were prepared by standard methods. **B.** Schematic diagram of stimulus paradigms used. Conditioning input stimuli (Strong input) were four trains of 100 Hz bursts. Each burst had 5 stimuli and the interburst interval was 200 ms. Each train lasted 2 seconds and had a total of 50 stimuli. Test input stimuli (Weak input) were four trains of shocks at 5 Hz frequency, each train lasting for 2 seconds. When these inputs were *in phase*, the test single shocks were superimposed on the middle of each burst of the conditioning input, as shown. When the test input was *out of phase*, the single shocks were placed symmetrically between the bursts.

(A)   Associative long-term potentiation

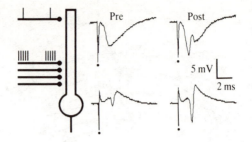

(B)   Associative long-term depression

(C)

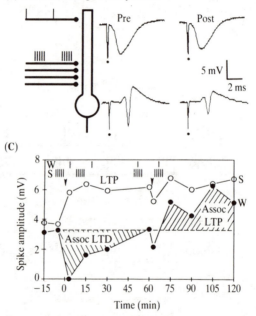

Figure 7.2 Associative LTP and associative long-term depression (LTD) of evoked extracellular potentials. **A.** Associative LTP of evoked EPSPs and population action potential responses in the test input. Test responses are shown before and 30 min after application of test stimuli in phase with the coactive conditioning input. **B.** Associative LTD of evoked EPSPs and population spike responses in the test input. Test responses are shown before and 30 min after application of test stimuli out of phase with the coactive conditioning input. **C.** Time course of the changes in population spike amplitudes for a typical experiment. Inset at the top shows the stimulus patterns for the test (T) and conditioning (C) inputs and arrows show the time of stimulation. Single responses from the conditioning input (open circles), show that the high- frequency bursts (5 pulses/100 Hz, 200 ms interburst interval as in Figure 7.1) elicited synapse-specific LTP independent of other input activity. Single responses from the test input (filled circles) show that stimulation of the test pathway out of phase with the conditioning one produced associative LTD (Assoc LTD) of this input. In-phase stimulation of the same pathway elicited **(cont. opposite)**

inhibitory post-synaptic potentials and after-hyperpolarization from mechanisms intrinsic to pyramidal neurons. This suggests that post-synaptic hyperpolarization coupled with pre-synaptic activation may trigger LTD. To test this hypothesis, we injected current through intracellular microelectrodes to hyperpolarize or depolarize the cell while stimulating a synaptic input. Pairing the injection of depolarizing current with the low-frequency stimulation led to LTP of the stimulated synapses (Figure 7.3A), while a response to a control input inactive during the stimulation did not change, as reported previously (Kelso *et al.*, 1986; Malinow & Miller, 1986; Gustafsson *et al.*, 1987). Conversely, prolonged hyperpolarizing current injection paired with the same low frequency stimuli led to induction of LTD in the stimulated pathway, but not in the unstimulated pathway (Figure 7.3B). The application of either depolarizing current, hyperpolarizing current, or the 5 Hz synaptic stimulation alone did not induce long-term alterations in synaptic strengths. Thus, the pairing of post-synaptic hyperpolarization and pre-synaptic activity is sufficient to induce LTD of the intracellular EPSPs in CA1 pyramidal neurons.

Associative LTP is believed to depend on the spread of current from conditioning synapses to test synapses in the dendritic tree, where the simultaneous depolarization of the post-synaptic membrane and activation of glutamate receptors of the N-methyl-D-aspartate (NMDA) subtype leads to LTP induction (Collingridge *et al.*, 1983; Harris *et al.*, 1984; Wigstrom & Gustafsson, 1984). Consistent with this hypothesis, we find that the NMDA receptor antagonist 2-amino-5-phosphonovaleric acid (AP5, 10μM) blocked the induction of associative LTP by the in-phase stimuli in CA1 pyramidal neurons. In contrast, the application of AP5 to the bathing solution at this same concentration did not affect associative LTD. Thus, the induction of associative LTD does not appear to involve the activation of the NMDA receptor.

These experiments confirm predictions made from the covariance model of information storage in neural networks (Sejnowski, 1977a,b). The plasticity is associative, long-lasting, and is produced when pre-synaptic activity occurs while the post-synaptic membrane is hyperpolarized. The other condition that should produce synaptic depression according to the predictions of the covariance model - the absence of pre-synaptic activity while the post-synaptic neuron is strongly depolarized - has also been found in the hippocampus (Levy & Steward, 1983; Lynch *et al.*, 1977). However, this heterosynaptic depression is not as long lasting as LTP and requires stronger stimulation. For example, the control stimulation of the strong pathway in our experiments did not produce measurable depression of the inactive test pathway. This may indicate that the algorithm for synaptic plasticity in the hippocampus only approximates the covariance.

(Fig. 7.2 cont.) associative LTP (Assoc LTP). The duration of associative LTD was at least 30 minutes and up to 3 hours following stimulation. The amplitude and duration of associative LTD or LTP could be increased by stimulating input pathways with more trains of shocks.

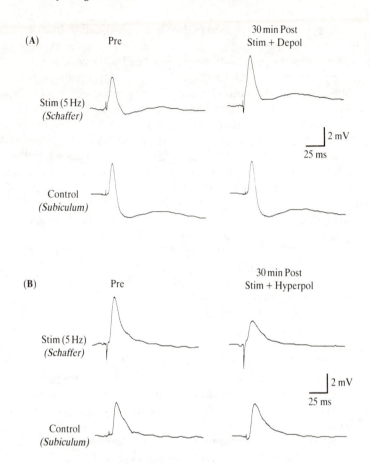

Figure 7.3 Pairing of post-synaptic hyperpolarization with stimulation of synapses on CA1 hippocampal pyramidal neurons produces LTD specific to the activated pathway, while pairing of post-synaptic depolarization with synaptic stimulation produces synapse-specific LTP. **A.** Intracellular evoked EPSPs are shown at stimulated (Stim 5 Hz) and unstimulated (Control) pathway synapses before and 30 min after pairing depolarizing current injection with 5 Hz synaptic stimulation (the constant +2.0 nA current produced a 20 mV depolarization of the soma without synaptic stimulation). The stimulated pathway exhibited associative LTP of the EPSP, while the control, unstimulated input showed no change in synaptic strength. **B.** Intracellular EPSPs are shown evoked at stimulated and control pathway synapses before and 30 min after pairing a 20 mV hyperpolarization at the cell soma with 5 Hz synaptic stimulation (the constant −1.0 nA current produced a 20 mV hyperpolarization of the soma in the absence of synaptic stimulation). The input (Stim 5 Hz) activated during the hyperpolarization showed associative LTD of synaptic evoked EPSPs, while synaptic strength of the silent input (Control) was unaltered. The cell fired action potentials during the depolarizing current injection, but not during injection of the hyperpolarizing current. In a previous study, hyperpolarizing current applied during high-frequency synaptic stimulation blocked LTP, but LTD of the synaptic input was not reported (Malinow & Miller, 1986). However, the input stimulus was typically 30 Hz or higher compared to the 5 Hz used in our experiment, so that the dendritic membrane potential during synaptic stimulation was probably significantly more positive at the 30 Hz rate.

7.4.2   Non-Hebbian and Hebbian synapses in area CA3

Area CA3 of the hippocampus exhibits two forms of LTP, one of which is dependent on NMDA receptors - the commissural pathway - and another that is not - the mossy fiber pathway (Harris *et al.*, 1984). We will summarize here our recent finding that both associative LTP and associative LTD can be induced in the commissural pathway, but neither can be elicited in the mossy fiber pathway of area CA3 (Chattarji *et al.*, 1989). The differences in the rules for plasticity in these pathways are likely to be related to the different functions that these pathways have in guiding the storage of information in the hippocampus: in particular, the mossy fiber pathway is non-Hebbian, but the commissural inputs are Hebbian.

In our experiments, extracellular field potential recordings were made in the CA3 pyramidal cell body and apical dendritic layers of rat hippocampal slices (Figure 7.4). Stimulating electrodes were placed on opposite sides of the hippocampal fissure and stimuli applied to separate Commissural/Schaffer collateral (COM) and mossy fiber (MF) afferents converging on CA3 pyramidal cells (Figure 7.4). The degree of potentiation or depression was evaluated by change in amplitude of the population spike and the peak initial slope of the compound excitatory post-synaptic potential (EPSP). In some control experiments, specific activation of mossy fibers was verified by inducing LTP of this pathway in the presence of AP5 (Harris *et al.*, 1984), which shows that this pathway is indeed the one that is independent of the activation of NMDA receptors. The same stimulus paradigm that was effective at eliciting associative LTP and associative LTD in area CA1 was used in area CA3.

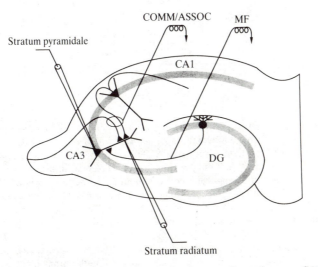

Figure 7.4 Hippocampal slice preparation and stimulus paradigms for area CA3. Schematic diagram of the *in vitro* hippocampal slice preparation showing recording sites in the CA3 pyramidal cell somatic (stratum pyramidale) and dendritic (stratum radiatum) layers, and stimulus sites activating Commissural/ Schaffer (COM) or mossy fiber (MF) afferents.

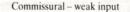

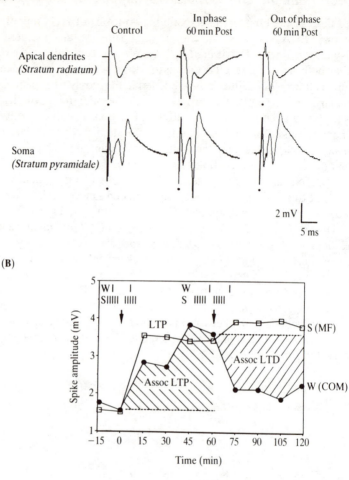

Figure 7.5 CA3 commissural synapses exhibit both associative LTP and associative LTD. **A**. When the COM side received a weak (W) input *in phase* with a strong (S) MF tetanus, the W site exhibited associative long-term potentiation (LTP) of both the synaptic EPSP in the apical dendritic layer (upper traces) and the population action potential in the cell soma layer (lower traces). This was followed by application of W stimuli to the COM site *out of phase* with the S stimuli to MF, which caused an associative long-term depression (LTD) seen as a marked reduction in the population spike amplitude with a lesser decrease in EPSP slope. Test responses are shown before (Control) and 60 min after application of weak stimuli in phase and out of phase with the strong MF input, respectively. **B**. Time course of the changes in population spike amplitude observed at each input for a typical experiment where synaptic strengths could be alternately enhanced and depressed in the same slice. Test responses from the strong input (S, open squares), show that the high-frequency bursts elicited LTP specific to MF synapses. Test responses from the weak input (W, filled circles) show that stimulation of the weak pathway in phase with the strong one produced associative LTP (Assoc LTP) of this input. Associative LTD of the same pathway was then elicited following out of phase stimulation.

In initial experiments, the commissural pathway was used as the test, or weak input site (W) and the mossy fiber pathway received the conditioning, or strong stimuli (S) (Figure 7.5). The weak stimulus train was first applied alone and did not itself induce long-lasting changes, following which strong site stimulation alone elicited homosynaptic LTP of the strong pathway without significantly altering weak input synaptic strength. However, when the commissural (COM) side received a weak input in phase with a strong mossy fiber (MF) tetanus, it elicited an associative long-term potentiation (LTP) of the weak input synapses, as shown in Figure 7.5A. Both the EPSP and population action potential (Figure 7.5A) were significantly enhanced for at least 60 min and up to 180 min following stimulation (Figure 7.5B).

In contrast, application of weak stimuli to the commissural site out of phase with the strong mossy fiber tetanus caused an associative long-term depression (LTD) of the weak input synapses (Figure 7.5A). There was a marked reduction in the population spike with smaller decreases in the EPSP. As in the experiments in area CA1 reported above, the stimulus patterns applied to each input were identical in these two experiments, and only the relative phase of the weak and strong stimuli was varied. Synaptic strengths could be alternately enhanced and depressed in the same slice, as is shown in Figure 7.5B.

In the second series of experiments, the stimulus paradigms were reversed so that the mossy fibers received the weak input and the strong tetanus was applied to commissural afferents. In contrast to commissural synapses, when the mossy fiber pathway received weak stimuli in phase with strong stimuli via the commissural input, mossy fiber synapses did not exhibit any associative potentiation of either synaptic EPSP or population spike (Figure 7.6A). Similarly, application of weak stimuli out of phase with strong stimuli also failed to elicit associative LTD of the EPSP or population spike (Figure 7.6). Finally, although a weak input to mossy fiber synapses failed to elicit either associative LTP or LTD, homosynaptic LTP was shown in response to a strong tetanus to mossy fiber afferents alone, verifying the intact LTP-generating mechanisms in these synapses.

Our studies of interactions between strong and weak inputs onto the same dendritic tree of hippocampal pyramidal cells of field CA3 suggest that these pyramidal cells receive two separate synaptic inputs that differ fundamentally in their processing capabilities. The CA3 commissural synapses, which depend on NMDA receptor activation for the induction of LTP, exhibit associative LTP when they receive weak stimuli positively correlated in time with a strong mossy fiber tetanus. This result supports evidence that these synapses show depolarization-dependent associativity, a property thought to derive from the voltage dependence of the NMDA receptor (Bliss & Lomo, 1973; Mayer *et al.*, 1984; Kelso *et al.*, 1986). When the same weak input stimulation of the CA3 commissural synapses is negatively correlated in time with the conditioning mossy fiber input, a long-term depression (LTD) of the test commissural input is induced, similar to our findings in CA1 (Stanton & Sejnowski, 1989).

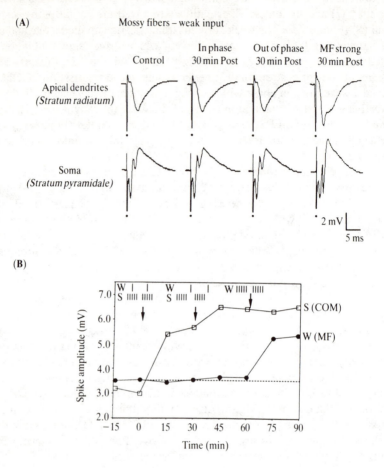

Figure 7.6 CA3 mossy fiber synapses do not exhibit either associative LTP or LTD. **A.** When the MF pathway received a weak stimuli (W) in phase with a strong stimulus (S) via the commissural input (COM), weak input MF synapses did not exhibit potentiation of either the synaptic EPSP in the apical dendritic layer or population spike in the cell body layer. Following this, application of W stimuli to the MF site out of phase with S stimuli to COM, also failed to elicit depression in population spike or EPSP. Finally, MF synapses did show homosynaptic LTP when presented with an S tetanus (MF Strong) to the MF pathway alone. Test responses are shown before (Control) and 30 min after application of in phase, out of phase and MF strong stimuli, respectively. **B.** Time course of the changes in population spike amplitude observed at each input for a representative experiment. Test responses from the strong input (S, open squares), show that the high-frequency bursts elicited homosynaptic LTP specific to COM synapses. Test responses from the weak input (W, filled circles) show that neither in phase nor out of phase stimulation elicited any potentiation or depression of this input. However, MF synapses did show homosynaptic LTP following the application of the strong bursts (S) to the MF pathway alone.

The rules for induction of long-term synaptic plasticity in mossy fiber inputs onto CA3 pyramidal neurons appear to be fundamentally different from those of commissural inputs. We have shown that a weak mossy fiber input failed to exhibit associative LTP when it was positively correlated in time with a strong commissural tetanus. This finding is in agreement with other studies (Kauer & Nicoll, 1989) and can be explained by the lack of NMDA receptors at this synapse (Monaghan & Cotman, 1985). The failure of these synapses to elicit associative LTD, however, is rather surprising, since results from similar experiments in area CA1 suggest that post-synaptic hyperpolarization coupled with pre-synaptic activation triggers associative LTD without requiring NMDA receptor activation (Stanton & Sejnowski, 1989). Our findings do not, however, rule out long-lasting potentiation or depression at these synapses that may require different stimulus patterns or important modulatory factors supplied by subcortical inputs to area CA3 (Hopkins & Johnston, 1984; Stanton & Sarvey, 1985).

7.5 Discussion

Most of the simplifying models of learning in neural networks leave out much of the biological detail, such as current spread in dendrites, active membrane conductances, and realistic patterns of connectivity. This does not mean that they cannot make contact with biological experiments, only that the predictions that come out of these models are necessarily broad, dealing with general relationships and not with specific details. These models can nonetheless suggest stimulus variables that should be explored and can help in interpreting the results.

For example, in our experiments on synaptic plasticity in the hippocampus, the covariance model suggested that negatively correlated inputs might be associated with synaptic depression, but did not provide the details of the stimulus paradigm (Sejnowski, 1977a,b). Thus, the choice of 100 Hz for the burst rate and 5 Hz for the burst repetition rate were determined by properties of the hippocampus and not the model. What the model did provide was the idea that synaptic depression comparable in magnitude and duration to LTP might be found in the hippocampus, and the general stimulus conditions that would be likely to characterize its induction. The covariance model pointed to negative temporal correlation between pre-synaptic and post-synaptic activity as a key variable and helped us design suitable patterns of stimuli.

Pyramidal cells in area CA3 have recurrent collaterals, which make it a good candidate area for a content-addressable associative memory (Kohonen, 1984; Hopfield, 1982; Rolls, 1987). The striking differences between synapses onto CA3 pyramidal neurons are likely to reflect their different roles in processing the flow of information from dentate granule cells to CA1 pyramidal neurons. Mossy fibers have a type of LTP that is non-associative and non-Hebbian. In contrast, the LTP and LTD exhibited by the commissural fibers to area CA3 are associative. Thus, the mossy fibers can 'instruct' the commissural inputs through associative interactions, but cannot themselves be influenced by information arriving from other pathways.

The recurrent collaterals of pyramidal cells within area CA3 have not been separately tested and it will be interesting to determine if they are of the associative or non-associative variety. It is also not known if there are associative interactions between mossy fiber synapses, though this would be unlikely given our present findings.

One of the consequences of having an associative mechanism that is pseudo-Hebbian rather than Hebbian (Kelso *et al.*, 1986), is that synapses on localized regions of a dendrite can interact with each other independently of processing occurring on other dendrites. The voltage-sensitive NMDA receptors which trigger LTP, effectively make each patch of dendrite a non-linear processing unit. This would greatly increase the amount of information that could be stored by a single neuron. The processing power of such a 'product' unit has been explored recently in the context of simplifying models by Durbin & Rumelhart (1989). More needs to be known about the timing relationships for LTP and LTD in the hippocampus, and also about the spatial integration possible within dendritic trees. Realistic models can help with sorting out these relationships, but only if enough data can be obtained to fully constrain the models.

The principles of neural representation and neural computation are likely to be different from the way that representation and computation are accomplished in digital computers (Churchland & Sejnowski, 1988). Discovering these principles, however, is a difficult undertaking that will require combined experimental and modeling techniques (Sejnowski *et al.*, 1989).

Acknowledgements

This research was supported by grants from the National Science Foundation and the Office of Naval Research to TJS. We have benefitted from discussion with Drs Thomas Brown, Charles Stevens, and Francis Crick.

References

Alkon D.L. (1987) **Memory Traces in the Brain**. Oxford University Press, Oxford.

Anderson J.A. (1970) Two models for memory organization using interacting traces. **Math. Biosci. 8**, pp. 137-160

Barrionuevo G. & Brown T.H. (1983) Associative long-term potentiation in hippocampal slices. **Proc. Nat. Acad. Sci. USA 80**, pp. 7347-7351

Bienenstock E.L., Cooper L.N. & Munro P.W. (1982) Theory for the development of neuron selectivity: orientation specificity and binocular interaction in visual cortex. **J. Neurosci. 2**, pp. 32-48

Bliss T.V.P. & Gardner-Medwin A. R. (1973) Long-lasting potentiation of synaptic transmission in the dentate area of the unanaesthetized rabbit following stimulation of the perforant path. **J. Physiol. (Lond.) 232**, pp. 357-374

Bliss T.V.P. & Lomo T. (1973) Long-lasting potentiation of synaptic transmission in the dentate area of the anaesthetized rabbit following stimulation of the perforant path. **J. Physiol. (Lond.) 232**, pp. 331-356

Brown T.H., Ganong A.H., Kariss E.W., Keenan C.L. & Kelso S.R. (1989) Long-term potentiation in two synaptic systems of the hippocampal brain slice. In: **Neural Models of Plasticity**. J.H. Byrne & W.O Berry (eds.) Academic Press, New York, in press.

Chattarji S., Stanton P.K. & Sejnowski T.J. (1989) Commissural synapses, but not mossy fiber synapses, in hippocampal field CA3 exhibit associative long-term potentiation and associative long-term depression. **Brain Res.** submitted.

Chauvet G. (1986) Habituation rules for a theory of the cerebellar cortex. **Biol. Cybern. 55**, pp. 201-209

Churchland P.S. & Sejnowski T.J. (1988) Neural representations and neural computations. In: **Neural Connections and Mental Computation**. L. Nadel (ed.) MIT Press, Cambridge, MA.

Collingridge G.L., Kehl S.L. & McLennan H. (1983) Excitatory amino acids in synaptic transmission in the Schaffer collateral-commissural pathway of the rat hippocampus. **J. Physiol. (Lond.) 334**, pp. 33-46

Crick F. (1989) The recent excitement about neural networks. **Nature 337**, pp. 129-132

Durbin R.M. & Rumelhart D.E. (1989) Product units for backpropagation networks. **Neural Computation 1**, pp. 133-142

Gray C.M. & Singer W. (1989) Neuronal oscillation in orientation columns of cat visual cortex. **Proc. Nat. Acad. Sci. USA 86**, pp. 1698-1702

Gray C.M., Konig P., Engel A.K. & Singer W. (1989) Oscillatory responses in cat visual cortex exhibit inter-columnar synchronization which reflects global stimulus properties. **Nature 338**, pp. 334-337

Gustafsson B., Wigstrom H., Abraham W.C. & Huang Y.Y. (1987) Long-term potentiation in the hippocampus using depolarizing current pulses as the conditioning stimulus to single volley synaptic potentials. **J. Neurosci. 7**, pp. 774-780

Harris E.W., Ganong A.H. & Cotman C.W. (1984) Long-term potentiation in the hippocampus involves activation of N-methyl-D-aspartate receptors. **Brain Res. 323**, pp. 132-137

Hebb D.O. (1949) **Organization of Behavior**. John Wiley & Sons, NY.

Hinton G.E. & Anderson J.A. (1989) **Parallel models of distributed memory**. Lawrence Erlbaum Press, Hillsdale, New Jersey.

Hopfield J.J. (1982) Neural networks and physical systems with emergent collective computational abilities. **Proc. Nat. Acad. Sci. USA. 79**, pp. 2554-2558

Hopkins W.F. & Johnston D. (1984) Frequency-dependent noradrenergic modulation of long-term potentiation in the hippocampus. **Science 226**, pp. 350-352

Kandel E.R., Klein M., Hochner B., Shuster M., Siegelbaum S.A., Hawkins R.D., Glanzman D.L. & Castellucci V.F. (1987) Synaptic modulation and learning: new insights into synaptic transmission from the study of behavior. In: **Synaptic Function**. pp. 471-518, G.M. Edelman, W.E. Gall & W.M. Cowan, (eds.) John Wiley & Sons, NY.

Katz B. & Miledi R. (1968) The role of calcium in neuromuscular facilitation. **J. Physiol. (Lond.) 195**, pp. 481-492

Kauer J.A. & Nicoll R.A. (1989) An APV-resistant non-associative form of long-term potentiation in the rat hippocampus. In: **Synaptic Plasticity in the Hippocampus**. Springer-Verlag, NY.

Kelso S.R., Ganong A.H. & Brown T.H. (1986) Hebbian synapses in hippocampus. **Proc. Nat. Acad. Sci. USA 83**, pp. 5326-5330

Klopf A.H. (1987) A neuronal model of classical conditioning. Air Force Wright Aeronautical Laboratories Technical Report **AFWAL-TR-87-1139**.

Kohonen T. (1970) Correlation matrix memories. **IEEE Trans. Comp. C-21**, pp. 353-359

Kohonen T. (1984) **Self-Organization and Associative Memory**. Springer Verlag, NY.

Larson J. & Lynch G. (1986) Induction of synaptic potentiation in hippocampus by patterned stimulation involves two events. **Science 232**, pp. 985-987

Levy W.B., Anderson J.A. & Lehmkuhle W. (1984) **Synaptic Change in the Nervous System**. Erlbaum, Hillsdale, New Jersey.

Levy W.B. & Steward O. (1979) Synapses as associative memory elements in the hippocampal formation. **Brain Res. 175**, pp. 233-245

Levy W.B. & Steward O. (1983) Temporal contiguity requirements for long-term associative potentiation/depression in the hippocampus. **Neurosci. 8**, pp. 791-797

Longuet-Higgins H.C. (1968) Holographic model of temporal recall. **Nature 217**, pp. 104-107

Lynch G.S., Dunwiddie T.V. & Gribkoff V.K. (1977) Heterosynaptic depression: a post synaptic correlate of long-term potentiation. **Nature 266**, pp. 737-739

Malinow R. & Miller J.P. (1986) Postsynaptic hyperpolarization during conditioning reversibly blocks induction of long-term potentiation. **Nature 320**, pp. 529-531

von der Malsburg C. (1973b) Self-organization of orientation sensitive cells in striate cortex. **Kybernetik 14**, p. 85.

Mayer M.L., Westbrook G.L. & Guthrie P.B. (1984) Voltage-dependent block by Mg^{2+} of NMDA responses in spinal cord neurons. **Nature 309**, pp. 261-263

McNaughton B.L., Douglas R.M. & Goddard G.V. (1978) Synaptic enhancement in fascia dentata: cooperativity among coactive afferents. **Brain Res. 157**, pp. 277-293

Monaghan D.T. & Cotman C.W. (1985) Distribution of N-methyl-D-aspartate-sensitive L-[^{3}H] glutamate-binding sites in rat brain. **J. Neurosci. 5**, pp. 2909-2919

Rolls E.T. (1987) Information representation, processing and storage in the brain: analysis at the single neuron level. In: **Neural and Molecular Mechanisms of Learning**. Springer-Verlag, Berlin.

Scharfman H. E. & Sarvey J. M. (1985) Postsynaptic firing during repetitive stimulation is required for long-term potentiation in hippocampus. **Brain Res. 331**, pp. 267-274

Sejnowski T.J. (1977a) Storing covariance with nonlinearly interacting neurons. **J. Math. Biol. 4**, pp. 303-321

Sejnowski T.J. (1977b) Statistical constraints on synaptic plasticity. **J. Theor. Biol. 69**, pp. 385-389

Sejnowski T.J., Koch C. & Churchland P.S. (1989) Computational neuroscience. **Science 241**, pp.1299-1306

Sejnowski T.J. & Tesauro G.J. (1989) The Hebb rule for synaptic plasticity: implementations and applications. In: **Neural Models of Plasticity.** pp. 94-103, J.H. Byrne & W.O. Berry (eds.), Academic Press, San Diego.

Stanton P.K. & Sarvey J.M. (1985) Depletion of norepinephrine, but not serotonin, reduces long-term potentiation in the dentate of rat hippocampal slices. **J. Neurosci. 5**, pp. 2169-2176

Stanton P.K. & Sejnowski T.J. (1989) Associative long-term depression in the hippocampus: induction of synaptic plasticity by Hebbian covariance. **Nature**, in press.

Steinbuch K. (1961) Die Lernmatrix. **Kybernetik 1**, pp. 36-45

Sutton R.S. & Barto A.G. (1981) Toward a modern theory of adaptive networks: expectation and prediction. **Psych. Rev. 88**, pp. 135-170

Tesauro G. (1986) Simple neural models of classical conditioning. **Biol. Cybern. 55**, pp. 187-200

Wigstrom H. & Gustafsson B. (1984) A possible correlate of the post-synaptic condition for long-lasting potentiation in the guinea pig hippocampus *in vitro*. **Neurosci. Lett. 44**, pp. 327-332.

8

The Representation and Storage of Information in Neuronal Networks in the Primate Cerebral Cortex and Hippocampus

Edmund Rolls

Summary

The ways in which information is represented, processed, and stored in neuronal networks in primates as shown by recordings from single neurons are considered.

1) Through the connected stages of the taste system of primates, neurons become more finely tuned to individual tastes, yet neurons which respond to only one taste are rare.

2) In the temporal lobe visual areas, which receive visual information after several prior stages of cortical processing, some neurons are found which are quite selective in that they respond to faces. However, even these neurons do not respond to the face of only one individual, but instead information about the individual is present across an ensemble of such cells.

3) It is suggested that ensemble encoding is used because this allows the emergent properties of completion, generalization, and graceful degradation to be generated in pattern association and auto-association matrix memory neuronal networks. It is suggested that nevertheless the representation is sparse, that is each pattern is represented by the firing of relatively small numbers of relatively finely tuned neurons, so that the patterns can be relatively orthogonal to each other, in order to minimize interference in the memory between the patterns and in order to increase the number of patterns which can be stored or associated. Given that the majority of neurons recorded in the cerebral cortex and hippocampal cortex of primates have positive responses, that is the response consists of an increase of firing rate from a low or zero spontaneous firing rate, the activity patterns for different inputs can only be relatively orthogonal to each other if the representation is sparse.

4) The hippocampal CA3 stage has recurrent collaterals which have Hebbian modifiability and a 4.3% contact probability. This network functional architecture suggests that it acts as an auto-association memory. It is suggested that this is the basis of episodic memories, which are formed in the

CA3 cells. Arbitrary association memories can be formed here because there is one auto-association matrix here, and because the hippocampus receives information from many cerebral cortical association areas. The dentate granule cells form the sparse representation required for the CA3 auto-association effect, and the CA1 cells prepare the memory for return to the cerebral cortex.

5) It is suggested that in the cerebral cortex, as well as in the hippocampus, competitive learning occurs in neuronal networks in order to build the finely tuned ensemble encoded representations required for association and auto-association memories in brain areas such as the amygdala and hippocampus to operate.

6) It is suggested that the backprojections to the cerebral cortex from the hippocampus and amygdala, and between adjacent areas of the cerebral cortex, are used to influence the storage of information in the cerebral cortex, as well as for recall, attention, and dynamic top-down processing.

7) These examples show that in the primate brain each neuron participates as part of an ensemble in a large network, the architecture of which specifies its functions and enables it to display important emergent properties. Moreover the coding of information in these systems appears to be appropriate for the networks to show these emergent properties, and is a compromise between fully distributed and fully localized (or 'grandmother cell' like).

The aims of this chapter are to consider how information is represented across populations of neurons in two sensory systems in the primate brain, the advantages of the representations found, and how these representations are built and memories are stored by neuronal networks. The sensory systems considered are the taste and visual systems.

8.1   Information representation in the taste system

In order to examine the representation of information in the taste system of primates, recordings of the responses of single neurons to the taste stimuli glucose, NaCl (salt), quinine (bitter), and HCl (sour) have been made at different levels of the taste system. It has been found that in the nucleus of the solitary tract, the first relay in the brain of the taste system, each neuron is not finely tuned to one of these tastants, but instead responds to several of the tastants (Scott *et al.*, 1986a). The breadth of tuning index (Smith & Travers, 1979) of these neurons, which takes a value of 1 if the neuron responds equally to all taste stimuli, and 0 if the neuron responds to only 1 stimulus, is shown in Figure 8.1, and confirms the broad tuning. Although responding to several tastants, the different neurons did respond with different relative responses to the different tastants, so that information was contained across an ensemble of these neurons about the nature of the tastant. It is suggested that the reason for this distributed representation early in the primate taste system is that this mode of encoding requires relatively few nerve fibres, and thus reflects efficient information transmission in the taste nerves. Because neurons are not tuned to only one stimulus, but instead each stimulus differentially activates its own set of graded filters, then fine, continuous, discriminations between the members of that set are enhanced, and potentially more discriminations are possible than with the one neuron/one stimulus type of encoding (see also, Erickson, 1963, 1982).

The nucleus of the solitary tract projects via the thalamic taste area to the primary taste cortex in the frontal operculum and the adjoining insula (Beckstead *et al.*, 1980). In these regions, gustatory areas were found, and it was discovered that the breadth of tuning of the neurons in these areas was finer than in the nucleus of the solitary tract (Scott *et al.*, 1986b; Yaxley *et al.*, 1989; see Figure 8.1). The primary taste cortex projects into a secondary cortical taste area in the caudolateral orbitofrontal cortex (Wiggins *et al.*, 1987), and here it was found that the tuning of gustatory neurons was even finer (Rolls *et al.*, 1989a; see Figure 8.1). This analysis shows that one change which takes place in the representation of information as it travels through the gustatory system is that the breadth of tuning of individual neurons becomes finer, that is, individual neurons become better able to differentiate between different stimuli, or, equivalently, the correlation between the responses of a given neuron to different stimuli becomes less.

Several reasons for this increase in the sharpness of tuning of neurons have been suggested (Rolls, 1987). The first is that when associations are made in simple pattern associator matrix memories (between for example taste and stimuli in another modality such as vision), it is useful to have relatively orthogonal representations, in order to minimize interference and increase capacity, as described below. It is of interest that in the taste system, the primary taste cortex is unimodal, so that associations between sensory modalities to form multimodal representations (between e.g. taste and vision) are only formed when a fine representation has been achieved by one or several stages of unimodal cortical processing. The second reason is that sensory-specific satiety appears to operate in the taste system, by habituation in the secondary taste cortex of neurons which respond relatively specifically to the taste of certain foods. This results in a reduction in the pleasantness of a food which has been eaten to satiety, but much less reduction in the pleasantness of the taste of other foods, and thus computes a function important in the control of feeding (Rolls *et al.*, 1989b), which could only be easily computed in this way with finely tuned neurons.

8.2 The fineness of tuning of neurons in the visual system

Given that neurons become more sharply tuned from stage to stage in the taste system, one may consider how specific the representations become at the end of sensory systems. Are 'grandmother cells' (Barlow, 1972) formed which are so specific that they might respond only for example to the sight of one's

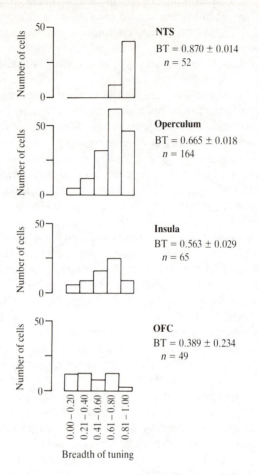

Figure 8.1 The breadths of tuning (BT) of neurons in different stages of the taste system. A value of 1 represents equal responses to all stimuli (i.e. very broad tuning), and a value of 0 represents a response to only 1 of the stimuli (see text). (The proportion of a neuron's total response that is devoted to each of the four basic stimuli was used to calculate its coefficient of entropy (H), used as the measure of breadth of tuning. The measure of entropy is derived from information theory, and is calculated as: $H = -k \sum_{i=1}^{n} p_i \log p_i$ where H = breadth of responsiveness, k = scaling constant (set so that $H = 1.0$ when the neuron responds equally well to all stimuli in the set of size n), p_i = the response to stimulus i expressed as a proportion of the total response to all the stimuli in the set.) The stimuli used were 1 M glucose, 1 M NaCl, 0.01 M HCl, and 0.001 M quinine HCl. NTS = nucleus of the solitary tract; OFC = caudolateral orbitofrontal cortex taste area.

grandmother? One way in which this has been investigated is by analysing the specificity of a very specific group of cells in the visual system which respond to faces (Perrett *et al.*, 1982; Rolls, 1984, 1989b). The question considered is whether information which could specify the face of one individual is represented by the firing of one neuron, or whether the pattern of firing of an ensemble is needed to enable identification of the individual being seen.

Neurons which respond preferentially or selectively to faces are found in certain areas of the temporal lobe visual cortex, which receive their inputs via a number of cortico-cortical stages from the primary visual (striate) cortex through prestriate visual areas (Seltzer & Pandya, 1978; Cowey, 1979; Desimone & Gross, 1979). The responses of these neurons to faces are selective in that they are 2-10 times as large to faces as to gratings, simple geometrical stimuli, or complex 3-D objects (Perrett *et al.*, 1982; Baylis *et al.*, 1985, 1987). They are probably a specialized population for processing information from faces, in that they are found primarily in architectonic areas TPO, TEa and TEm, and are not just the neurons with the most complex types of response found throughout the temporal lobe visual areas (Baylis *et al.*, 1987). The advantage of such a specialized system in the primate may lie in the importance of rapid and reliable recognition of other individuals using face recognition so that appropriate social and emotional responses can be made (Rolls, 1984, 1989b).

In experiments to determine how information which could be used to specify an individual is represented by the firing of these neurons, it has been shown that in many cases (77% of one sample), these neurons are sensitive to differences between faces (Baylis *et al.*, 1985), but that each neuron does not respond to only one face. Instead, each neuron has a different pattern of responses to a set of faces, as illustrated by the breadths of tuning in Figure 8.2. In that each neuron does not respond to only one face, and in that a particular face can activate many neurons, these are not gnostic or 'grandmother' cells (Barlow, 1972). Instead they use ensemble encoding. However, in that their responses are relatively specialized for the class 'faces' and within this class, they could contribute to relatively economic coding of information over relatively few cells (Barlow, 1972). (The data shown in Figure 8.2 are only for neurons specialized for the class 'faces'. Within this class, some of the neurons are tuned for expression and not identity, so that probably only the more selective neurons in Figure 8.2 provide information about identity - see Rolls *et al.*, 1989c). It may be emphasized that the output of such an ensemble of neurons would be useful for distinguishing between different faces. This is shown by the values of d' in Figure 8.2, which indicate that there are for many neurons 1-3 standard deviations between the response of the neuron to the most effective and to the least effective face. The appropriateness of these neurons for distinguishing between faces is enhanced by their relative constancy of response over some physical transforms, such as size, contrast, and color (Perrett *et al.*, 1982; Rolls & Baylis, 1986; Rolls, 1989b).

It is unlikely that there are further processing areas beyond those described where ensemble coding changes into grandmother cell encoding, in that

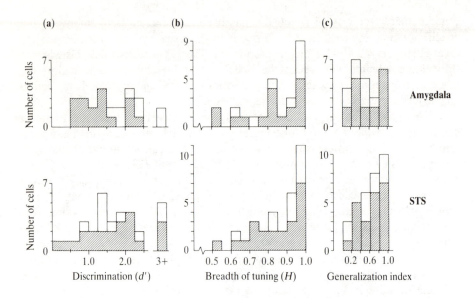

Figure 8.2 a: The discriminatability indices (d', the number of standard deviations between the response of the neuron to the most effective and to the least effective face) and **b:** the breadths of tuning indices calculated across the standard set of faces for cells recorded in the cortex in the superior temporal sulcus. **c:** shows the generalization indices, that is the proportion of the stimulus set of faces to which each neuron responded with firing greater than half its maximal response rate. (After Baylis *et al.*, 1985.) Comparable recordings from the amygdala show that ensemble encoding is used there too. (After Leonard *et al.*, 1985.) (The shading indicates data useful for a within-monkey comparison.)

anatomically there do not appear to be a whole further set of purely unimodal cortical visual processing areas present in the brain; and from the temporal lobe visual areas such as those described, outputs are taken to limbic and related regions such as the amygdala and via the entorhinal cortex to the hippocampus. Indeed, tracing this pathway onwards, Leonard *et al.* (1985) have found a population of neurons with face-selective responses in the amygdala, and in the majority of these neurons, different responses occur to different faces, with ensemble not gnostic encoding still being present. After interfacing with limbic circuits in this way, there is evidence that there are further links which may be important in the behavioral output via the connections of the amygdala to the ventral striatum (which includes the nucleus accumbens), for in the ventral striatum a small number of neurons are found which also respond to faces (see Rolls & Williams, 1987).

The advantages of the quite finely tuned representations found in the visual and taste systems, which are still ensemble encoded, can be appreciated by considering the operation of pattern association matrix memories (see Kohonen, 1988; Rolls, 1987). (In a typical pattern association matrix memory used to investigate the properties of neuronal networks found in the brain, the firing rates of the input axons and output neurons and the synaptic weights might take continuously variable positive values, the synaptic rule might be Hebbian, and the output neurons might have a sigmoid output activation function.) In order to derive the benefits of information storage in a matrix memory, such as completion, generalization, and graceful degradation, it is essential that each individual object in the environment (such as a particular grandmother) be represented by the firing pattern of an ensemble of neurons. This is because completion, generalization, and graceful degradation rely on some of the neurons which represented the original object or event being activated by the incomplete event, by the similar event, or after some of the synapses or neurons in the network have been destroyed. On the other hand, each event must not be represented over a very large population of neurons which overlaps almost completely with the population activated by a different event, for if this were the case then the matrix memory would display great interference and would be a very inefficient memory storage system. Given that neurons have positive firing rates which appear in many parts of the brain against a very low or zero level of spontaneous firing, the only way in which the relatively orthogonal representations required can be formed is by making the number of neurons active for any one input stimulus relatively low (see e.g. Jordan, 1986). With sparse representations a large number of different patterns can be stored in the memory. These two arguments above lead to the conclusion that in a matrix memory system, each event must be represented across an ensemble of neurons, but that the ensemble must be of limited size. In such an ensemble, in which information was represented which could individuate an event (e.g. the face of a particular person), it would be expected that each neuron would be tuned to differentiate quite sharply between the different members of the set of individual stimuli represented in that matrix, but would typically respond to more than one member of the set of stimuli. That is, neurons which responded only to one object or event would not be useful in a matrix memory system. This theoretical analysis thus explains the utility of the type of information representation across the neurons in the cortex in the superior temporal sulcus of the monkey, where it is found that each neuron typically responds to a limited subset of the stimuli (which in this case are faces) which are effective for activating the different neurons in this region (see above), and the utility of the representations built in the other sensory system considered, the taste system.

It is also of great interest to note that the representation which leaves at least some parts of the visual system is appropriate in another way for interfacing to other modalities via an association memory. The representation is appropriate in that some neurons provide an object-based rather than a viewer-based response to a stimulus. This means that objects or persons and their actions can be more economically represented without the need for multiple views which would further burden an associative memory. The evidence that an object-based description is provided by at least some neurons comes from recordings made from some of the face-selective neurons in the cortex in the superior temporal sulcus and inferior temporal cortex of the macaque. It has been shown that some of the neurons with responses selective for faces only respond if the face is moving (Perrett *et al.*, 1985). We took advantage of the fact that these neurons respond to moving faces to investigate whether the encoding of faces by these neurons is in viewer-centered or object-centered coordinates (Hasselmo *et al.*, 1989). For 10 neurons it has been shown that the neuron responds to particular movements which can only be described in object-centered coordinates. For example, four neurons responded vigorously to a head undergoing ventral flexion, irrespective of whether the view of the head was full face, of either profile, or even of the back of the head. These different views could only be specified as equivalent in object-centered coordinates. Further, for all of the neurons that were tested in this way, the movement specificity was maintained across inversion, responding for example to ventral flexion of the head irrespective of whether the head was upright or inverted. In this procedure, retinally encoded or viewer-centered movement vectors are reversed, but the object-centered description remains the same. It was of interest that the neurons tested generalized across different heads performing the same movements (Hasselmo *et al.*, 1989).

Further evidence supporting the hypothesis that some of the neurons in this region use object-centered descriptions, is that their selectivity between the faces of different individuals is maintained across anisomorphic transforms of the stimulus. For example, some neurons reliably responded differently to the faces of two different individuals independently of viewing angle. However, in most cases (16/18 neurons) although the identity of the face was reflected in the neuronal response, the response was not perfectly view-independent, and viewing angle also influenced the response. It is possible that these latter neurons represent an intermediate stage in the computation of object-centered descriptions (Hasselmo *et al.*, 1989).

Thus ensemble encoded representations - which are in at least some cases representations of objects - leave sensory systems and are projected to multimodal areas. The significance of this, it is suggested, is that these representations are appropriate as inputs to pattern associator matrix memories (see Kohonen, 1988; Rumelhart & McClelland, 1986; and Rolls, 1987, for further details of these memories.) There are several parts of the brain where different multimodal association memories are formed. One is the amygdala, which is involved in associations of stimuli to primary reinforcers (Rolls, 1985, 1986). Another is the hippocampus, which is important in forming memories of past episodes, for which it is suggested that auto-association is important, as described next.

8.3 The processing and storage of information in memory - the role of the hippocampus

Given that information is processed in sensory systems to produce ensemble encoded representations of events, we may next ask how memories of these events, which may involve multimodal inputs, are formed and stored. We may also ask whether the regions of the brain which organize these multimodal memories also influence how the representations are built in the primarily unimodal sensory pathways, so that the representations formed there may reflect, for example, their utility to the organism, and not just all possible features.

It is known that damage to certain regions of the temporal lobe in man produces anterograde amnesia, evident as a major deficit following the damage in learning to recognise new stimuli, and to remember events which have happened since the damage which produced the amnesia (Scoville & Milner, 1957; Milner, 1972; Squire, 1986; Squire & Zola-Morgan, 1988). The anterograde amnesia is attributed to damage to the hippocampus, which is within the temporal lobe, and to its associated pathways such as the fornix (Scoville & Milner, 1957; Milner, 1972; Gaffan, 1974, 1977; Zola-Morgan *et al.*, 1986; Squire *et al.*, 1989). Episodic memory, for example memory for what was eaten for lunch the day before, where, and with whom, is severely impaired in anterograde amnesia. Memory for events which occurred before the damage to the brain can be relatively spared in anterograde amnesia (especially if the events occurred many years before the brain damage) (Squire, 1986; Squire & Zola-Morgan, 1988; Zola-Morgan *et al.*, 1986), so that it appears possible that the hippocampus is necessary for the process of storing information (in another brain region), but is not itself the final site of long term memories.

Given this evidence which implicates the hippocampus in the storage of information in the brain, we now consider the neural networks in the hippocampus, the computations they may perform, and how these computations may be important in the long term storage of information in the brain. This analysis shows how in mammals it is possible to understand computations which have emergent properties as the result of operations performed by large numbers (e.g. 10 000 - 200 000) of relatively simple and similar neurons which are connected to form a network. Moreover, the analysis illustrates how different functional architectures of these neuronal networks result in quite different forms of computation.

8.3.1 Computational theory of the hippocampus

A schematic diagram of the connections of the hippocampus is shown in Figure 8.3. In primates, major input connections are from the association areas of the cerebral cortex, including the parietal cortex (which processes spatial information), the temporal lobe visual and auditory areas, and the frontal cortex. Within the hippocampus, there is a three stage sequence of processing, consisting of the dentate granule cells (which receive from the entorhinal cortex via the perforant path), the CA3 pyramidal cells, and the CA1 pyramidal cells. Outputs return from the hippocampus to the cerebral cortex via the subiculum, entorhinal cortex, and parahippocampal gyrus.

One major feature of hippocampal neuronal networks is the recurrent collateral system of the CA3 cells, formed by the output axons of the CA3 cells having a branch which returns to make synapses with the dendrites of the other CA3 cells, as shown in Figure 8.3. The contact probability of an axon with one of the dendrites is relatively high, 4.3% in the rat, calculated on the basis that there are 180 000 CA3

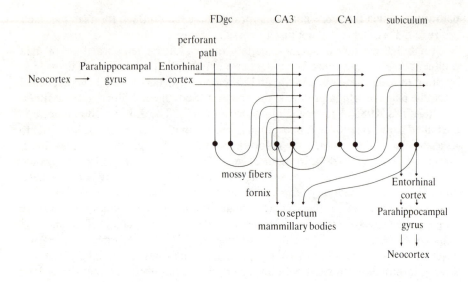

Figure 8.3 Representation of connections within the hippocampus. Inputs reach the hippocampus via the parahippocampal gyrus and entorhinal cortex through the perforant path which makes synapses with the dendrites of the dentate granule cells and also with the apical dendrites of the CA3 pyramidal cells. The dentate granule cells project via the mossy fibers to the CA3 pyramidal cells. The well developed recurrent collateral system of the CA3 cells is indicated. The CA3 pyramidal cells project via the Schaffer collaterals to the CA1 pyramidal cells, which in turn have connections to the subiculum, and thus via the entorhinal cortex and parahippocampal gyrus back to the cerebral cortex. FDgc - dentate granule cells.

cells and that approximately 7700 synapses per CA3 pyramidal cell are likely to be devoted to recurrent collaterals (Rolls, 1989a,c). It is remarkable that the contact probability is so high, and also that the CA3 recurrent collateral axons travel so widely in all directions that they can potentially come close to almost all other CA3 neurons (D.G.Amaral, personal communication; Squire *et al.*, 1989; Rolls, 1989a,c). Further, there is evidence from studies of long term potentiation that the synapses in the recurrent collateral system are Hebb modifiable, that is that they become stronger when there is strong conjunctive post-synaptic and pre-synaptic activity (Ganong *et al.*, 1986). (This has been confirmed to date primarily for the commissural part of this system, but it is a strong prediction that it can be demonstrated also for the recurrent collateral part of the system.) This functional anatomy immediately suggests that this is an auto-association (or auto-correlation) matrix memory. The auto-association arises because the output of the matrix, expressed as the firing rate of the CA3 pyramidal cells, is fed back along the horizontally running axons so that the pattern of activity in this part of the matrix (the CA3 pyramidal cells) is associated with itself (see e.g. Kohonen *et al.*, 1981; Kohonen, 1988; Rolls, 1987; Gardner-Medwin, 1976). Consistent with this suggestion about the computational role of the CA3 system of the hippocampus, it is known that the probability of contact of the neurons in an auto-association matrix must not be very low if it is to operate usefully (see Marr, 1971). It is suggested below that the systems level function of this auto-association memory is to enable events occurring conjunctively in quite different parts of the association areas of the cerebral cortex to be associated together to form a memory which could well be described as episodic. Each episode would be defined by a conjunction of a set of events, and each episodic memory would consist of the association of one set of events (such as where, with whom, and what one ate at lunch on the preceding day). The importance of the hippocampus in episodic memory may arise from the fact that in one part of it, the CA3 region, there is one association matrix with a relatively high contact probability which receives information originating in many different areas of the cerebral cortex.

One reason why there may not be more cells in the CA3 region is that it is important that the connectivity be kept relatively high so that any event represented by the firing of a sparse set of CA3 cells can be associated with any other event represented by a different set of CA3 cells firing. Because each CA3 pyramidal cell has a limited number of synapses (cf. fan-in) (perhaps 10 000, see above), the total number of cells in the auto-association memory cannot be increased beyond the limit set by the fan in and the connectivity. The advantages of sparse encoding and a well interconnected matrix are that a large number of different (episodic) memories can be stored in the CA3 system, and that the advantageous emergent properties of a matrix memory, such as completion, generalization, and graceful degradation (see Kohonen *et al.*, 1977, 1981; Kohonen, 1988; Rolls, 1987) are produced efficiently. Completion may operate particularly effectively here with a sparse representation, because it is under these conditions that the simple auto-correlation effect can reconstruct the whole of one pattern without interference, which would arise if too high a proportion of the input neurons was active. Another effect of the auto-association matrix is that the central tendency of a pattern of activity which is noisy is learned, thus achieving useful prototype extraction (McClelland & Rumelhart, 1988).

The means by which the efficiently encoded (i.e. with little redundancy) yet sparse representation in CA3 neurons which is required for the auto-association to perform well is achieved is, it is suggested, a function of the mossy fiber inputs to the CA3 cells described next, as well as of an orthogonalizing function of competition between the dentate granule cells described later.

The mossy fiber system connects the granule cells of the dentate gyrus to the CA3 pyramidal cells of the hippocampus. In the rat, each mossy fiber forms approximately 14 'mosses' or contacts with CA3 cells, there are 1×10^6 dentate granule cells and thus 14×10^6 mosses onto 0.18×10^6 CA3 cells (D. Amaral, personal communication), and thus each CA3 pyramidal cell may be contacted by approximately 80 dentate granule cells. This means that (in the rat) the probability that a CA3 cell is contacted by a given dentate granule cell is 80 synapses / 10^6 granule cells = 8×10^{-5}. These mossy fiber synapses are very large, and probably therefore strong so that even with such a relatively small number on each CA3 cell dendrite (and a much smaller number active at any one time), the mossy fiber synapses can have an important influence on the cell. One computational effect which can be achieved by this low probability of contact of a particular dentate granule cell with a particular pyramidal cell is pattern separation. This is achieved in the following way. Consider a pattern of firing present over a set of dentate granule cells. The probability that any two CA3 pyramidal cells receive synapses from a similar subset of the dentate granule cells is very low (because of the low probability of contact of any one dentate granule cell with a pyramidal cell), so that each CA3 pyramidal cell effectively samples a very small subset of the active granule cells. It is therefore likely that each CA3 pyramidal cell will respond differently to the others, so that in this way pattern separation is achieved. (The effect is similar to codon formation described in other contexts by Marr, 1970.) The advantage of a low number of inputs, is that the thresholds of the post-synaptic cells need not be set with great accuracy for pattern separation to be achieved, and for sparse, relatively orthogonal, patterns to be formed (within the limits set by the relative numbers of dentate granule and CA3 cells shown in Table 8.1), which are required if the auto-association matrix memory formed by the CA3 cells is to operate with usefully large memory capacity, and with minimal interference (see Kohonen *et al.*, 1977; Rolls, 1987). As the neurons have positive firing rates, the only way in which relatively orthogonal representations can be formed is by making the number of neurons active for any one input stimulus relatively low (see e.g. Jordan, 1986). An advantage of the modifiability of the mossy fiber synapses may be that CA3 neurons learn to respond to just those subsets of activity which happen to occur in dentate granule cells, so that cells are used efficiently. Even if these mossy fiber synapses are not modifiable, the mossy fiber system would still achieve pattern separation and form sparse representations.

Table 8.1

	Rat	Monkey	Man
Entorhinal Cortex		4.0×10^6	
Dentate Granule cells	1.00×10^6	5.0×10^6	8.8×10^6
CA3/CA2	0.18×10^6	0.9×10^6	2.5×10^6
CA1	0.25×10^6	1.4×10^6	6.0×10^6

Contact probability of a granule cell with a CA3 cell = 0.008% (rat)
    (via mossy fibers)
Contact probability of a CA3 cell with a CA3 cell = 4.3% (rat)
    (via recurrent collaterals)

It is notable that in addition to the mossy fiber inputs, the CA3 pyramidal cells also receive inputs directly from perforant path fibers (see Figure 8.3). This is not a sparse projection, in that each pyramidal cell may receive in the order of 2300 such synapses. (This is calculated using the evidence that of 15 mm of total dendritic length with 10 000 spines, approximately 3.5 mm (range 2.5-4.5 mm) is in the lacunosum moleculare and thus receives inputs from the perforant path; D.G.Amaral, personal communication). What would be the computational effect of this input together with the very sparse, but large and thus strong, synapses from the mossy fibers? One effect is that the mossy fiber input would largely determine the response of the CA3 cell. However each CA3 cell would show cooperative Hebbian learning between its activation by the mossy fiber input and the direct perforant path input, allowing the direct input to specify more exactly the response of the CA3 cell, and after learning to elicit the response normally produced by the mossy fibre input if this was absent.

The other way in which it is suggested that a sparse representation is prepared for the CA3 neurons is by competitive learning at the dentate granule stage (see Figure 8.3). Architecturally, there is one major set of input axons, the perforant path fibers, which connect via a synaptic matrix with the dentate granule cells. A version of this represented as a simplified matrix is shown in Figure 8.4. The matrix is clearly very different from an association matrix memory, in that in the hippocampal system there is no unconditioned stimulus which forces the output neurons to fire (see Rolls, 1987). Nor is there a climbing fiber for each output cell which could act as a teacher as in the cerebellum (see Ito, 1984). There is thus no teacher apparent, so that this appears to be an example of an unsupervised learning system (see further Rolls, 1989). The following describes one mode of operation for such a network. Later, properties of the hippocampus which suggest that it may operate in this way are discussed.

Consider a matrix memory of the form shown in Figure 8.4 in which the strengths of the synapses between horizontal axons and the vertical dendrites are initially random (postulate 1). Because of these random initial synaptic weights, different input patterns on the horizontal axons will tend to activate different output neurons (in this case, granule cells). The tendency for each pattern to select or activate different neurons can then be enhanced by providing mutual inhibition between the output neurons, to prevent too many neurons responding to that stimulus (postulate 2). This competitive interaction can be viewed as enhancing the differences in the firing rates of the output cells (cf. the contrast enhancement described by Grossberg, 1982). Synaptic modification then occurs according to the rules of long term potentiation in the hippocampus, namely that synapses between active afferent axons and strongly activated post-synaptic neurons increase in strength (see Bliss & Lomo, 1973; Andersen, 1987; McNaughton, 1984; Levy, 1985; Kelso *et al.*, 1986; Wigstrom *et al.*, 1986) (postulate 3). The effect of this modification is that the next time the same stimulus is repeated, the neuron responds more (because of the strengthened synapses), more inhibition of other neurons occurs, and then further modification to produce even greater selectivity is produced. The response of the system as a categorizer thus climbs over repeated iterations. One effect of this observed in simulations is that a few neurons then obtain such strong synaptic weights that almost any stimulus which has any input to that neuron will succeed in activating it. The solution to this is to limit the total synaptic weight that each output (post-synaptic) neuron can receive (postulate 4). In simulations this is performed by normalizing the sum of the synaptic weights (or the

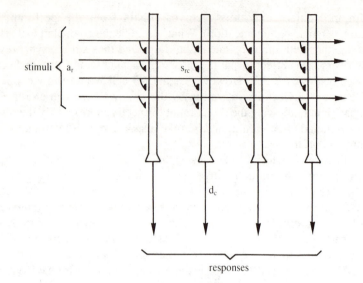

Figure 8.4 A matrix for competitive learning in which the input stimuli are presented along the rows of the input axons (a_r) which make modifiable synapses (s_{rc}) with the dendrites of the output neurons, which form the columns (d_c) of the matrix. The connections necessary for competition require inhibitory interneurons not shown in the diagram.

length of the synaptic weight vector) on each neuron to a constant (e.g. 1.0) (see von der Malsburg, 1973; Rumelhart & Zipser, 1986). This has the effect of distributing the output neurons evenly between the different input patterns received by the network. In the brain the normalization of the synaptic weight vector on each dendrite may be approximated by using a modified Hebbian rule which produces some decrease in synaptic strength if there is high pre-synaptic activity but post-synaptic activation below a certain threshold which can alter as a function of the average activation of the neuron (see Bienenstock *et al.*, 1982; Bear *et al.*, 1987), and we (E.T. Rolls, G. Littlewort, R. Payne & A. Bennett) have found that the use of such a learning rule does indeed abolish the need for explicit normalization of the synaptic weight vectors on each dendrite, that is for a separate process to implement postulate 4 above. It is in any case not physiologically unreasonable to postulate that the total synaptic strength onto a post-synaptic neuron is somewhat fixed (Levy & Desmond, 1985).

A simulation of the operation of such a competitive neuronal network is shown in Figure 8.5. (In the simulation the firing rates and the synapses could take continuous positive values; the competition was implemented by raising the output vector to the power required to produce a given breadth of tuning, set for example to 0.5, followed by normalization to a given maximum and minimum firing rate;

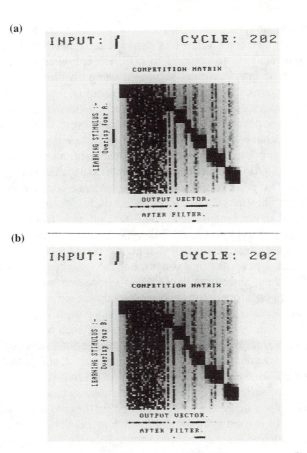

Figure 8.5 Simulation of learning in a competitive matrix memory. The architecture is as shown in Figure 8.4, except that there are 64 horizontal axons and 64 vertical dendrites which form the rows and columns respectively of the 64 x 64 matrix of synapses. The strength of each synapse, which was initially random, is indicated by the darkness of each pixel. The activity of each of the 64 input axons is represented in the 64 element vector at the left of the diagram by the darkness of each pixel. The output firing of the vertical neurons is represented in the same way by the output vectors at the bottom of the diagram. The upper output vector is the result of multiplying the input stimulus through the matrix of synaptic weights. The vector resulting from the application of competition between the output neurons (which produces contrast enhancement between the elements or neurons of the vector) is shown below by the vector labelled 'after filter'. The state of the matrix is shown after 202 cycles in each of which stimuli with eight of 64 active axons were presented, and the matrix allowed to learn as described in the text. The stimuli were presented in random sequence, and consisted of a set of vectors which overlapped in 0, 1, 2, 3, 4, 5, or 6 positions with the next vector in the set. The columns of the matrix were sorted after the learning to bring similar columns together, so that the types of neuron formed, and the pattern of synapses formed on their dendrites, can be seen easily. The dendrites with random patterns of synapses have not been allocated to any of the input stimuli. It is shown that application of one of the input stimuli (overlap four A) or vectors which overlapped in 4 of 8 positions with another stimulus (overlap four B) produced one pattern of firing of the output neurons, and that application of input stimulus overlap four B produced a different pattern of firing of the output neurons. Thus the stimuli were correctly categorized by the matrix as being different.

and the lengths of the synaptic weight vectors were normalized after the weights had been modified by a Hebbian rule.) It is shown that the network effectively selects different output neurons to respond to different combinations of active input horizontal lines. It thus performs a type of categorization, in which different complex input patterns are encoded economically onto a few output lines. It should be noted that this categorization finds natural clusters in the input events; it orthogonalizes the categories, in that overlap in input events can become coded onto output neurons with less overlap, and in that many active input lines may be coded onto few active output lines; and does not allocate neurons to events which never occur (see Marr, 1970, 1971; Rumelhart & Zipser, 1985; Grossberg, 1982, 1987). It may be noted that there is no special correspondence between the input pattern and which output lines are selected. It is thus not useful for any associative mapping between an input and an output event, and is thus different from associative matrix memories (Rolls, 1987). Instead, this type of matrix finds associations or correlations between input events (which are expressed as sets of simultaneously active horizontal input lines or axons), allocates output neurons to reflect the complex input event, and stores the required association between the input lines onto the few output neurons activated by each complex input event. It thus acts as a categorizer, which removes redundancy present in the input vectors, and forms new output representations which are more orthogonal to each other than are the input vectors. It thus helps to form the sparse representations required for the CA3 neurons, so that large numbers of memories can be stored, and so that the emergent properties of the auto-association effect in the CA3 neurons can operate effectively.

It is thus suggested that the sparse yet efficient (i.e. with little redundancy) representation in CA3 neurons which is required for the auto-association to perform well is produced in two ways by the stage which precedes the CA3 neurons, that is by the orthogonalizing function of competition between the dentate granule cells, and by the low contact probability in the mossy fiber-CA3 connections. The function of the CA1 stage which follows the CA3 cells is considered next.

The connections of the CA3 cells to the CA1 pyramidal cells are shown in Figure 8.3. The connections are of the form shown in Figure 8.4. It is suggested that the CA1 cells provide a stage of competitive learning which operates as follows on the inputs received from the CA3 cells. Consider the operation of auto-association across the CA3 neurons. Several sparse patterns of firing occur together on the CA3 neurons, and become associated together to form an episodic memory. It is essential for this operation that several different sparse representations are present conjunctively in order to form the association which implements the episodic memory. Moreover, when completion operates in the CA3 auto-association system, all the neurons firing in the original conjunction can be brought into activity by only a part of the original set of conjunctive events. For these reasons, a memory in the CA3 cells consists of several simultaneously active, different, sparse ensembles of activity. It is suggested that the CA1 cells, which receive these groups of simultaneously active ensembles, can detect the correlations of firing which represent the episodic memory, and allocate by competitive learning a relatively few neurons to represent each episodic memory. The episodic memory would thus consist in the CA3 cells of groups of active cells, each representing one of the subcomponents of the episodic memory (including context), whereas the whole episodic memory would be represented not by its parts, but as a single collection of active cells, at the CA1 stage, with the redundancy implicit in the CA3 representation removed. It is suggested below that one role which these economical (in terms of the number of activated fibers) and relatively orthogonal signals have, is to guide information storage or consolidation in the cerebral cortex. To understand how the hippocampus may perform this function for the cerebral cortex, it is necessary to turn to a systems level analysis to show how the computations performed by the hippocampus fit into overall brain function. It may be noted that by forming associations of events derived from different parts of the cerebral cortex (the CA3 stage), and by building new economical representations (with low redundancy) of the conjunctions detected (the CA1 stage), the hippocampus provides an output which is suitable for directing the long term storage of information.

8.3.2   *Systems level theory of hippocampal function*

First, the anatomical connections of the primate hippocampus with the rest of the brain will be considered, in order to provide a basis for considering how the computational ability of the hippocampus could be used by the rest of the brain. Then the responses shown by single hippocampal neurons will be described to provide evidence of its systems level function.

The hippocampus receives inputs via the entorhinal cortex (area 28) and the parahippocampal gyrus from many areas of the cerebral association cortex, including the parietal cortex which is concerned with spatial functions, the visual and auditory temporal association cortical areas, and the frontal cortex (see Figure 8.6) (Van Hoesen & Pandya, 1975; Van Hoesen *et al.*, 1975; Van Hoesen, 1982; Amaral, 1987; Rolls, 1989a,c). In addition, the entorhinal cortex receives inputs from the amygdala. There are also subcortical inputs to the hippocampus, for example via the fimbria/fornix from the cholinergic cells of the medial septum and the adjoining limb of the diagonal band of Broca. The hippocampus in turn projects back via the subiculum, entorhinal cortex, and parahippocampal gyrus (area TF-TH), to the cerebral cortical areas from which it receives inputs (Van Hoesen, 1982) (see Figures 8.6 & 8.3). Thus the hippocampus can potentially influence the neocortical regions from which it receives inputs. A second efferent projection of the hippocampal system reaches the supplementary motor cortex via the subiculum, the fimbria/fornix, mammillary bodies, anterior thalamus, and the cingulate cortex, providing a potential route for the hippocampus to influence motor output (Van Hoesen, 1982). It is suggested that functions of the hippocampus in for example conditional spatial response learning utilize this output path to the motor system.

During the performance of an object-place memory task, for which the primate hippocampus is needed, it has been found that not only do some hippocampal neurons respond to certain positions in space, but that others respond

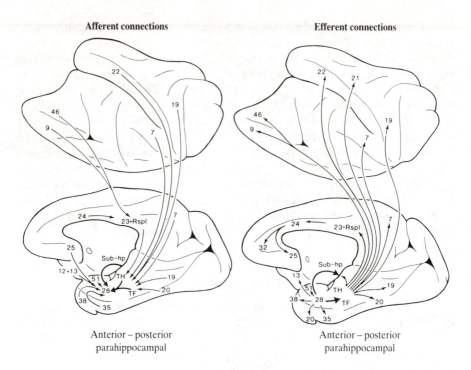

Figure 8.6 Connections of the primate hippocampus with the neocortex (from Van Hoesen, 1982). A medial view of the macaque brain is shown below, and a lateral view is shown inverted above. The hippocampus receives its inputs via the parahippocampal gyrus, areas TF and TH, and the entorhinal cortex, area 28. The return projections to the neocortex (shown on the right) pass through the same areas. (The hippocampus is behind area 28 in the diagram.) Cortical areas 19, 20 and 21 are visual association areas, 22 is auditory association cortex, 7 is parietal association cortex, and 9, 46, 12 and 13 are frontal cortical association areas.

only when novel stimuli are shown in a particular place. These neurons thus responded to a combination of information about the stimulus being shown and about position in space (Rolls *et al.*, 1989a). Further, in tasks in which monkeys had to learn which spatial response to make to different stimuli, that is to acquire associations between visual stimuli and spatial responses, 14% of the neurons responded to particular combinations of stimuli and responses (Miyashita *et al.*, 1989). (The representation was quite sparse, in that the proportion of neurons responding to any one combination of a stimulus and a response was much lower than 14%, which is the total proportion of hippocampal neurons which were activated across all stimulus-response combinations in the task.) These neurophysiological findings provide support for the computational model described above, for they show that combinations of events received by the hippocampus from different parts of the brain do activate single hippocampal neurons, as predicted from the convergence of inputs received from the cerebral cortex onto single hippocampal neurons. Moreover, particular combinations of events come as a result of learning to activate hippocampal neurons (Cahusac *et al.*, 1989), consistent with the synaptic modifiability which is part of the model. The model is also supported by evidence that during the learning of conditional spatial responses some hippocampal neurons start, but then stop showing differential responses to the different stimuli, consistent with competitive interactions between hippocampal neurons during learning so that only some hippocampal neurons become allocated to any one learned conjunction of events (Cahusac *et al.*, 1989).

The analyses above have shown that the hippocampus receives from high order areas of association cortex; is able by virtue of the large number of synapses on its dendrites and the CA3 auto-association effect to detect conjunctions of events even when these are widely separated in information space, with their origin from quite different cortical areas; allocates neurons to code efficiently for these conjunctions probably using a competitive learning mechanism (CA1); and has connections back to the areas of the cerebral cortex from which it receives, as well as to subcortical structures via the fimbria/fornix system. What could be achieved by this system? It appears that the very long term storage of information is not in the hippocampus, at least in man, in that the retrograde amnesia produced by damage to the hippocampal system in man is not always severe, and in that very old memories (e.g. for events which occurred 30 years previously) are not destroyed (Squire, 1986, 1987; Squire & Zola-Morgan, 1988). On the other hand, the hippocampus does appear to be necessary for the storage of certain types of information (characterized by the description 'declarative', or knowing that, as contrasted with 'procedural', or knowing how, which is spared in amnesia). Declarative memory includes what can be declared or brought to mind as a proposition or an image. Declarative memory includes episodic memory, that is memory for particular episodes, and semantic memory, that is memory for facts (Squire & Zola-Morgan, 1988; Squire *et al.*, 1989). How could the hippocampus then be involved in the storage of information?

The suggestion which is made on the basis of these and other findings described above is that the hippocampus is specialized to detect the best way in which to store information, and then directs memory storage there by the return paths to the cerebral cortex. It is suggested that the CA3 auto-association system is ideal for remembering particular episodes, for perhaps uniquely in the brain it provides a single auto-association matrix which receives from many different areas of the cerebral association cortex. It is thus able to make almost any arbitrary association, including associating the context in which a set of events occurred. This auto-association type of memory is also what is required for paired-associate learning, in which arbitrary associations must be made between words, and an impairment of which is almost a defining test of anterograde amnesia. Impairment of this ability to remember episodes by using the CA3 auto-association matrix memory may also underlie many of the memory deficits produced by damage to the hippocampal system. For example, conditional spatial response learning (see Miyashita *et al.*, 1989) may be impaired by hippocampal damage because a monkey or human cannot make use of the memory of the episode of events on each particular trial, for example that a particular stimulus and a particular response were made, and reward was received. Similarly, object-place memory tasks, also impaired by hippocampal damage, require associations to be made between particular locations and particular objects - again a natural function for an auto-association memory. Further, the difficulty with memory for places produced by hippocampal damage (see Barnes, 1988) may be because a place is normally defined by a conjunction of a number of features, environmental cues or stimuli, and this type of conjunction is normally made by the auto-association memory capability of the hippocampus (see further Rolls *et al.*, 1989a). (It should be noted that associations to primary reinforcing stimuli do not require the hippocampus. Associations to primary reinforcers seem to require the amygdala - see Rolls, 1985, 1986.) Clearly the hippocampus, with its large number of synapses on each neuron, its potentiation type of learning, and its CA3 auto-association system is able to detect when there is conjunctive activation of arbitrary sets of its input fibers, and is able, as indicated both theoretically and by recordings made in the behaving monkey, to allocate neurons economically (i.e. with relatively few neurons active) to code for each complex input event (by the output or CA1 stage). Such output neurons could then represent an efficient way in which to store information, in that complex memories with little redundancy would have been generated. It should be noted that this theory is not inconsistent with the possibility that the hippocampus provides a working memory, in that in the present theory the hippocampus sets up a representation using Hebbian learning which is useful in determining how information can best be stored in the neocortex, and this representation could provide a useful working memory. It may be that by understanding the operations performed by the hippocampus at the neuronal network level, it can be seen how the hippocampus could contribute to several functions which are not necessarily inconsistent.

The question then arises of where the long term storage occurs, and how it may be directed by the hippocampus. Now the hippocampus is reciprocally connected via the subiculum and entorhinal cortex with the parahippocampal gyrus, which in turn is reciprocally connected with many high order areas of association neocortex (see Figure 8.6). It is therefore possible that the actual storage takes place in the parahippocampal gyrus, and that this might be particularly appropriate for multimodal memories. However, having detected that, for example, a visual stimulus is regularly associated with an event in another modality such as a movement, it might be useful to direct the unimodal representation of that visual image, so that it is stored efficiently and can provide a useful input to the multimodal conjunction store. Thus return pathways (via e.g. the parahippocampal gyrus) to unimodal cortex (for example inferior temporal visual cortex, area TE) might, it is suggested, be used to direct unimodal storage also, by contributing to detection of the most economical way in which to store representations of stimuli.

The question of how the hippocampal output is used by the neocortex (i.e. cerebral cortex) will be considered next. Given that the hippocampal output returns to the neocortex, a theory of backprojections in the neocortex will be needed. This is developed next. By way of introduction to this, it may be noted that which particular hippocampal neurons happen to represent a complex input event is not determined by any teacher or forcing (unconditioned) stimulus. Thus the neocortex must be able to utilize the signal rather cleverly. One possibility is that any neocortical neuron with a number of afferents active at the same time as hippocampal return fibers in its vicinity are active, modifies its responses so that it comes to respond better to those afferents the next time they occur. This learning by the cortex would involve a Hebbian-like learning mechanism. It may be noted that one function served by what are thus in effect backprojections from the hippocampus is some guidance for or supervision of neocortical learning. It is a problem of unsupervised learning systems that they can remove redundancy efficiently by detecting local conjunctions, but that these local conjunctions are not necessarily those of most use to the whole system. It is exactly this problem which it is proposed the hippocampus helps to solve, by detecting useful conjunctions globally (i.e. over the whole of information space), and then directing storage locally at earlier stages of processing so that filters are built locally which provide representations of input stimuli which are useful for later processing.

8.4   Theoretical significance of backprojections in the neocortex

The forward and backward projections which will be considered are shown in Figure 8.7 (for further anatomical information see Peters & Jones, 1984). In primary sensory cortical areas, the main extrinsic 'forward' input is from the thalamus, and ends in layer 4, where synapses are formed onto spiny stellate cells. These in turn project heavily onto pyramidal cells in layers 3 and 2, which in turn send projections forward to terminate strongly in layer 4 of the next cortical layer (on small pyramidal cells in layer 4 or on the basal dendrites of the layer 2 and 3 (superficial) pyramidal cells). (Although the forward afferents end strongly in layer 4, the forward afferents have some synapses also onto the basal dendrites of the layer 2 pyramidal cells, as well as onto layer 6 pyramidal cells and inhibitory interneurons.) Inputs reach the layer 5 (deep) pyramidal cells from the pyramidal cells in layers 2 and 3 (Martin, 1984), and it is the deep pyramidal cells which send backprojections to end in layer 1 (predominantly) of the preceding cortical area (see Figure 8.7), where there are apical dendrites of pyramidal cells. There are few current theories about the functions subserved by the cortico-cortical backprojections, even though there are almost as many backprojecting as forward projecting axons. It is important to note that in addition to the axons and their terminals in layer 1 from the succeeding cortical stage, there are also axons and terminals in layer 1 in many stages of the cortical hierarchy from the amygdala and (via the subiculum, entorhinal cortex and parahippocampal cortex) from the hippocampal formation (see Figure 8.7) (Turner, 1981; Van Hoesen, 1981; Amaral & Price, 1984; Amaral, 1986, 1987). Now the amygdala and hippocampus are stages of information processing at which the different sensory modalities (such as

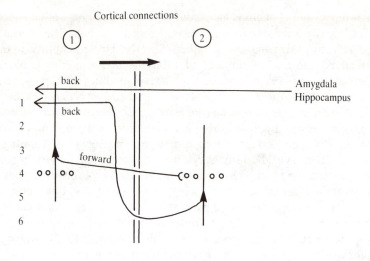

Figure 8.7 Schematic diagram of forward and backward projections in the neocortex. The arrow from left to right connecting cortical areas 1 and 2 shows the forward direction. The superficial pyramidal cells (triangles) in layers 2 and 3 project forward to terminate in layer 4 of the next cortical area. The deep pyramidal cells in the next area project back to layer 1 of the preceding cortical area, in which there are apical dendrites of pyramidal cells. The hippocampus and amygdala also are the source of backprojections which end in layer 1. Spiny stellate cells are represented by small circles in layer 4. See text for further details.

vision, hearing, touch, and taste for the amygdala) are brought together, so that correlations between inputs in different modalities can be detected in these regions, but not at prior cortical processing stages in each modality, as these cortical processing stages are unimodal. Now, as a result of bringing together the two modalities, significant correspondences between the two modalities can be detected. One example might be that a particular visual stimulus is associated with the taste of food. Another example might be that another visual stimulus is associated with painful touch. Thus at these stages of processing, but not before, the significance of for example visual and auditory stimuli can be detected and signalled, and sending this information back to the neocortex thus can provide a signal which indicates to the cortex that information should be stored, but even more than this, provides a signal which could help the neocortex to store the information efficiently.

The way in which backprojections could assist learning in the cortex can be considered using the architecture shown in Figure 8.8. The (forward) input stimulus occurs as a vector applied to (layer 3) cortical pyramidal cells through modifiable synapses in the standard way for a competitive net. (If it is a primary cortical area, the input stimulus is at least partly relayed through spiny stellate cells, which may help to normalize and orthogonalize the input patterns in a preliminary way before the patterns are applied to the layer 3 pyramidal cells. If it is a non-primary cortical area, the cortico-cortical forward axons may end more strongly on

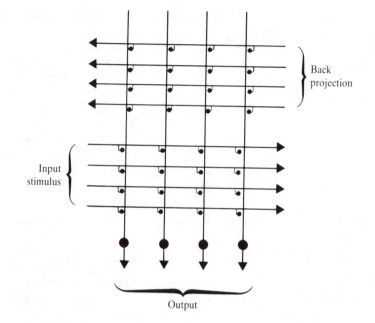

Figure 8.8 The architecture used to simulate the properties of backprojections. The forward ('input stimulus') and backprojected axons make Hebbian modifiable synapses onto the same set of vertical dendrites, which represent cortical pyramidal cells.

the basal dendrites of neurons in the superficial cortical layers.) The lower set of synapses on the pyramidal cells would then start by competitive learning to set up representations on the lower parts of these neurons which would represent correlations in the input information space, and could be said to correspond to features in the input information space, where a feature is defined simply as the representation of a correlation in the input information space.

Consider now the application of one of the (forward) input stimulus vectors with the conjunctive application of a pattern vector via the backprojection axons with terminals in layer 1. Given that all the synapses in the matrix start with random weights, some of the pyramidal cells will by chance be strongly influenced both by the (forward) input stimulus and by the backprojecting vector. These strongly activated neurons will then compete with each other as in a standard competitive net, to produce contrast enhancement of their firing patterns. (The relatively short-range (50 μm) excitatory operations produced by bipolar and double bouquet cells, together with more widespread (300 - 500 μm) recurrent lateral inhibition produced by the smooth non-pyramidal cells and perhaps the basket cells, may be part of the mechanism of this competitive interaction.) Next, Hebbian learning takes place as in a competitive net, with the addition that not only the synapses between forward projecting axons and active post-synaptic neurons are modified, but also the synapses in layer 1 between the backward projecting axons and the (same) active post-synaptic neurons are modified.

This functional architecture has the following properties. First, the backprojections, which are assumed to carry signals which are relatively information-rich (i.e. non-redundant) (see Rolls, 1987) and orthogonal to each other as a result of the conjunctions formed by the hippocampus, amygdala, or next cortical stage, help the neurons to learn to respond differently to (and thus separate) input stimuli (on the forward projection lines) even when the input stimuli are very similar. This is illustrated in the simulation shown in Figure 8.9, in which it is shown that even input stimuli which overlap in six positions out of eight, can be easily learned as separate if presented conjunctively with different orthogonal backprojecting 'tutors'. (For a similar idea on the guidance of a competitive learning system see Rumelhart & Zipser, 1986.) Another way in which the learning of pyramidal cells can be influenced is that if two relatively different input stimuli are being received, but the same backprojecting signal occurs with these two somewhat different forward inputs, then the pyramidal cells will be guided by the tutor to build the representation of the forward input stimuli on the same pyramidal cells. If the representations of the forward inputs built by modification of the synapses on the pyramidal cells are considered as vectors in a multidimensional space, then the representations in this case will be forced towards each other as a result of the operation of the common backprojecting tutor.

In the cerebral cortex, the backprojecting tutors can be of two types. One originates from the amygdala and hippocampus, and by benefiting from cross-modal comparison, can provide an orthogonal backprojected vector. This backprojection moreover may only be activated if the multimodal areas detect that the visual stimulus is significant, because, for example, it is associated with a pleasant taste. This provides one way in which guidance can be provided for a competitive learning system as to what it should learn, so that it does not attempt to lay down representations of all incoming sensory information, but only those shown to be significant as a result of comparison made with inputs originating in a different modality. Another way for this important function to be achieved is by activation of neurons which 'strobe' the cortex when new or significant stimuli are shown. The cholinergic system originating in the basal forebrain (which itself receives information from the amygdala), and the noradrenergic input to layer 1 of the cortex from the locus coereleus may also contribute to this function (see Bear & Singer, 1986; Rolls, 1987). However, in that there are relatively few neurons in these basal forebrain and noradrenergic systems, it is suggested that these projections only provide a simple 'strobe' (see Rolls, 1987). In contrast there are sufficient axons in the backprojecting systems from the hippocampus and amygdala to carry pattern-specific information, so that the hypothesis presented here is therefore that these backprojections guide how information is consolidated, by influencing how information is stored on pyramidal cells in the way described above. The situations in which the amygdala and hippocampal backprojections guide learning (and also recall and attention as discussed below) are probably different in the following way. It is suggested that the amygdala is particularly involved when associations are made between a neutral stimulus (such as a visual stimulus) and a reinforcing stimulus (arising from for example the taste or touch inputs it receives) (see Rolls, 1985, 1986). In contrast, it is suggested that the hippocampus is particularly involved when conjunctions must be detected between spatial inputs (received by the major inputs of the hippocampus which originate from the parietal cortex) and its other inputs (from for example the inferior temporal visual cortex), in for example conditional spatial and object-place learning tasks (see above and Rolls, 1989).

The second type of backprojection is that from the next cortical area in the hierarchy. This next cortical area operates in the same manner, and because it is a competitive system, is able to further categorize or orthogonalize the stimuli it receives. This next cortical stage then projects back these more orthogonal representations as tutors to the preceding stage, to effectively build better filters at the preceding stage for the diagnosis of the categories being found at the next stage.

A second property of this architecture is that it provides for recall. Recall of a previously stored representation by another stimulus or event occurs in the following way. If only the tutor is presented, then the neurons originally activated by the forward projecting input stimuli are activated. This occurs because the synapses from the backprojecting axons onto the pyramidal cells have been modified only where there was conjunctive forward and backprojected activity during learning. A simulation of this is shown in Figure 8.9. Consider the situation when in the visual system the sight of food is forward projected onto pyramidal cells, and conjunctively there is a backprojected signal elicited by the taste of the food and originating from a multimodal area such as the amygdala. Neurons which have conjunctive inputs from these two stimuli set up representations of both, so that later if a backprojected signal produced by the taste occurs, then the visual neurons originally activated by the sight of that food will be activated, and thus recall of the visual representation is achieved. In this way many of the low-level details of the original visual stimulus can be recalled. Evidence that during recall relatively early cortical processing stages are activated comes from cortical blood flow studies in man, in which it has been found for example that quite early visual cortical association areas are activated during recall of visual (but not auditory) information (Roland *et al.*, 1980; Roland & Friberg, 1985). Recall could operate as a result of signals backprojected directly from the amygdala or parahippocampal gyrus, or indirectly through series of back-connected cortical stages.

A third property of this architecture is that attention could operate from higher to lower levels to selectively facilitate only certain pyramidal cells by using the backprojections. Indeed, the backprojections described could produce many of the 'top-down' influences which are common in perception. A fourth property is that semantic priming could operate by using the backprojecting neurons to provide a small activation of just those neurons in earlier stages which are appropriate for responding to that semantic category of input stimulus.

A fifth property of such a return mechanism would be a positive feedback effect which would result in better storage in the cerebral cortex in the long term. This would operate so that when a useful tutor had been built at a higher level this

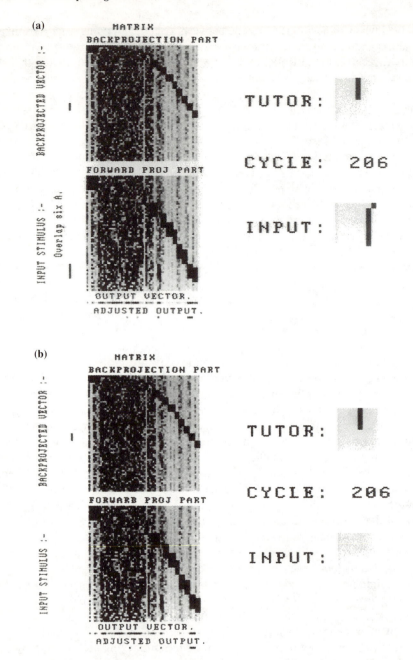

Figure 8.9 Simulation of neocortical backprojection learning matrix. Conventions as in Figure 8.5. During learning, both a forward input (chosen from the same set as used in Figure 8.5) and a backprojected vector which was orthogonal to the other backprojected vectors were presented simultaneously, as shown in Figure 8.9a. After 206 cycles with input stimulus and backprojected tutor pairs chosen in random sequence, the synapses had modified as shown. In Figure 8.9b & 8.9c it is

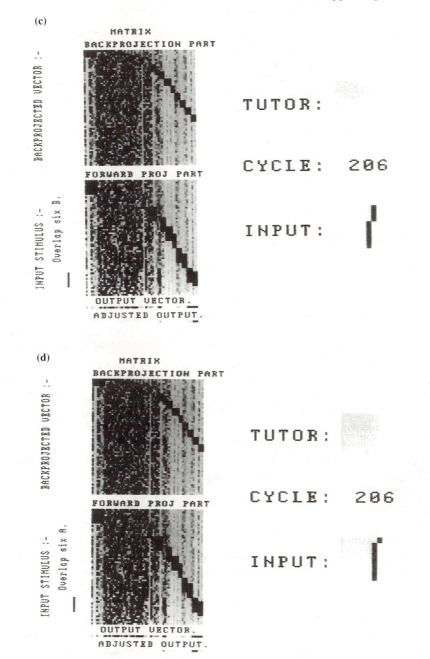

shown that two quite similar input stimuli (overlap six A & six B) produce different outputs. The learning has been guided by the backprojected tutors presented during learning. In Figure 8.9d it is shown that if only the tutor originally paired with input stimulus overlap six A is presented, then recall of the output vector normally recognized by input stimulus overlap six A occurs.

would influence the earlier stage(s) so that a better filter would be built at the earlier level. This is turn would lead to formation of an even better tutor at the higher stage, and so on repeatedly. This might provide a neurophysiological and computational basis for any gradient of retrograde amnesia which may occur for the period just before disruption of temporal lobe function (Squire, 1986; Squire & Zola-Morgan, 1988). A sixth property of the backprojections is that they might assist the stability of the preceding competitive networks by providing a relatively constant guiding signal as a result of associations made at a higher stage, to for example, an unconditioned taste or somatosensory input. A seventh property of such a return mechanism would be a dynamic (short term), positive feedback effect by which higher levels might affect the tuning of lower levels to help the system settle into the best fit to multiple constraints. An eighth property of the backprojection system is that it can speed the rate of learning above that possible in a simple competitive learning system.

This theory of the functions of backprojections in the cerebral cortex requires a large number of backprojecting axons, as pattern-specific information (used to guide learning by providing a set of mutually orthogonal guidance signals, or to produce recall) must be provided by the backprojections. It also solves the de-addressing problem in that the hippocampus does not need to know exactly where in the cortex information should be stored. Instead, the backprojection signal spreads widely in layer 1, and the storage site is simply on those neurons which happen to receive strong (and precise) forward activity as well as backprojected activity, so that Hebbian learning by conjunction occurs there. This scheme is consistent with neocortical anatomy, in that it requires the same pyramidal cell to receive both forward and (more diffuse) backprojected activity, which the arrangement of pyramidal cells with apical dendrites which extend all the way up into layer 1 achieves (see Peters & Jones, 1984). Indeed, in contrast to the relatively localized terminal distributions of forward cortico-cortical and thalamo-cortical afferents, the cortico-cortical backward projections which end in layer 1 have a much wider horizontal distribution, of up to several mm (Amaral, 1986, 1987). The suggestion is thus that this enables the backward projecting neurons to search over a larger number of pyramidal cells in the preceding cortical area for activity which is conjunctive with their own. It is also of interest that the theory utilizes a Hebbian learning scheme which provides for learning to occur when conjointly there is forward and backprojected input to a pyramidal cell resulting in sufficient post-synaptic activation to provide for modification of synapses which happen to be active. This provides the opportunity to make it clear that the theoretical ideas introduced here make clear predictions which can be empirically tested. For example, the theory of backprojections just proposed predicts that the backprojections in the cerebral cortex have modifiable synapses on pyramidal cells in the previous cortical area. If this were found not to be the case in empirical tests, then the theory would be rejected.

The ideas introduced here also have many theoretical implications. One is that if the backprojections are used for recall, as seems likely as discussed above (see also Roland & Friberg, 1985), then this would place severe constraints on their use for functions such as error backpropagation. Error backpropagation is an interesting and powerful algorithm in parallel distributed processing networks for setting the weights in hidden units (i.e. nodes in layers which are not input and output layers) to allow networks to learn useful mappings between input and output layers (Rumelhart, Hinton & Williams, 1986). However, the backprojections in the architecture in which this algorithm is implemented have very precise functions in conveying error from the output layer back to the earlier, hidden, layers. It would be difficult to use the weights (synaptic strengths) from the backprojecting neurons to neurons in earlier layers both to convey the error correctly, and to have the appropriate strengths for recall.

In conclusion, in this paper experimental evidence on and theoretical approaches to the function of the hippocampus and of backprojections in the cerebral cortex have been considered. Theories of how the hippocampus functions and of the functions of back-projections in the neocortex have been proposed. The theories are at the level of neuronal networks, and are based partly on evidence on the fine architecture of the networks, on the rules of synaptic modifiability incorporated, and on the systems level connections. It is suggested that this approach will be useful in future in linking anatomical evidence on structure to physiological evidence on modifiability, understanding the global properties of the networks, and thus understanding the role of the networks in brain function and behavior.

Acknowledgements

The author has worked on some of the experiments and neuronal network modelling described here with A. Bennett, G.C. Baylis, P. Cahusac, D. Cohen, J. Feigenbaum, M. Hasselmo, R. Kesner, G. Littlewort, Y. Miyashita, H. Niki, R. Payne, T. Scott and S. Yaxley and their collaboration is sincerely acknowledged. Discussions with David G. Amaral of the Salk Institute, La Jolla, were also much appreciated. This research was supported by the Medical Research Council.

References

Amaral D.G. (1986) Amygdalohippocampal and amygdalocortical projections in the primate brain. In **Excitatory Amino Acids and Epilepsy**, pp. 3-17, R. Schwarz & Y. Ben-Ari (eds.) Plenum, New York.

Amaral D.G. (1987) Memory: anatomical organization of candidate brain regions. In **Handbook of Neurophysiology. Section 1: The Nervous System. Vol. V. Part 1** pp. 211-294 American Physiological Society, Washington, DC.

Amaral D.G. & Price J.L. (1984) Amygdalo-cortical projections in the monkey (*Macaca fascicularis*). **J. comp. Neurol. 230**, pp. 465-496

Andersen P.O. (1987) Properties of hippocampal synapses of importance for integration and memory. In **New Insights into Synaptic Function**. pp. 403-429, G.M. Edelman, W.E. Gall & W.M. Cowan (eds.) Neuroscience Research Foundation, Wiley, NY.

Barlow H.B. (1972) Single units and sensation: a neuron doctrine for perceptual psychology? **Perception 1**, pp. 371-394

Barnes C.A. (1988) Spatial learning and memory processes: the search for their neurobiological mechanisms in the rat. **TINS 11**, pp. 163-169

Baylis G.C., Rolls E.T. & Leonard C.M. (1985) Selectivity between faces in the responses of a population of neurons in the cortex in the superior temporal sulcus of the monkey. **Brain Res. 342**, pp. 91-102

Baylis G.C., Rolls E.T. & Leonard C.M. (1987) Functional subdivisions of temporal lobe neocortex. **J. Neurosci. 7**, pp. 330-342

Bear M.F. & Singer W. (1986) Modulation of visual cortical plasticity by acetylcholine and noradrenaline. **Nature 320**, pp. 172-176

Bear M.F., Cooper L.N. & Ebner F.B. (1987) A physiological basis for a theory of synapse modification. **Science 237**, pp. 42-48

Beckstead R.M., Morse J.R. & Norgen R. (1980) The nucleus of the solitary tract in the monkey: Projections to the thalamus and brainstem nuclei. **J. comp. Neurol. 190**, pp. 259-282

Bienenstock E.L., Cooper L.N. & Munro P.W. (1982) Theory for the development of neuron selectivity: orientation specificity and binocular interaction in visual cortex. **J. Neurosci. 2**, pp. 32-48

Bliss T.V.P. & Lomo T. (1973) Long-lasting potentiation of synaptic transmission in the dentate area of the anaesthetized rabbit following stimulation of the perforant path. **J. Physiol. 232**, pp. 331-356

Cahusac P.M.B., Rolls E.T., Miyashita Y. & Niki H. (1989) Modification of the responses of hippocampal neurons in the monkey during the learning of a conditional response task. **J. Neurosci.** in press.

Cowey A (1979) Cortical maps and visual perception. **Quart. J. Exp. Psychol. 31**, pp. 1-17

Desimone R. & Gross C.G. (1979) Visual areas in the temporal lobe of the macaque. **Brain Res. 178**, pp. 363-380

Erickson R.P. (1963) Stimulus encoding in topographic and nontopographic modalities: On the significance of the activity of individual sensory neurons. **Psychol. Rev. 75**, pp. 447-465

Erickson R.P. (1982) The across-fiber pattern theory: an organizing principle for molar neural function. **Contributions to Sensory Physiology 6**, pp. 79-110

Gaffan D. (1974) Recognition impaired and association intact in the memory of monkeys after transection of the fornix. **J. comp. Physiol. Psychol. 86**, pp. 1100-1109

Gaffan D. (1977) Monkey's recognition memory for complex pictures and the effects of fornix transection. **Quart. J. Exp. Psychol. 29**, pp. 505-514

Ganong A.H., Harris E.W., Monaghan D.T., Watkins J.C. & Cotman C.W. (1986) Evidence for both NMDA- and non-NMDA-receptor mediated LTP: analysis with D-AP5 and new more potent NMDA antagonist. **Soc. Neurosci. Abstr. 12**, p. 61

Gardner-Medwin A.R. (1976) The recall of events through the learning of associations between their parts. **Proc. Roy. Soc. Lond. B. 194**, pp. 375-402

Grossberg S. (1982) **Studies of Mind and Brain**. Reidel, NY.

Grossberg S. (1987) Competitive learning: from interactive activation to adaptive resonance. **Cognitive Science 11**, pp. 23-63

Hasselmo M.E., Rolls E.T., Baylis G.C. & Nalwa V. (1989) Object-centered encoding by face-selective neurons in the cortex in the superior temporal sulcus of the monkey. **Exp. Brain Res.**, in press.

Ito M. (1984) **The Cerebellum and Neural Control**. Raven Press,NY.

Jordan M.I. (1986) An introduction to linear algebra in parallel distributed processing. In **Parallel Distributed Processing**, Vol. 1. Foundations, pp. 365-442, D.E. Rumelhart & J.L. McClelland (eds.) MIT Press, Cambridge, Mass.

Kelso S.R., Ganong A.H. & Brown T.H. (1986) Hebbian synapses in the hippocampus. **Proc. Nat. Acad. Sci. 83**, pp. 5326-5330

Kohonen T. (1988) **Self-Organization and Associative Memory**. 2nd Edition. Springer-Verlag, Berlin.

Kohonen T., Lehtio P., Rovamo J., Hyvarinen J., Bry K. & Vainio L. (1977) A principle of neural associative memory. **Neurosci. 2**, pp. 1065-1076

Kohonen T., Oja E. & Lehtio P. (1981) Storage and processing of information in distributed associative memory systems. In **Parallel Models of Associative Memory**, pp. 105-143, G.E. Hinton & J.A. Anderson (eds.) Erlbaum, Hillsdale, New Jersey.

Leonard C.M., Rolls E.T., Wilson F.A.W. & Baylis G.C. (1985) Neurons in the amygdala of the monkey with responses selective for faces. **Behav. Brain Res. 15**, pp. 159-176

Levy W.B. (1985) Associative changes in the synapse: LTP in the hippocampus. In **Synaptic Modification, Neuron Selectivity, and Nervous System Organization**, pp. 5-33, W.B. Levy, J.A. Anderson & S. Lehmkuhle (eds.) Erlbaum, Hillsdale, New Jersey.

Levy W.B. & Desmond N.L. (1985) The rules of elemental synaptic plasticity. In **Synaptic Modification, Neuron Selectivity, and Nervous System Organization**, pp. 105-121, W.B. Levy, J.A. Anderson & S. Lehmkuhle (eds.) Erlbaum, Hillsdale, New Jersey.

von der Malsburg C. (1973) Self-organization of orientation-sensitive columns in the striate cortex. **Kybernetik 14**, pp. 85-100

Marr D. (1970) A theory for cerebral cortex. **Proc. Roy. Soc. B 176,** pp. 161-234

Marr D. (1971) Simple memory: a theory for archicortex. **Phil. Trans. Roy. Soc. B 262**, pp. 23-81

Martin K.A.C. (1984) Neuronal circuits in cat striate cortex. In **The Cerebral Cortex**, Vol. 2, Functional properties of cortical cells. pp. 241-285, E.G. Jones & A. Peters (eds.) Plenum, NY.

McClelland J.L. & Rumelhart D.E. (1988) **Explorations in Parallel Distributed Processing**. MIT Press, Cambridge, Mass.

McNaughton B.L. (1984) Activity dependent modulation of hippocampal synaptic efficacy: some implications for memory processes. In **Neurobiology of the Hippocampus,** pp. 233-252, W. Seifert (ed.) Academic Press, London.

Milner B. (1972) Disorders of learning and memory after temporal lobe lesions in man. **Clinical Neurosurgery 19**, pp. 421-446

Miyashita Y., Rolls E.T., Cahusac P.M.B., Niki H. & Feigenbaum J.D. (1989) Activity of hippocampal formation neurons in the monkey related to a conditional response task. **J. Neurophysiol.**, in press.

Perrett D.I., Rolls E.T. & Caan W. (1982) Visual neurons responsive to faces in the monkey temporal cortex. **Exp. Brain Res. 47**, pp. 329-342

Perrett D.I., Smith P.A.J., Mistlin A.J., Chitty A.J., Head A.S., Potter D.D., Broennimann R., Milner A.D. & Jeeves M.A. (1985) Visual analysis of body movements by neurons in the temporal cortex of the macaque monkey: a preliminary report. **Behav. Brain Res. 16**, pp. 153-170

Peters A. & Jones E.G. (1984) **The Cerebral Cortex,** Vol. 1, Cellular Components of the Cerebral Cortex. Plenum, New York.

Roland P.E., Vaernet K. & Lassen N.A. (1980) Cortical activations in man during verbal report from visual memory. **Neurosci. Lett. Suppl. 5**, S478

Roland P.E. & Friberg L. (1985) Localization of cortical areas activated by thinking. **J. Neurophysiol. 53**, pp. 1219-1243

Rolls E.T. (1984) Neurons in the cortex of the temporal lobe and in the amygdala of the monkey with responses selective for faces. **Human Neurobiology 3**, pp. 209-222

Rolls E.T. (1985) Connections, functions and dysfunctions of limbic structures, the prefrontal cortex, and hypothalamus. In **The Scientific Basis of**

Clinical Neurology, pp. 201-213, M. Swash & C. Kennard (eds.) Churchill Livingstone, London.

Rolls E.T. (1986) A theory of emotion, and its application to understanding the neural basis of emotion. In **Emotions. Neural and Chemical Control**, pp. 325-344, Y. Oomura (ed.) Japan Scientific Societies Press, Tokyo & Karger, Basel.

Rolls E.T. (1987) Information representation, processing and storage in the brain: analysis at the single neuron level. In **The Neural and Molecular Bases of Learning**, pp. 503-540, J.-P. Changeux & M. Konishi (eds.) Wiley, Chichester.

Rolls E.T. (1989a) Functions of neuronal networks in the hippocampus and neocortex in memory. In **Neural Models of Plasticity: Theoretical and Empirical Approaches**. J.H. Byrne & W.O. Berry (eds.) Academic Press, New York.

Rolls E.T. (1989b) Visual information processing in the primate temporal lobe. In **Models of Visual Perception: from Natural to Artificial**. M. Imbert (ed.) Oxford University Press, Oxford.

Rolls E.T. (1989c) Parallel distributed processing in the brain: implications of the functional architecture of neuronal networks in the hippocampus. In **Parallel Distributed Processing: Implications for Psychobiology and Neurobiology**. R.G.M. Morris (ed.) Oxford University Press, Oxford.

Rolls E.T., Baylis G.C. & Leonard C.M. (1985) Role of low and high spatial frequencies in the face-selective responses of neurons in the cortex in the superior temporal sulcus. **Vision Res. 25**, pp. 1021-1035

Rolls E.T. & Baylis G.C. (1986) Size and contrast have only small effects on the responses to faces of neurons in the cortex of the superior temporal sulcus of the monkey. **Exp. Brain Res. 65**, pp. 38-48

Rolls E.T. & Williams G.V. (1987) Sensory and movement-related neuronal activity in different regions of the primate striatum. In **Basal Ganglia and Behavior: Sensory Aspects and Motor Functioning**. pp. 37-59, J.S. Schneider & T.I. Lidsky (eds.) Hans Huber, Bern.

Rolls E.T., Baylis G.C. & Hasselmo M.E. (1987) The responses of neurons in the cortex in the superior temporal sulcus of the monkey to band-pass spatial frequency filtered faces. **Vision Res. 27**, pp. 311-326

Rolls E.T., Miyashita Y., Cahusac P.M.B., Kesner R.P., Niki H., Feigenbaum J. & Bach L. (1989a) Hippocampal neurons in the monkey with activity related to the place in which a stimulus is shown. **J. Neurosci.**, in press.

Rolls E.T., Sienkiewicz Z.J. & Yaxley S. (1989b) Hunger modulates the responses to gustatory stimuli of single neurons in the orbitofrontal cortex. **European J. Neurosci.**, in press.

Rolls E.T., Baylis G.C., Hasselmo M. & Nalwa V. (1989c) The representation of information in the temporal lobe visual cortical areas of macaque monkeys. In **Seeing Contour and Colour**. J.J. Kulikowski & C.M. Dickinson (eds.) Manchester University Press, Manchester.

Rumelhart D.E. & McClelland J.L. (1986) **Parallel Distributed Processing**, Vol. 1. Foundations. MIT Press, Cambridge, Mass.

Rumelhart D.E. & Zipser D. (1986) Feature discovery by competitive learning. In **Parallel Distributed Processing**, Vol. 1. Foundations, pp. 151-193, D.E. Rumelhart & J.L. McClelland (eds.) MIT Press, Cambridge, Mass.

Rumelhart D.E., Hinton G.E. & Williams R.J. (1986) Learning internal representations by error propagation. In **Parallel Distributed Processing**, Vol. 1. Foundations, pp. 318-362, D.E. Rumelhart & J.L. McClelland (eds.) MIT Press, Cambridge, Mass.

Scott T.R., Yaxley S., Sienkiewicz Z.J. & Rolls E.T. (1986a) Taste responses in the nucleus tractus solitarius of the behaving monkey. **J. Neurophysiol. 55**, pp. 182-200

Scott T.R., Yaxley S., Sienkiewicz Z.J. & Rolls E.T. (1986b) Gustatory responses in the frontal opercular cortex of the alert cynomolgus monkey. **J. Neurophysiol. 56**, pp. 876-890

Scoville W.B. & Milner B. (1957) Loss of recent memory after bilateral hippocampal lesions. **J. Neurol. Neurosurg. Psychiat. 20**, pp. 11-21

Seltzer B. & Pandya D.N. (1978) Afferent cortical connections and architectonics of the superior temporal sulcus and surrounding cortex in the rhesus monkey. **Brain Res. 149**, pp. 1-24

Smith D.V. & Travers J.B. (1979) A metric for the breadth of tuning of gustatory neurons. **Chemical Senses and Flavour 4**, pp. 215-229

Squire L. (1986) Mechanisms of memory. **Science 232**, pp. 1612-1619

Squire L.R. & Zola-Morgan S. (1988) Memory: brain systems and behavior. **TINS 11**, pp. 170-175

Squire L.R., Shimamura A.P. & Amaral D.G. (1989) Memory and the hippocampus. In **Neural Models of Plasticity: Theoretical and Empirical Approaches**, J. Byrne & W.O. Berry (eds.) Academic Press, NY.

Turner B.H. (1981) The cortical sequence and terminal distribution of sensory related afferents to the amygdaloid complex of the rat and monkey. In **The Amygdaloid Complex**, pp. 51-62, Y. Ben-Ari (ed.) Elsevier, Amsterdam.

Van Hoesen G.W. (1981) The differential distribution, diversity and sprouting of cortical projections to the amygdala in the rhesus monkey. In **The Amygdaloid Complex**, pp. 79-90, Y. Ben-Ari (ed.) Elsevier, Amsterdam.

Van Hoesen G.W. (1982) The parahippocampal gyrus. New observations regarding its cortical connections in the monkey. **TINS 5**, pp. 345-350

Van Hoesen G.W. & Pandya D.N. (1975) Some connections of the entorhinal (area 28) and perirhinal (area 35) cortices in the monkey. I. Temporal lobe afferents. **Brain Res. 95**, pp. 1-24

Van Hoesen G.W., Pandya D.N. & Butters N. (1975) Some connections of the entorhinal (area 28) and perirhinal (area 35) cortices in the monkey. II. Frontal lobe afferents. **Brain Res. 95**, pp. 25-38

Wiggins L.L., Rolls E.T. & Baylis G.C. (1987) Afferent connections of the caudolateral orbitofrontal cortex taste area of the primate. **Soc. Neurosci. Abstr. 13**, p. 1406

Wigstrom H., Gustaffson B., Huang Y.-Y. & Abraham W.C. (1986) Hippocampal long-term potentiation is induced by pairing single afferent volleys with intracellularly injected depolarizing currents. **Acta Physiol. Scand. 126**, pp. 317-319

Yaxley S., Rolls E.T. & Sienkiewicz Z.J. (1989) Gustatory responses of single neurons in the insula of the macaque monkey. **J. Neurophysiol.**, in press.

Zola-Morgan S., Squire L.R. & Amaral D.G. (1986) Human amnesia and the medial temporal region: enduring memory impairment following a bilateral lesion limited to field CA1 of the hippocampus. **J. Neurosci. 6**, pp. 2950-2957

9
The Computational Unit as an Assembly of Neurones: an Implementation of an Error Correcting Learning Algorithm

Ian McLaren

9.1   Introduction

There is a consensus amongst animal learning theorists that a learning rule of an error correcting nature is required; i.e. that learning should be governed by the difference between what is required (in terms of some variable such as associative strength) and what currently exists (Rescorla & Wagner, 1972; Mackintosh, 1975; Pearce & Hall, 1980). This class of rule is also favoured in modelling humans' cognitive abilities (McClelland & Rumelhart, 1985; Rumelhart & McClelland, 1986), and is recognized as possessing a number of computational advantages over the various Hebbian rules (for a discussion see Stone, 1986, and the next section). One particular error correcting algorithm, a generalization of the delta rule known as back propagation (Rumelhart *et al.*, 1986), is probably the current market leader in connectionist modelling.

Whilst much of the impetus towards using error correcting algorithms comes from psychology, the trend in the neurobiological modelling of learning seems to be more in favour of the Hebbian type of rule (Levy & Desmond, 1985), with the extent to which any two units' activities are correlated over time governing the learning between them (Hebb, 1949). This is not to say that neurobiologists deny the importance of the behavioural data, rather that there is an implicit assumption that error correcting circuits of some kind can be constructed from the more fundamental Hebbian elements, and that as a consequence the disagreement on the type of rule is more apparent than real (for an excellent case in point see Anderson, 1985). This chapter examines that assumption critically, and assesses the feasibility of constructing error correcting units from simpler components.

The themes of neurobiological plausibility, computational analysis and goodness of fit to the behavioural data are interwoven in this chapter. The behavioural and computational motivation for taking learning to be error correcting is briefly touched upon before considering some of the more Hebbian candidates for the role of basic learning element suggested by neurobiology. A computational analysis of the requirements for the construction of an error correcting assembly indicates that Hebbian elements are unsuitable for this task. A learning element that overcomes some of the difficulties faced by the earlier candidates is then discussed, starting with some neurobiological motivation for this type of element, and then demonstrating how it can be used to build an error correcting assembly. The chapter concludes with an examination of the assembly's neurobiological plausibility.

9.2   Error correction and learning

The first step is briefly to make the case for an error correcting rule. Many of the learning rules proposed by psychologists have, broadly speaking, been error correcting (e.g. Bush & Mosteller, 1955); in that the change in the variable tracking the learning has been proportional to its difference from some target value or asymptote. An important development in animal learning, initiated by Rescorla & Wagner, was to have the asymptote specified by the unconditioned stimulus (US, the motivationally significant stimulus), so that it set the target for the associative strength that the conditioned stimulus (CS, the typically neutral stimulus preceding the US) had to acquire to the US. The classic work of Kamin, and Rescorla and Wagner strongly suggests that this type of rule is required to explain the behavioural data. Kamin (1968) was the first to report the phenomenon of blocking in Pavlovian conditioning. In this procedure CS1 is paired repeatedly with a US, and after the CS1-US association has been conditioned to near asymptote, a new stimulus, CS2, is presented in compound with CS1 on further conditioning trials. Reduced to its bare essentials, the finding is that the subject shows little evidence of forming an association between CS2 and the US when tested in isolation after the compound conditioning; although the procedure would have produced substantial conditioning of the CS2-US association in the absence of pre-training, the CS1 has blocked it by virtue of its prior association with the US.

Rescorla & Wagner (1972) put forward the following learning algorithm as an explanation of the blocking phenomenon:

$$dv_i = ab(q - \Sigma v_j) \tag{9.1}$$

where v is an associative strength (and summation is over all CS's present), dv_i the change in associative strength for a given CS on a trial, q an asymptote dependent on the US used, and a and b learning rate parameters reflecting the salience of the CS and US respectively. This is an error correcting rule with (as Sutton & Barto, 1981, note) strong similarities to the rule developed by Widrow & Hoff (1960) and discussed by McClelland & Rumelhart (1985) as the delta rule. Note that, once the sum of the v's reaches asymptote, learning stops and the system maintains the current value of v, a critically important feature of this type of rule. The asymptote represents a desired target value for v, and the discrepancy between v and asymptote acts as an error signal controlling the change in v. Rescorla (1971) has performed a number of experiments to test this algorithm; for example, manipulations to make the error large and positive, resulting in extremely rapid learning. The Rescorla-Wagner model has proved very successful in accounting for a large body of data, and whilst certainly incorrect in its simple form (cf.

phenomena such as latent inhibition, Lubow & Moore, 1959) can be developed into a general associative system of considerable power (McLaren *et al.*, 1989).

Quite apart from a good fit to behaviour, error correcting rules have computational advantages over their Hebbian counterparts. They are, under at least some conditions, able to store more information for a given size of network and are also more powerful, in that they can normally be expected to arrive at some least-squares solution to a problem (Stone, 1986). These desirable properties have led to their widespread use in various guises: the perceptron (Rosenblatt, 1962) provides one example from the pattern recognition domain, whilst McClelland & Rumelhart (1985) have used a delta rule system to model the acquisition of concepts. A final advantage is the existence of a generalization of this type of rule to multi-layer networks (Rumelhart *et al.*, 1986).

It seems then, that some type of error correcting architecture is indicated. Here I focus on the case of a general purpose associative system, in which the processing units themselves are error correcting: i.e. each unit sets its own required (asymptotic value of) input from other units in the system based on information it receives from outside the system. It is important to understand that by unit is meant whatever computational machinery constitutes a processor in the system, without necessarily identifying a unit with a single neurone. On the contrary, as the learning rules considered will not themselves be error correcting at the level of the individual neurone: construction of the processing units will proceed via embedding the particular mechanism for synaptic plasticity under consideration in an assembly of neurones with fixed synaptic weights. Error correction then becomes a property of the assembly, rather than of the individual neurones that constitute that assembly.

9.3   The basic learning element

In order to construct such an assembly, however, it is necessary to specify the basic learning element. Neurobiological evidence suggests that learning occurs via changes in synaptic efficiency at certain 'plastic' synapses, and that the rules governing the change are essentially Hebbian. By this is meant that the change in synaptic strength depends in some fashion on both the pre-synaptic and post-synaptic firing rates (or some other measure of activity). A review of the evidence will not be attempted here, though work on LTP in the hippocampus (Levy, 1985) and maturation of the visual cortex (Singer, 1985) may be cited as supporting this conjecture in mammals. Given the assumption of a Hebbian type mechanism for synaptic plasticity, the next step is an examination of Hebbian rules and the feasibility of constructing error correcting assemblies from elements employing them.

The neurones S and R are the input and receptor neurones respectively, with no connotations of a stimulus-response reflex intended. If A_s, A_r stand for the activity of neurones S and R in Figure 9.1, and w is the synaptic strength or weight from S to R and t is time, then the basic Hebb (1949) rule is:

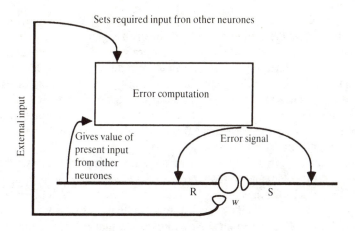

Figure 9.1 A schematic representation of an assembly that computes an error signal. w is the strength of the plastic synaptic connection between S and R, with the circle (shown large for emphasis) on R being the post-synaptic site. The other (fixed strength) synapse delivers an external input to R.

$$dw/dt = A_s A_r \mu \quad \text{where } \mu \text{ is a positive constant} \tag{9.2}$$

A number of variants on this basic rule have been proposed. For example:

$$dw/dt = A_s A_r \mu - A_s \beta \quad \text{where } \beta \text{ is a positive constant} \tag{9.3}$$

whereby activation of S alone weakens the pathway as found in habituation (see Chapter 1 in Horn, 1985) is a possible candidate. A further modification of the basic Hebbian rule is to make changes in the strength of a synapse dependent on its current strength. Levy & Desmond (1985), for example, give:

$$dw/dt = gF\{A_r\}(hA_s - w) \tag{9.4}$$

where g, h are positive constants, and F some monotonic function, increasing with increasing A_r. They also suggest a variety of equations to govern changes in the strength of inhibitory synapses. Whatever the details of the rule used, as long as it is essentially Hebbian then error correction is hard, if not impossible, to achieve. Apart from the S and R neurones Figure 9.1 also depicts in abstract terms the information required for error correction. A signal external to the system sets the input that the R neurone requires from all the other S neurones synapsing on it (only one is shown in the figure for clarity). The R neurone itself must signal the current value of the input from the S neurones to some other system (shown as a box), which uses this information in conjunction with its copy of the external signal to compute the error signal for R. This error signal must then be fed back to R or S (or both) to control learning.

The problem for any Hebbian system is that it does not have enough components to meet these requirements. If the error signal sets the activity of R so as to control changes in w then this is incompatible with that same activity representing the summed input received by R from the S neurones. If, however, the error signal were to control learning via S's activity, then this would interfere with its representing variations in the input from that S neurone to R. Allowing the changes made to synaptic weights to depend on their current value only worsens the situation, as now a separate error signal for each S neurone would be necessary to control learning appropriately.

The conclusion that can be drawn from a more detailed analysis than space allows here is that elements of the type considered so far are, to say the least, not ideal building blocks for the construction of error correcting assemblies. Given this, it is tempting to assume that the basic learning element is error correcting in itself *, making an assembly unnecessary. Note, however, that the basic element would now require a number of components or component processes in order to represent the information necessary for error correction. The point here is that it is not enough to state that any system is error correcting without showing how the error signal is computed, represented, and made available to control learning. Thus error correction can either be based on intra-elemental components or processes, a possibility not considered further here, or implemented by learning element(s) embedded in an assembly of other elements; though this would not seem to be possible in the case of any of the learning elements considered up to this point.

How then are we to proceed? The use of more complex functions within rules of the type discussed so far does not seem to offer much hope of success. Our arguments have been based on the quantities available to represent information, and the main problem is that there have simply not been enough of them to stand for the variables required. Now, however, let us consider a type of rule that may be characterized as quasi-Hebbian and that does not suffer from this failing. This class of rule is distinguished by there being some third component added to the two-component (S and R) system discussed up to this point, and in one form was proposed by Kandel & Tauc (1965) as a 'pre-synaptic facilitation mechanism'.

A good example of this type of system has been suggested as the learning mechanism in *Aplysia californica*, by Hawkins *et al.* (1983), and is shown in Figure 9.2.

In this case the site of plasticity is pre-synaptic and requires a special arrangement of synapses, as shown in the figure. Three types of event may be distinguished. If the S neurone alone fires then the synaptic strength of the S-R connection (w) decreases, which manifests behaviourally as habituation. If the F

---

* A rule put forward by Konorski (1948) may fall into this class. He proposed that an excitatory synapse be strengthened when pre-synaptic activation was paired with an increasing post-synaptic activation, and that pre-synaptic activity in conjunction with decreasing post-synaptic activity would result in the strengthening of an inhibitory connection, there being separate systems of inhibitory and excitatory links. Preliminary results using these rules do suggest that they are capable of implementing a form of error correction. Note, however, that intra-neural components or processes are needed to detect the rates of change of activation of a neurone.

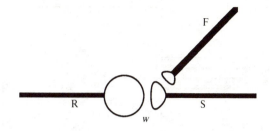

Figure 9.2 The synaptic arrangement found in *Aplysia*. F is the new facilitatory component that is thought to modulate pre-synaptic processes controlling the strength of the S-R synapse.

(facilitator) neurone fires on its own then w increases somewhat, corresponding to sensitization. On those occasions on which S fires followed by an F spike at an appropriate interval, then a dramatic increase in w occurs, termed pairing specific enhancement (PSE). Gluck & Thompson (1987) have modelled this type of system in a recent paper, implementing sensitization and PSE via an eligibility trace (after Sutton & Barto, 1981) which grows in strength after an S firing, peaks, then decays away until reset by another S spike. The level of the eligibility trace determines how effective an F spike is in increasing w. My argument is that, with modifications, this basic learning element can be used in an assembly with other neurones to implement error correction. A more general treatment of this class of rule and some speculation as to possible members of this class follows the derivation of the required assembly. Before introducing the assembly, however, a more quantitative account of the basic learning rule is needed. In order to achieve error correction whilst employing a neural arrangement of the *Aplysia* type, it was found necessary to introduce some modifications and further assumptions in the treatment of this learning element. A major modification is to ignore sensitization: whereas before, a firing of the F neurone on its own could increase the synaptic weight w, now, in the absence of an appropriately timed S spike, a firing of the F neurone has negligible effect. In practical terms all that is required is that intense stimulation of the F neurone is necessary to produce behavioural sensitization, and that this level of activity will never be reached by F in the normal course of the assembly's operation. Another assumption is that the increment or decrement to w for a given event be of constant magnitude, though not the same constant in each case. This gives a learning rule of the form:

$$dw/dt = A_S A_f \mu - A_S \beta \quad \text{where } \mu \text{ and } \beta \text{ are positive constants} \tag{9.5}$$

if the activation of any neurone is interpreted as an average firing rate. Implicit in this rule is the assumption that the temporal window after an S spike, in which an F spike must fall to give PSE, is of short duration, so that the chances of F firing more than once in it are negligible, and hence $A_S A_f$ is the correct expression for the expected number of PSE events in a second. Thus the $A_S A_f \mu$ term represents the

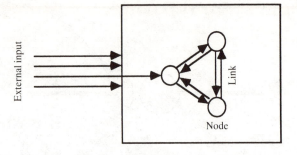

Figure 9.3 The delta rule. External input arrives from outside the system, is not itself mediated by plastic connections and sets the required internal input for a given node. Internal input is that arriving from other nodes in the system, generally via plastic links which are unidirectional. The nodes take activation values that determine the output along a link in conjunction with the strength of a link.

increase in the synaptic weight due to PSE events, and the $A_s\beta$ term represents the decrease in w due to S firing, which occurs irrespective of PSE. Note that changes in w make no direct reference to its current value. Given Equation 9.5, it can be seen that for maintenance, i.e. for $dw/dt = 0$, $A_f = \beta/\mu$, a value independent of A_s. In fact A_s plays a part in controlling the rate of learning, but not its direction as it cannot be less than zero, given the interpretation of activation as an average firing rate. These are the key results that make the construction of an error correcting assembly possible. The activations themselves are assumed to be linear functions of their inputs with a lower bound of zero (an assumption discussed in detail in a later section), that is:

$$A = k(\text{total input}) \quad \text{where } k \text{ is a positive constant.} \tag{9.6}$$

9.4 An error correcting assembly

Having defined the learning rule to be used at the neural level, it only remains to specify the error correcting rule to be instantiated by the assembly prior to consideration of the assembly itself. The learning rule implemented here is the delta rule referred to earlier, particularly the version of it discussed by McClelland & Rumelhart (1985). Figure 9.3 gives a schematic representation of a typical system employing this rule.

External input, e, is that input arising from outside the system (box), with the external input to the ith node being denoted by e_i. Each node has an activation, a, and the jth node has activation a_j. The activation is generally some monotonically increasing function of its total input. Each node transmits activation via links from that node to other nodes, and the summed input received by the ith node from other nodes is termed i_i, the internal input. Each link has a certain strength, w, and the

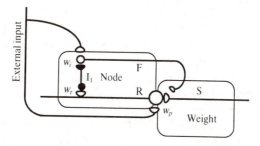

Figure 9.4 An error correcting assembly for excitatory associations. The various w's stand for the synaptic weights with the subscripts generally indicating the neurone making the synapse: only w_p can vary. The weights for the synapses from the neurone carrying external input are not given, instead the total external input received by R and F is simply taken to be e. No weight is specified for the F synapse either, as it has a special facilitatory function. The inhibitory interneurone, I_1, is shown in solid black.

link from node j to node i is defined here as w_{ij}. The activation transmitted along w_{ij} is $w_{ij}a_j$. The internal input is then:

$$i_i = \Sigma w_{ij}a_j \quad \text{with summation over } j. \tag{9.7}$$

The error signal for the ith node, Δ_i, is given by $e_i - i_i$, and the learning rule is:

$$dw_{ij}/dt = s\Delta_i a_j \quad \text{where } s \text{ is a positive constant.} \tag{9.8}$$

That is, w_{ij} changes so as to reduce Δ_i, taking into account how active the node at the input end of the link is.

Equation 9.8 gives the computational target: the assembly must change the strengths of its incoming connections in accordance with this formula if it is to instantiate the delta rule using neurone-like elements. The first derivation will be of an error correcting assembly that allows only excitatory associations; mathematical details are given in the appendix. The assembly is shown in Figure 9.4. For simplicity only one incoming connection is shown; our arguments apply equally well with an arbitrary number of connections since the effects of each are simply summed. Note that the main difference from Figure 9.1 is that a means of allowing the error signal to control learning is now possible, with the F neurone performing this function.

The box labelled 'NODE' contains the components that compute Δ, i, and a; i.e. those quantities that define a node's state. In fact, one may loosely speak of F computing Δ, I_1 computing i and R computing a. The R neurone is shown as receiving external input so that it can represent that input. This has the consequence that activation of R by internal input alone is readily interpretable, the system is indicating that it expects the external input to R to be forthcoming. The output of R can then be taken by other systems as measuring whether a certain external input is present or expected. This treatment follows that of McClelland & Rumelhart (1985) in which nodal activation was determined by the sum of the external and internal inputs, and provides the basis for implementation of the 'stimulus substitution' principle in animal learning theory. The box labelled 'WEIGHT' contains the components implementing a variable w. External input is shown arriving via another neurone; however, rather than specify a synaptic strength and activation function for this neurone, the total external input received by R will be termed e. To gain some feel for how the assembly works, imagine an e to be applied and S to be active. If R is not receiving enough input from S to match e, then it will be less active than it should be, and will fail to inhibit F enough to keep its activation below $ß/\mu$. Hence w_p will increase, at a rate governed by both A_s and A_f. Eventually R will receive sufficient input for A_r to be large enough to bring A_f down to $ß/\mu$ and learning will stop. If S is subsequently active on its own, then extinction will take place. A_f will be zero so each S spike decrements w_p until it reaches zero. The e applied must always be enough to raise A_f above $ß/\mu$ (on its own) for this assembly to work properly, but as $ß/\mu$ will be small this is a minor restriction.

As shown in the appendix, the learning rule for this assembly is:

$$dw_p/dt = A_s \mu k_f (e - i)/2 \quad \text{with } k_f \text{ a positive constant, and } i = w_p A_s \qquad (9.9)$$

which is the correct form for the delta rule. In the course of the derivation a constant input, c, is introduced for the F neurone which effectively sets its spontaneous firing rate. The inclusion of a c term is not strictly necessary in order to have an error correcting rule for this excitatory case, but it does make the algebra tidy. Such a term is necessary, however, if inhibitory learning is to be implemented as well. The revised assembly that achieves this is shown in Figure 9.5.

Two new components are needed, the synapse from S onto I_2, and I_2 and its synapse onto R, with the (fixed) synaptic strength of I_2 assumed equal to that of I_1, i.e. w_i. The net result is Equation 9.9 again. The difference is that inhibitory learning can now occur, as can be seen by considering the case of R being activated via internal input only. If the external input is zero then F will be completely inhibited ($A_f = 0$), instead of firing at its spontaneous rate (which is set at $ß/\mu$ so that dw_p/dt equals zero when F receives zero net input), and the various w_p's with active S neurones will decrease. If w_p and w_s are initially set so that the net input delivered by an S neurone is zero (see discussion in appendix), then decreasing w_p will cause this S neurone to exert an inhibitory effect on R when subsequently activated: in fact the arrangement labelled 'WEIGHT' is now most easily understood as having an effective weight of $w_p - w_s$, and, given an initial effective value of zero, any decrease in w_p must make this effective weight negative. Note that this implementation of inhibitory learning only requires variation in excitatory synapses, and that requiring F to have a baseline rate of activity allows the activation of R by internal input only to have the correct effect on F, and hence on w_p. When the net input to R is zero, the spontaneous rate of F will allow non-zero values of w_p to be maintained, whereas without it they would extinguish to zero. Essentially, the baseline rate of F allows it to both detect cases when the internal input exceeds the

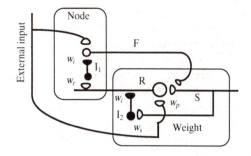

Figure 9.5 A development of the assembly shown in Figure 9.4 that permits inhibitory associations to be formed as well. For simplicity, both inhibitory neurones are assumed to have the same characteristics, though this is not a necessary assumption. The effective weight for the S-R connection is now $w_p - w_s$, if I_2 is taken as simply reversing the sign of the input from S.

external input (negative error) and to maintain the status quo whenever the error is zero.

When both the R and S neurones are externally activated then the w_p's will increase and S may make the transition from inhibitor to excitor. As things stand, however, there is one anomalous feature of this assembly's behaviour: inhibitors will not extinguish. If an S that has an inhibitory effect on R is activated in isolation, then A_r will remain at zero, A_f at β/μ and no change in w_p will take place. This could be remedied by postulating a base rate for A_r as well as A_f, then an inhibitory influence could be explicitly registered by R at all times and inhibitors would extinguish, implementing the delta rule in full. A threshold below which input had no effect on a neurone would also be needed to prevent all connections from spontaneously extinguishing. Given that the available evidence suggests that inhibitors do not extinguish (Zimmer-Hart & Rescorla, 1974), however, there seems little reason to add these modifications.

A number of simulations have been run on this assembly. Rather than use continuous activation values in the model, stochastic firing rates were adopted in an attempt at greater realism. In this case the variables in the equations are interpreted as average values of the quantities represented, with A_f, for example, now standing for the expected firing rate of F in our derivation. When running the simulation, F fires at random with an average firing rate that depends on its input and characteristics. The system was able to display simple conditioning, extinction, blocking and inhibitory learning, confirming the analytic treatment given here.

9.5 Neurobiological plausibility

Having constructed an error correcting assembly, some further consideration of the assumptions made in this enterprise is indicated. From a computational standpoint the most restrictive may be the requirement for an activation that is a linear function of input. It is well known that a delta rule employing a linear activation function is limited in the types of problem that it can solve, mainly because no benefit can be derived from the construction of multilayer networks (Rumelhart *et al.*, 1986). A strictly linear activation function is not neurobiologically plausible either. This requirement can be relaxed somewhat without destroying this assembly's ability to error correct. The inclusion of a low threshold, i.e. a threshold that the input to the neurone must exceed for it to become active, does not disrupt the system's performance to any great extent. Two possibilities arise, distinguished by the effects of the threshold on the response of F to input, as this is the neurone whose behaviour at low input values is critical. Given that F already has a baseline rate, it might be thought that any input would affect this rate as in some sense F was already over threshold, in which case error correction proceeds as before. If this is not assumed to be the case, and F maintains its baseline rate until input is above threshold, then the assembly will still error correct, though not to asymptote. The internal input will approach to within some constant from *e* and learning will then cease. This constant can be made small if the threshold itself is small, an assumption that seems to conflict with the observation that neurones cannot typically fire another cell on their own, at least in cerebral cortex. The apparent conflict can be resolved by assuming that a large number of inputs are active to any given assembly during learning, and hence that the synaptic strength developed by any one neurone is sufficiently small that that neurone's input to the assembly is sub-threshold.

If the inputs to the neurones were high enough to cause them to saturate, however, then the assembly's error correction would deteriorate. In this case the behaviour of the neurones other than F is crucial. Either the neurones' activation functions are linear over their operating range, with at most weak non-linearities towards the top end; or as the neurones saturate then synaptic transmission becomes more effective in such a way that the output of a neurone remains a linear function of its input *. Under the latter circumstances the activation function could be highly non-linear and the assembly would still error correct perfectly.

The assumption of negligible sensitization, constant increments in synaptic strength and short eligibility period for PSE may well be incorrect for *Aplysia*. One response is to investigate to what extent all these requirements can be relaxed. However, the derivation here is by way of an existence proof that an error correcting assembly can be constructed from this *type* of rule; it is not meant to imply that the synaptic arrangement employed by *Aplysia* is a strong candidate for implementing plasticity in cerebral cortex. It is nevertheless interesting to pursue the question of computational and neurobiological plausibility, if only to establish reference points for future discussion.

---

* Strong non-linearities at the top end of a neurone's range could be countenanced as long as the neurone's behaviour became linear as the error approached zero. This could be the case if this type of assembly was implemented in a system of the type envisaged by McLaren *et al.* (1989), as the activations in such a system are in large part determined by the error. The R and I neurones would approach their final activities from above, making it plausible to suppose that at asymptote their activations would be in the linear part of the neurones' dynamic range.

Other assumptions were made in the course of the derivation, and some of the more mathematically based ones are discussed in the appendix. In turning to the issue of the plausibility of this type of approach to computation in cerebral cortex, however, new problems emerge. Assuming for the moment that the elemental learning rule is correct, the assembly nevertheless violates a number of anatomical constraints, perhaps the most important of which is the requirement that there be no 'sign change' neurones (Crick & Asanuma, 1986). These are neurones whose only function is to receive input from one neurone and output to one other, effectively multiplying the input by some negative constant. The assembly currently does have inhibitory neurones that take one input and deliver one output and hence are exactly the sort of sign changer not apparently found in cerebral cortex. This problem can be circumvented, however, by the arrangement shown in Figure 9.6. Here there is just one inhibitory interneurone that accepts inputs from all incoming S neurones (though only one is shown in the figure) as well as the R neurone, and synapses on all incoming S neurones as well as R and F. The inhibitory interneurone now integrates several inputs and delivers several outputs, and hence can no longer be characterized as a sign changer. Each S now has to synapse on F. The neurone transmitting *e* is exempted from these arrangements, but this is reasonable as it is a distinctly different component bringing in a signal from outside the system. F is not shown as synapsing on I either, but it is plausible that F might be a special case that did not make such connections. Even if it were to synapse on I, however, it would make no crucial difference to the performance of the assembly. Broadly speaking, the wiring requirements for this assembly are that all afferents (except *e*) synapse on I which in turn synapses on everything (except *e*) nearby. F must make a facilitatory synapse at each excitatory synapse on R (excepting those made by *e*) and all afferents must synapse on F. These are fairly loose constraints, which can in large part be implemented by making the region over which synaptic contacts are made fairly small, so that connections are local. The abandonment of sign change neurones does seem to enhance the plausibility of the assembly in a number of ways.

The assembly functions as follows. If F and R are externally activated conjointly with S then I becomes active also. The net effect of S on F is zero, its excitatory influence being cancelled out via its input to I, and the net effect of S on R is determined by w_p. If w_p is large enough then it more than compensates for the S input to I, and R becomes more active, delivering more input to I which suppresses F. Learning ceases when the net input to F is zero, which will be when the internal input to R matches the external input. The synapse from I back onto R simply alters the constant of proportionality relating R's activation to input, and has no deeper significance. If now the R neurone were to be activated by S without there being a simultaneously applied *e*, then I would become sufficiently excited to inhibit F below its baseline rate. As a consequence w_p would decrease until R was no longer active, resulting in the extinction of S or, if other S neurones whose effective weights were already zero were involved, in the development of conditioned inhibition.

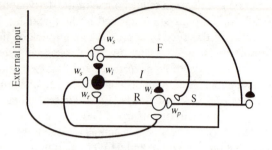

Figure 9.6 A version of the assembly without sign change inhibitory neurones. All synapses from a given neurone are shown as having the same strength irrespective of the type of neurone receiving the synapse. This convention is adopted for ease of exposition, and is not crucial to the derivation given. It is necessary, however, that the strength of the synapse from an S neurone onto F be some fixed multiple of the synaptic weight for that same S neurone projecting onto I, if these two inputs from S to F, one direct and one via I, are to cancel out all the S.

The derivation proceeds much as before, arriving at Equation 9.9 once again (see appendix). There are, however, some new emergent properties of this assembly. The fact that I projects onto each S afferent raises the possibility that any S neurone's activity could be influenced by other S neurones' activities via the common inhibitory interneurone, which would be undesirable as the S neurones also act as R neurones, and hence require their activations to reflect the internal input they are receiving. This problem can be avoided by postulating either that the inhibitory effects of I are local to the branch of the S neurone that it synapses onto or that separate linking excitatory neurones are involved. What is certain, however, is that the inputs to a given R neurone will compete with one another, via I, with the stronger ones tending to suppress the weaker *.

Conclusions

I have attempted to provide an existence proof that at least one class of elemental learning rule can be used to construct an error correcting assembly, by demonstrating how this can be done in one particular case. The key feature of the rule that makes this construction feasible seems to be the existence of the separate F component used to code the error signal. Clearly it would be of great interest if a member of this type of rule could be identified that was also a realistic candidate for implementing plasticity in cerebral cortex. Potentially there is one such candidate, which somewhat paradoxically stems from an essentially Hebbian mechanism

---

* The implementation of lateral inhibition between inputs to a neurone is novel in modelling learning though common in modelling perception. It may have implications for phenomena such as overshadowing and external inhibition which are not considered in this chapter.

proposed to account for LTP in the hippocampus (see Gustafsson & Wigstrom, 1988, for a review). This mechanism makes use of NMDA receptors, which require the simultaneous occurrence of two events to function, allowing calcium influx into the neurone and hence, it is hypothesized, learning to take place. The two prerequisites for action are that the cell containing the receptor must be appreciably depolarized and that glutamate must arrive at the receptor site. This dual requirement means that this mechanism could be employed (in principle) to instantiate the type of rule under consideration. Either the glutamate or depolarization requirement must be placed under the control of an F neurone, with the other requirement being met by the S neurones. Thus, when the facilitator fires it can be responsible either for depolarizing the R neurone or for sending glutamate to appropriate receptor sites. Taking the latter alternative, then the S neurone must be able to depolarize the R neurone using a different neurotransmitter(s). The former alternative seems a little odd, since if the R neurone is depolarized by F, this seems to mean that S cannot depolarize it, but surely such depolarization is necessary if R is to register input. In this case it would seem that self-potentiation of S-R synapses would occur, though Gustafsson & Wigstrom (1988) have argued that this need not be the case.

The comments in the last paragraph have been of a highly speculative nature, though it is intriguing to note that two of the most thoroughly researched mechanisms for synaptic plasticity do seem to have at least the potential to construct error correcting assemblies of the type considered here; and that whether the mechanism involved is essentially pre-synaptic or post-synaptic the crucial common feature is the dual control of plasticity. Interestingly, an assembly employing this type of rule need violate none of the criteria laid down by Crick & Asanuma (1986) for neural plausibility. There is no requirement that all the S and R neurones interconnect, the connectivity of a system is a separate question that determines its architecture rather than constraining it at the level of the assembly. It is also not required that a neurone be able to fire another by itself. A high connectivity coupled with a threshold below which input is ineffective, will tend to ensure that one cell will not be able to fire another on its own. The weights achieved by individual neurones will tend to be too small to allow any one neurone to produce a supra-threshold output. This will make the error correction of the assembly more rough and ready but still quite viable. A final consideration is of the types of neurones found in cerebral cortex and their relative proportions. Apart from noting that 'local' excitatory and inhibitory neurones exist in satisfying numbers along with pyramidal neurones suitable for transmitting *e*, it is difficult to make a detailed assessment of the assembly's plausibility, due to our lack of knowledge of the proportions of different cell types and the undoubted fact that cerebral cortex must contain many types of computational machinery.

Acknowledgements

The work reported here was supported by a Science and Engineering Research Council studentship. I am deeply indebted to A. Dickinson, N.J. Mackintosh and S. Monsell for their comments on an earlier draft.

9.6 Appendix

The treatment here will be rather general so as to make explicit the constraints required for the assembly to give a good implementation of the delta rule. My first derivation is for the assembly shown in Figure 9.5. The total internal input received by R is i, where:

$$i = \Sigma A_{sj} w_{pj} \quad \text{with summation over } j \tag{9.6.1}$$

This is simply the sum of all the inputs from the S neurones to R, with each input given by the product of the S neurone's activity and the strength of the synapse it makes on R. Note that the first subscript always indicates the type of neurone or structure involved, whilst the second denotes a particular member of that set. The activation of R is given by:

$$A_r = k_r(e + i) \quad \text{where } k_r \text{ is a positive constant} \tag{9.6.2}$$

with the sum of e and i representing the total input to the neurone. The external input is taken as e, rather than including parameters for the synapses that the neurone carrying external input makes on R and F. Similarly, the equation for the inhibitory interneurone is:

$$A_i = k_i A_r w_r \quad \text{where } k_i \text{ is a positive constant} \tag{9.6.3}$$

and where $A_r w_r$ is the input from R to I. Lastly, the activation of F:

$$A_f = k_f(e - A_i w_i + c) \quad \text{where } k_f \text{ and } c \text{ are positive constants} \tag{9.6.4}$$

with $-A_i w_i$ the input from the inhibitory neurone and c a constant that sets a baseline or spontaneous rate for F, whose significance will become clear in due course. Substituting Equation 9.6.2 into 9.6.3, and then 9.6.3 into 9.6.4:

$$A_f = k_f(e - k_i w_i k_r w_r(e + i) + c) \tag{9.6.5}$$

and taking $k_i w_i k_r w_r = 1/2$, this gives:

$$A_f = k_f(e - i + 2c)/2 \tag{9.6.6}$$

so that the activity of F is controlled by $e - i$ or Δ. The learning rule for a given plastic synapse, w_{pj}, connecting the jth S neurone to R is:

$$dw_{pj}/dt = A_{sj}A_f\mu - A_{sj}\beta \qquad (9.6.7)$$

as given in the main text. Substituting for A_f:

$$dw_{pj}/dt = A_{sj}((\mu k_f(e - i + 2c)/2) - \beta) \qquad (9.6.8)$$

If $\mu k_f s$ is taken to equal β, and $e - i$ termed Δ:

$$dw_{pj}/dt = A_{sj}\mu k_f\Delta/2 \qquad (9.6.9)$$

which is the correct form for the delta rule. The c term allows the algebra to be exact, though the assembly would error correct without it. A baseline rate for F is necessary, however, for the assembly shown in Figure 9.5 to function properly. The equation for the new inhibitory neurone I_2 is:

$$A_{i2} = k_i\Sigma A_{sj}w_{sj} \quad \text{with summation over } j, \qquad (9.6.10)$$

$A_{sj}w_{sj}$ being the input it receives from the jth S neurone and taking I_1 and I_2 to have the same parameters. This leads to the internal input, i, being given by the difference between that arriving directly from the S neurones and that arriving via I_2:

$$i = \Sigma A_{sj}w_{pj} - A_{i2}w_i \quad \text{with summation over } j \qquad (9.6.11)$$

and taking $k_i w_i = 1$:

$$i = \Sigma A_{sj}(w_{pj} - w_{sj}) \qquad (9.6.12)$$

so that the effective weight for the jth S neurone is given by $w_{pj} - w_{sj}$. It is desirable to have the input from any S neurone set to zero initially, which can be achieved by setting w_{pj}(initial) equal to w_{sj}. Equation 9.6.2 now holds, and the derivation proceeds as before. The baseline rate for F allows it to explicitly register i in the absence of e, and to maintain positive values of w_{pj} when the net input to R is zero. Without this spontaneous activity of F the w_{pj} would tend towards zero whenever the S neurones were activated, eventually causing them to develop a net inhibitory influence over R.

A number of assumptions were made in the course of the derivations which require some discussion. Taking w_{pj}(initial) to equal w_{sj} plausibly implies that the only difference between the two S-R synapses is the presence of F conferring plasticity. Taking $k_i w_i = 1$ is sensible in that it requires a relationship between two parameters which apply to the same structure. Given that $k_i w_i k_r w_r$ is one half, this implies that $k_r w_r = 1/2$, another relation between parameters governing the same structure. Minor violations of these requirements will not have serious consequences. If w_{pj}(initial) does not exactly match w_{sj} then it will tend to adjust itself appropriately with experience, and if the relationships between the k's and w's are not quite right then this will change the asymptotic i value, so that it no longer matches e but some multiple of e. Nevertheless the assembly will still error correct. Turning to the requirement that the baseline activity of F be ß/µ, this is necessary for learning rate to be proportional to Δ, but if A_f(baseline) ≥ ß/µ then the assembly will error correct with an asymptotic $i \geq e$.

The final assembly considered here is shown in Figure 9.6. The equations unique to this assembly are:

$$A_i = k_i(A_r w_r + \Sigma A_{sj} w_{sj}) \qquad \text{with summation over } j \qquad (9.6.13)$$

$$A_f = k_f(e + \Sigma A_{sj} w_{sj} - A_i w_i + c) \quad \text{with summation over } j \qquad (9.6.14)$$

$$i = \Sigma A_{sj} w_{pj} - A_i w_i \qquad \text{with summation over } j \qquad (9.6.15)$$

with A_r given by Equation 9.6.2. Substituting Equation 9.6.13 into 9.6.15, taking $k_i w_i = 1$ and simplifying:

$$i = \Sigma A_{sj}(w_{pj} - w_{sj}) - A_r w_r$$

The $A_r w_r$ term is somewhat inconvenient. Substituting into Equation 9.6.2 gives:

$$A_r = k_r(e + \Sigma A_{sj}(w_{pj} - w_{sj}) - A_r w_r)$$

and redefining i as:

$$i = \Sigma A_{sj}(w_{pj} - w_{sj}) \qquad (9.6.16)$$

and simplifying results in:

$$A_r = k_r(e + i)/(1 + k_r w_r) \qquad (9.6.17)$$

Substituting in A_f :

$$A_f = k_f(e + \Sigma A_{sj} w_{sj} - k_i w_i \Sigma A_{sj} w_{sj} - k_i w_i A_r w_r + c)$$

as $k_i w_i = 1$, and using Equation 9.6.17 with $k_r w_r$ now set to one:

$$A_f = k_f(e - i + 2c)/2 \qquad (9.6.18)$$

as before; and hence Equation 9.6.9 holds. A new feature is that each S neurone receives an input from I, so that unless the excitatory input to that neurone exceeds that from I then its activation will be zero. The S neurones compete, via I, to be active, with the stronger suppressing the weaker.

References

Anderson J.A. (1985) What Hebb synapses build. In: **Synaptic modification, neuron selectivity, and nervous system organisation.** pp. 153-174. W.B. Levy, J.A. Anderson & S. Lehmkuhle (eds.) LEA, Hillsdale, NJ.

Bush R.R. & Mosteller F. (1955) **Stochastic models for learning.** Wiley, NY.

Crick F.H.C. & Asanuma C. (1986) Certain aspects of the anatomy and physiology of the cerebral cortex. In **Parallel distributed processing Vol. II.** pp. 333-371. J.L. McClelland & D.E. Rumelhart (eds.) Bradford Books, Cambridge, Mass.

Gluck M.A. & Thompson R.F. (1987) Modelling the neural substrates of associative learning and memory: a computational approach. **Psych. Rev. 94**, pp. 176-191

Gustafsson B. & Wigstrom H. (1988) **TINS 11**, pp. 156-162

Hawkins R.D., Abrams T.W., Carew T.J. & Kandel E.R. (1983) A cellular mechanism of classical conditioning in *Aplysia*: activity-dependent amplification of presynaptic facilitation. **Science 219**, pp. 400-405

Hebb D.O. (1949) **The organization of behaviour.** Wiley, NY.

Horn G. (1985) **Memory, imprinting and the brain.** Clarendon Press, Oxford.

Kamin L.J. (1968) 'Attention-like' processes in classical conditioning. In: **Miami symposium on the prediction of behaviour: aversive stimulation.** pp. 9-33. M.R. Jones (ed.) University of Miami Press.

Kandel E.R. & Tauc L. (1965) Mechanism of heterosynaptic facilitation in the giant cell of the abdominal ganglion of *Aplysia depilans.* **J. Physiol. 181**, pp. 28-47

Konorski J. (1948) **Conditioned reflexes and neuron organisation.** Cambridge University Press, Cambridge.

Levy W.B. (1985) Associative changes at the synapse: LTP in the hippocampus. In **Synaptic modification, neuron selectivity, and nervous system organisation.** pp. 5-34. W.B. Levy, J.A. Anderson & S. Lehmkuhle (eds.) LEA, Hillsdale, NJ.

Levy W.B. & Desmond N.L. (1985) The rules of elemental synaptic plasticity. In **Synaptic modification, neuron selectivity, and nervous system organisation.** pp. 105-122. W.B. Levy, J.A. Anderson & S. Lehmkuhle (eds.) LEA, Hillsdale, NJ.

Lubow R.E. & Moore A.U. (1959) Latent inhibition: the effect of nonreinforced pre-exposure to the conditioned stimulus. **J. comp. Physiol. Psychol. 52**, pp. 415-419

Mackintosh N.J. (1975) A theory of attention: variations in the associability of stimuli with reinforcement. **Psych. Rev. 82**, pp. 276-298

McClelland J.L. & Rumelhart D.E. (1985) Distributed memory and the representation of general and specific information. **JEP: general 114**, pp. 159-188

McLaren I.P.L., Kaye H. & Mackintosh N.J. (1989) An associative theory of the representation of stimuli: applications to perceptual learning and latent inhibition. In: **Parallel distributed processing - implications for psychology and neurobiology.** R.G.M. Morris (ed.) Oxford University Press, Oxford. In press.

Pearce J.M. & Hall G. (1980) A model for Pavlovian learning: variations in the effectiveness of conditioned but not of unconditioned stimuli. **Psych. Rev. 87**, pp. 532-552

Rescorla R.A. (1971) Variations in the effectiveness of reinforcement and nonreinforcement following prior inhibitory conditioning. **Learning and Motivation 2**, pp. 113-123

Rescorla R.A. & Wagner A.R. (1972) A theory of Pavlovian conditioning: Variations in the effectiveness of reinforcement and nonreinforcement. In: **Classical conditioning II: current research and theory.** pp. 64-99. A.H. Black & W.F. Prokasy (eds.) Appleton-Century-Crofts, NY.

Rosenblatt F. (1962) **Principles of neurodynamics.** Spartan, NY.

Rumelhart D.E., Hinton G.E. & McClelland J.L. (1986) A general framework for parallel distributed processing. In: **Parallel distributed processing Vol. I.** pp. 45-76. D.E. Rumelhart & J.L. McClelland (eds.) Bradford Books, Cambridge, Mass.

Rumelhart D.E., Hinton G.E. & Williams R.J. (1986) Learning internal representations by error propagation. In: **Parallel distributed processing Vol. I.** pp. 318-362. D.E. Rumelhart & J.L. McClelland (eds.) Bradford Books, Cambridge, Mass.

Rumelhart, D.E. & McClelland, J.L. (1986) On learning the past tenses of English verbs. In **Parallel distributed processing Vol. II.** pp. 216-271. J.L. McClelland & D.E. Rumelhart (eds.) Bradford Books, Cambridge, Mass.

Singer W. (1985) Hebbian modification of synaptic transmission as a common mechanism in experience-dependent maturation of cortical functions. In: **Synaptic modification, neuron selectivity, and nervous system organisation.** pp. 35-64. W.B. Levy, J.A. Anderson & S. Lehmkuhle (eds.) LEA, Hillsdale, NJ.

Stone G.O. (1986) An analysis of the delta rule and the learning of statistical associations. In: **Parallel distributed processing Vol. I.** pp.444-459. D.E. Rumelhart & J.L. McClelland (eds.) Bradford Books, Cambridge, Mass.

Sutton R.S. & Barto A.G. (1981) Toward a modern theory of adaptive networks: expectation and prediction. **Psych. Rev. 88**, pp. 135-170

Widrow G. & Hoff M.E. (1960) Adaptive switching circuits. **Institute of radio engineers, western electronic show and convention, convention record, part 4**, pp. 96-104

Zimmer-Hart C.L. & Rescorla R.A. (1974) Extinction of Pavlovian conditioned inhibition. **J. comp. Physiol. Psych. 86**, pp. 837-845

10
Behavioral Choice - In Theory and In Practice

William Kristan, Shawn Lockery, George Wittenberg &
Garrison W. Cottrell

Summary

We are studying the neuronal basis of behavioral choice in the medicinal
leech. We are characterizing the neuronal circuitry responsible for each of three
behaviors: local bending, shortening and swimming. All three behaviors can be
elicited by the same mechanosensory neurons and use the same set of motor
neurons. In preliminary studies, we have recorded the activity of identified
interneurons involved in one of these behaviors during the expression of another.
To understand the role of these neurons, we used back-propagation to generate
networks that simulate local bending and shortening. These studies suggest that the
same interneurons may be involved in several behaviors, and that behavioral choice
can involve circuit interactions of a kind not previously considered.

10.1 Introduction

Animals may respond to the same stimulus in different ways for a variety of
reasons, including their developmental state, affect or previous experience (Toates,
1980). This type of behavioral choice has been studied behaviorally in a number of
animals (Davis, 1979; Toates & Halliday, 1980). The neuronal basis of such
behaviors has been most effectively studied in invertebrates, because the activity of
identifiable neurons can be recorded, even intracellularly, during the performance of
complex behaviors (Selverston, 1985). Two major issues have been addressed in
these studies. The first is whether the individual circuits generating the patterned
activity for each of two or more behaviors (i.e. their *pattern generators*) are
completely separate sets of neurons or whether they share some of the same
neurons. One way to pursue the issue of behavioral choice is to determine whether a
given neuron is used in only a single behavior (i.e. it is *committed* to that behavior)
or whether, instead, it participates in two or more behaviors (i.e. it is *multifunctional*) (Kristan et al., 1988). The second issue is to characterize how the
circuits interact. Several possibilities are shown schematically in Figure 10.1.

For three of the cases shown (A, B & D), two separate pattern generators are indicated, one that feeds onto motor neurons that generate behavior X and the other that activates motor neurons producing behavior Y. In each of these cases, the interneurons in these pattern-generating circuits are committed to behaviors X and Y respectively. In the fourth case (C), at least some of the pattern-generating neurons are involved in both behaviors; i.e. they are multifunctional. One way to distinguish among the various cases - a way that is physiologically tractable - is to ask what the neurons in circuit Y do when behavior X is produced. These responses are indicated by the activity profiles shown to the right of each circuit. At the time indicated by the arrow, a stimulus is given which sometimes elicits behavior X and other times behavior Y; for this discussion, we are interested only in the case when behavior X is elicited. In Figure 10.1A, when behavior X occurs, neurons in circuit X inhibit those in circuit Y, hence the activity in circuit Y neurons decreases. In Figure 10.1B, circuit Y is active during behavior X but behavior Y is not seen. This might occur for any of several reasons: neurons between the Y circuit and the motor neurons may be inhibited by circuit X (case a); behavior X may incorporate the motor pattern for behavior Y into its own pattern (case b); or behavior Y may be expressed but be so weak compared to behavior X that it is not seen (case c). The circuits shown in Figure 10.1C also produce increased activity in the neurons producing behavior Y during the expression of behavior X, but for a different reason than in Figure 10.1B. Here both behaviors X and Y are produced by the same set of interneurons, but in different patterns of activation. This is a more difficult case to deal with, both conceptually and physiologically. It is, however, the type of circuitry that appears to underlie local bending and shortening in the leech. As will be discussed in Section 10.3, simulations show that this sort of interaction can produce qualitatively different behaviors from the same set of interneurons. Finally, a number of combinations of the previous possibilities are possible. One such combination is shown in Figure 10.1D, in which part of the circuit for behavior Y is inhibited by X and the rest of it is incorporated into behavior X.

From previous studies, there is no single mechanism of behavioral choice, nor are there any obvious rules. For instance, an early investigation of the choice between striking toward or retracting away from a food stimulus by the sea slug *Pleurobranchaea* (Kovac & Davis, 1980) concluded that the pattern generators for the two behaviors are separate and that the choice of behaviors is likely to be made by inhibition, as in Figure 10.1A. A similar conclusion was reached in studies of competing behaviors in the locust (Ramirez & Pearson, 1988). Other studies, however, have concluded that two competing behaviors, such as swallowing and regurgitation (McClellan, 1982a,b; Croll *et al.*, 1985a,b) or backward vs. forward walking (Kovac, 1974) use essentially the same pattern generator, with small modifications of a few of the elements. In these cases, the pattern generators for the competing behaviors are both rhythmic and the differences are simply a variation in the phasing of the muscle contractions. These studies would, therefore, suggest a

(A) Circuit *X* inhibits circuit *Y*

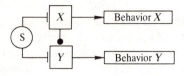

(B) Circuit *X* blocks the expression of *Y*

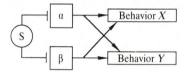

(C) Behaviors *X* and *Y* use same set of neurons

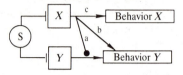

(D) Example of combined mechanisms

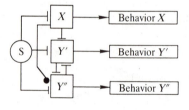

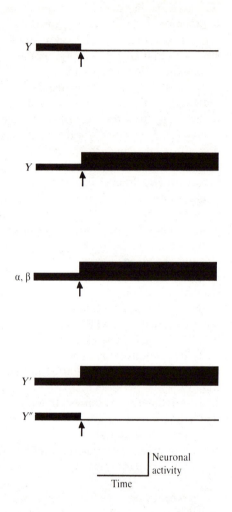

Figure 10.1 A number of circuit interactions that could be responsible for behavioral choice. In all cases, a stimulus is applied to the *X* and *Y* pattern-generating circuits and behavior *X* alone is elicited. To the right of each drawing of the circuits is a representation of the activity of circuit *Y* before and after the stimulus, indicated by the upward arrows. T-bars at the ends of lines indicate excitatory connections, black circles indicate inhibitory connections, and arrows indicate complex effects. **A.** By its inhibitory connection, circuit *X*, when activated, shuts off circuit *Y*. As a result, the activity of the neurons on circuit *Y* decreases. **B.** Circuit *X* does not affect circuit *Y*, so that circuit *Y* is activated by the same stimulus that produces behavior *X*. However, circuit *X* can have several effects on the expression of behavior *Y*. **(a)** Circuit *X* may inhibit the output of circuit *Y*, so that behavior *Y* is not expressed. **(b)** Circuit *X* may incorporate behavior *Y* into its own expression. For example, stretch reflexes (a behavior *Y*) are incorporated into more complex acts such as walking (behavior *X*). **(c)** Behavior *X* might be so large that behavior **(cont. opposite)**

mechanism of choice more like Figure 10.1B. Finally, a study of the choice between swimming and withdrawing from a tactile stimulus (a non-rhythmic response) showed that withdrawal used a subset of the central pattern-generating interneurons that are used for swimming (a rhythmic behavior) in the sea slug *Tritonia* (Getting & Dekin, 1985); this is similar to the case represented by Figure 10.1D.

We undertook our studies on the medicinal leech to determine which functional or behavioral constraints, if any, favor one mechanism of behavioral choice over another. In what follows, we discuss our physiological approach and summarize our progress. On the assumption that choices between different pairs of behaviors can be accomplished by a variety of mechanisms, we will next compare the advantages of related mechanisms. Our thinking in this regard has been aided considerably by the use of back propagation networks (Rumelhart *et al.*, 1986). This approach has been used with some success by others in modeling sensory processing (Lehky & Sejnowski, 1988; Zipser & Andersen, 1988) in higher animals. In applying this approach to the comparatively simple nervous system of the leech, we can more readily test the predictions of the model. As discussed in Section 10.2.2, such models are capable of producing behavioral choice under different stimulus conditions. The models produced interesting suggestions about what kinds of interneurons might be involved in behavioral choice.

10.2 Our approach to studying behavioral choice

Our goal is to determine the physiological basis of behavioral choice; we are approaching this problem in three steps:

1) Description of the physiological basis of three different behaviors: local bending, shortening, and swimming.

2) Recording from identified interneurons involved in one behavior while the other two are being performed.

3) Characterization of the connections among the interneurons to determine the basis for choosing one over another.

(Fig. 10.1 Cont.) Y, even though it occurs, cannot be detected. Note that in both (b) and (c) behavior Y occurs, but that only behavior X is detectable. C. In this case, there are no neurons completely committed to either behavior; i.e. all interneurons contribute to both behaviors. Behavioral choice must therefore come about by the level or pattern of activity in the intermediate circuit. In this type of organization, all the cells active during behavior X must also be active during behavior Y. D. This system incorporates some of the features of the other three. Circuit X activates part of the Y circuit and inhibits the remaining part. In this way, some of the neurons in the Y circuit, namely the Y' neurons, increase their activity during behavior X whereas the others (the Y'' neurons) decrease their activity.

In parallel, we will assemble models that produce each of the individual behaviors and make choices between the behaviors, to better understand the functional significance of the kinds of physiological connections found. This section summarizes our progress to date in each of these efforts.

10.2.1   The neuronal basis of individual behaviors

The leech

Leeches are annelids, similar to earthworms but with specialized structures called suckers at each end. The body plan is tubular, with a body wall composed primarily of muscles overlaid by skin enclosing an internal space filled with viscera. Unlike earthworms, the number of segments is fixed at 32. The central nervous system, reflecting the segmentation, is composed of 32 ganglia, one per segment, with 4 ganglia fused to form an anterior brain and 7 fused to form a posterior brain; the remaining 21 midbody ganglia are, for the most part, identical to one another (Muller *et al.*, 1981). Each ganglion contains the somata of about 400 neurons (Macagno, 1980). Because most of these are bilaterally paired, the functional unit of the leech nervous system is about 200 neurons.

Of the 200 neurons, 7 are mechanosensory neurons: 3 respond to light touch (T cells), 2 to pressure (P cells) and 2 to pain (N cells, for nociceptive) (Nicholls & Baylor, 1968). Each of these has a well defined receptive field on one side of its segment, and secondary fields in the adjacent segment on each side. (Because we took care not to activate these secondary fields in the present studies, their effects can be ignored.) The three behaviors under consideration are produced primarily by the longitudinal musculature, aligned parallel to the long axis of the body; contraction of this muscle causes shortening of the body tube along this axis. There are 8 excitatory motor neurons to these muscle fibers on each side of each segment and 4 inhibitory ones (Stuart, 1970; Ort *et al.*, 1974). Each excitatory motor neuron causes the contraction of a localized strip of muscle in its own segment. For the present purposes, these motor neurons can be divided into two types: dorsal excitors (DE), which cause a U-shaped bend of the body, and ventral excitors (VE), which cause an inverted U. The dorsal and ventral excitors, when activated together, cause the segment to shorten.

Characterization of individual behaviors in terms of motor neuron patterns

Local bending behavior   Lightly touching the external surface of the leech evokes a U-shaped bend away from the source of the point of contact (Kristan *et al.*, 1982). One such response is shown in Figure 10.2A, in which a dorsal touch caused the dorsal surface to shorten and the ventral surface to lengthen. This bending is local in two senses. First, only the segment being stimulated plus perhaps the segments on either side participate in the response. Second, whole-

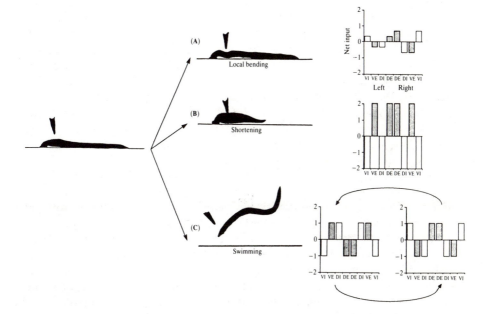

Figure 10.2 Three behaviors of the medicinal leech in response to mechanical stimulation. In all cases, a blunt probe was applied to the dorsal surface, near the posterior end of the leech. The graphs to the right of each response indicate the net input to the four pairs of motor neurons in each segment that contribute to the behavior, in arbitrary units; positive values indicate excitation and negative values indicate inhibition. **A.** A very gentle touch typically elicits a local bending response, consisting of a contraction of the dorsal surface and a relaxation of the ventral surface. This pulls the touched area of skin away from the site of touch. This response is caused by activation of DE and VI, along with the inhibition of DI and VE. **B.** A stronger prod elicits a shortening response, brought about by the simultaneous shortening of many of the segments in the body. The records to the right show that this behavior is caused by contraction of both sets of excitors, DE and VE, and the inhibition of both inhibitors, DI and VI. **C.** Sometimes, the same type of stimulus that elicits shortening may instead, as in this case, elicit swimming. The undulatory behavior is caused by a phasic activation of each of the four types of motor neurons.

body behaviors, such as crawling, can take place at the same time that local bending occurs in a small part of the animal. The local bending response is caused by a concomitant activation of the dorsal longitudinal muscles and a relaxation of the ventral longitudinal muscles in the segment stimulated. As shown on the right side of Figure 10.2A, the dorsal muscle activation is caused by the excitation of the dorsal excitor (DE) motor neurons and the inhibition of the dorsal inhibitors (DI). The ventral muscle relaxation is caused by inhibition of the ventral excitors (VE) and excitation of the ventral inhibitors (VI). Each segment is, in fact, capable of bending in any of four directions: down, as demonstrated in Figure 10.2A; up (away from a ventral touch); and laterally left or right, away from a touch to either side. In each case the appropriate sets of longitudinal motor neurons are used.

The intensity of mechanical stimulation required to evoke local bending activates T cells at moderate rates and P cells at low rates (Kristan *et al.*, 1982). Activating T cells by themselves at the rates observed during a local bend produces almost no response, whereas activating P cells at the observed rates produces nearly the whole response (Kristan, 1982). Therefore, the P cells provide the major share of the excitation driving this behavior.

Shortening behavior   Strong mechanical stimulation of the skin elicits a response that spreads well beyond the stimulated segment. This response consists of a *co-contraction* of the dorsal and ventral longitudinal muscles of many segments, causing the animal to shorten and, because the back sucker is usually tightly attached to a surface, to pull away from the stimulus (Figure 10.2B). The strength of stimulation required to evoke the shortening response activates T cells and P cells much more intensely than in local bending (Kristan *et al.*, 1982). The shortening response is graded with the intensity of the stimulus: the segments near the site of stimulation shorten more vigorously and more segments are recruited as stimulus intensity increases.

In local bending, stimulation of the dorsal, lateral and ventral surfaces each produce a different pattern of motor activity. In shortening, the situation is quite different; no matter where the stimulus is placed, the response of the motor neurons is the same: all the excitatory motor neurons (DE's *and* VE's) are excited and all the inhibitors (DI's *and* VI's), are inhibited. This means that shortening involves the same sensory and motor neurons as local bending, but that, somehow, increased T and P cell activation switches the motor activity from the local bending to the shortening pattern. A major goal of our study of behavioral choice is to understand the neuronal mechanisms responsible for this switch.

Swimming behavior   At levels of mechanical stimulation that cause shortening of most of the body, another response sometimes occurs (Figure 10.2C). The leech first flattens and elongates (using another set of muscles, the 'flatteners'), then swims (Kristan *et al.*, 1974). Swimming is achieved by alternating contraction and relaxation of dorsal and ventral longitudinal muscles in each segment, with the same pattern occurring slightly later in each successively more posterior body segment. This produces a sinusoidal undulation that propels the leech forward.

The same sensory and motor neurons are used in swimming as in the other two behaviors, but there the similarities end. First, the motor neurons are activated in a radically different pattern. Second, swimming is inherently a whole-body response, with no variation in the number of participating body segments (Kristan *et al.*, 1974). Finally, swimming cannot occur at the same time as either of the other two behaviors, although it sometimes occurs after them. For instance, in response to a strong mechanical stimulus, shortening can precede swimming (Kristan *et al.*, 1982).

10.2.2 *Neuronal circuits responsible for the three behaviors*

Because all three behaviors use the same sensory and motor neurons, the differences between the behaviors must be at the level of the interneurons involved in generating the motor patterns. In order to identify and characterize these interneurons, parts of the isolated central nervous system and a variety of semi-intact preparations have been used (Ort *et al.*, 1974; Kristan & Calabrese, 1976; Kristan, 1982; Brodfuehrer & Friesen, 1986b; Friesen, 1989). What is known about these neuronal circuits is shown in Figure 10.3.

Neuronal circuit for local bending

A previous study (Kristan, 1982) concluded that the mechanosensory neurons responsible for local bending (and, hence, all the other behaviors we are considering) do not make monosynaptic connections with the motor neurons responsible for this behavior, but that the synaptic latencies were consistent with a disynaptic connection. In considering local bending in response to a dorsal touch, the simplest explanation (as shown in Figure 10.3A) is that a single local bend interneuron makes all the connections responsible for producing the local bending motor pattern. We know now that this is not correct: rather there are several interneurons in each segment that have the appropriate connections to be local bend interneurons (Lockery & Kristan, 1988). As yet we do not know whether these interneurons make connections with each other or whether they form instead completely parallel pathways to the motor neurons.

Neuronal circuit for shortening

Our work to date has established that the major sensory and motor neurons involved in shortening are those used in local bending (Wittenberg & Kristan, 1987, 1988). In particular, activation of the T and P cells at moderate frequencies activates the DE and VE motor neurons simultaneously while inactivating the DI and VI cells (Figure 10.3B). Because this pattern is unique to shortening and because shortening always involves muscle contractions in many segments, the interneuronal pool for this behavior must be different, at least in part, from the pool that produces local bending. The search for this circuit has just begun. We are

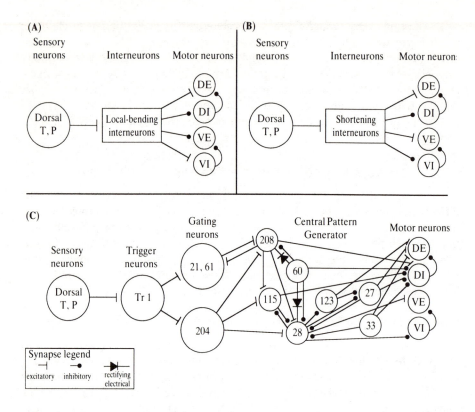

Figure 10.3 Neuronal circuitry responsible for behaviors. In all cases the motor neurons involved project to longitudinal muscle. A. Local bending. In response to stimulation of the dorsal T and P cells, interneurons excite the dorsal excitor (DE) and ventral inhibitor (VI), and inhibit the dorsal inhibitor (DI) and ventral excitor (VE). B. Shortening. A stronger stimulation of the same sensory neurons causes interneurons to excite both excitors and inhibit both inhibitors. C. Swimming. There is a complex network of identified neurons which initiate and pattern the motor output of swimming. This is a summary of all connections found either within a single ganglion, or between neurons in different ganglia.

looking for interneurons that (1) are active during the shortening response, (2) receive strong input from P cells, and (3) produce a purely excitatory effect on DE or VE motor neurons.

Neuronal circuit for swimming

Based upon work in several laboratories over the last fifteen years, we now know most of the cell-to-cell connections in the interneuronal circuit for swimming (Stent *et al.*, 1978; Kristan & Weeks, 1983; Friesen, 1989). Unlike the other behaviors, which are potentially generated by a simple, one-layered interneuronal system, in swimming the shortest path from the T and P cells is by way of three levels of interneurons (Figure 10.3C). The first interneuronal level is a group of trigger neurons that are activated monosynaptically by P cells (Brodfuehrer & Friesen, 1986a,b). A brief burst of impulses in these trigger neurons activates swim-initiating interneurons of several sorts. Cells 204 and 205 are unpaired swim-initiating interneurons that extend over many segments (Weeks & Kristan, 1978; Weeks, 1982a,b), and cells 21 and 61 are paired neurons with shorter axons that reach only two ganglia in each direction (Nusbaum & Kristan, 1986). These swim-initiating interneurons directly excite some of the pattern-generating interneurons (Nusbaum *et al.*, 1987). The pattern-generating neurons form a highly interconnected network. Many of the connections are reciprocal and inhibitory, between neurons in both the same and adjacent ganglia (Friesen *et al.*, 1978; Weeks, 1982a,b; Friesen, 1985; Friesen, 1989). This pattern of inhibitory contacts, along with an underlying tonic activation, cause the pattern-generating neurons to fire in bursts that alternate with silent periods of inhibition. Many of the pattern-generating interneurons connect directly to the DE, DI, VE and VI motor neurons (Poon *et al.*, 1978). The pattern of activity in the interneurons which connect to the motor neurons results in the swimming motor pattern, an undulatory wave that progresses from anterior to posterior.

10.2.3 Activity of interneurons in the 'wrong' behavior

We have begun to study the activity of interneurons known to participate in one behavior while another is being performed. Examples of the results are shown in Figure 10.4. In Figure 10.4A, one of the swim-initiating interneurons, cell 204, was recorded intracellularly while a T and a P cell were activated at a frequency sufficient to produce shortening. The fact that this neuron is inhibited by this stimulus is not surprising because this neuron, by itself, can initiate swimming, a behavior incompatible with shortening. What was unexpected was that the inhibition of cell 204 was short-lived, and that it was actually excited for part of the time that shortening was occurring. This may be the basis for the behavioral observation that swimming sometimes occurs after shortening. It may also mean that cell 204 can participate in shortening as well as swimming (Kristan *et al.*, 1988); i.e. that this interneuron is not committed to a single behavior.

In Figures 10.4B-D, a recently identified local bend interneuron, cell 218 (Lockery & Kristan, 1988), was recorded after stimulation that sometimes produced shortening. The recordings in Figure 10.4B show that this interneuron is activated strongly by the P cell that innervates the dorsal skin in cell 218's own segment. This input, at low frequencies of P cell stimulation, produces only a local bending response (Figure 10.4B); at higher frequencies of P cell activity, shortening was elicited as indicated by the extracellular recordings (Figure 10.4C). Cell 218 received essentially identical input during shortening as in local bending, even though the motor response was quite different. To see whether cell 218 receives input related to shortening *per se*, we produced shortening in another way, by stimulating nerves in a more posterior ganglion (Figure 10.4D). Such stimuli

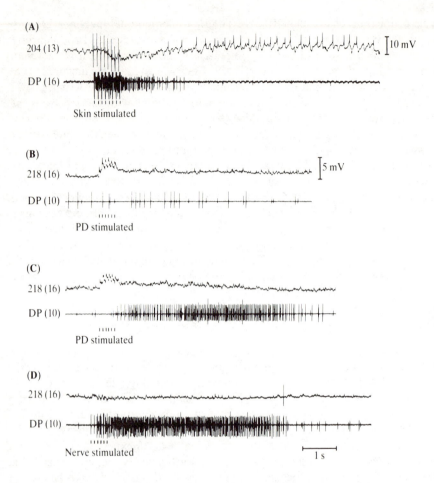

Figure 10.4 Recordings from interneurons known to be involved in one behavior while a second is elicited. In all cases, the top trace is an intracellular recording from an interneuron and the bottom trace is an extracellular recording from a nerve, the DP, in which the largest impulses are from a single dorsal excitatory (DE) motor neuron. **A**. Recording from cell 204, known to be involved in the initiation of swimming, during a shortening response. The burst of impulses in the DP recording indicate that shortening has occurred. The response was triggered by stimulation of the T and P mechanosensory neurons in segment 16 by way of a suction electrode attached to a piece of skin left attached to an otherwise isolated nerve cord. **B-D**. Recordings from cell 218, known to be involved in the local bending response, during stimulation intended to elicit shortening. All recordings are from the same cell 218 in an isolated nerve cord. **B**. Intracellular stimulation of a dorsal P cell (i.e. PD) produced excitation of the cell 218 but, as indicated by the nerve recording, did not produce a shortening response. **C**. An identical train of PD impulses this time did produce a shortening response; the activation of cell 218 was essentially identical to that in part **B**. **D**. Stimulation of two DP nerves in ganglion 17 produced a shortening response similar to that in **C**, but without any net input onto cell 218. The time calibration applies to all panels.

produced little response in cell 218, even though there was a brisk shortening response, as evidenced by the nerve recording.

These recordings indicate that cell 218 is unaffected by expression of the shortening response, as shown conceptually in Figure 10.1B. There are several mechanisms which could account for this: the shortening response may be sufficiently strong that the weak local bend may not be visible; or cell 218's activity may be negated by shortening interneurons, acting on this cell's output terminals, on its target motor neurons, or on the longitudinal muscles. Further physiological experiments are necessary to make these distinctions. However, we can rule out the possibility that shortening turns off the activity of cell 218 (i.e. Figure 10.1A), a mechanism that does seem to be used during shortening to keep swimming from being activated. Hence, it appears that the shortening pattern generator accomplishes behavioral choice over local bending and swimming by different mechanisms.

10.3 Network modeling of leech behavioral circuits

Description of the model

To expand the range of conceptually plausible circuits underlying behavioral choice we have used a back-propagation trained network (Rumelhart & McClelland, 1986) of idealized neurons that incorporates important circuit properties derived from our neurophysiological studies. We hope that such an exercise, in remaining close to the physiological facts, will make useful predictions regarding the actual organization of the nervous system of the leech. We began our simulation studies by training a simple feed-forward network of sensory, motor and interneurons to produce local bends appropriate to the site of stimulation. This network was trained to two intensity levels that corresponded to mild and moderate tactile stimuli. We next trained an identical network to produce both local bending and (to strong stimuli) shortening, and compared the functional organization of the two networks.

The modeled network was three-layered. The first, or input, layer represented the two dorsal and two ventral sensory cells which make the most important contribution to the behavior of each body segment (Figure 10.5A). In local bending, sensory cells do not directly activate motor neurons. We therefore added a single layer of hidden units (or interneurons) between the input and output units. A single layer is a close approximation to the actual circuitry since the sensory to motor neuron latency is probably disynaptic (Kristan, 1982). The eight output units represented left and right, dorsal and ventral motor neurons with excitors and inhibitors arranged in pairs. At the start of training, each hidden unit received input from every input unit and projected to every output unit.

In an effort to make our simulations as realistic as possible, we added fixed inhibitory connections from inhibitory motor neurons to excitatory motor neurons (Granzow *et al.*, 1985), and synapses from input units were constrained to be excitatory (Lockery and Kristan, 1988) whereas connections to output units could be excitatory or inhibitory (Poon *et al.*, 1978). The output of each hidden unit ranged from 0 to 1. It was computed as a sigmoidal function of the weighted sum of the inputs, plus a fixed bias term. The bias value was chosen so that, in the absence of input, the output of each hidden unit was negligible. This was done to reflect the fact that, in one well characterized synapse in the network, synaptic transmission is minimal in the absence of pre-synaptic input (Granzow *et al.*, 1985). In most network models, a neuron's output is represented by its firing rate. It appears, however, that synaptic output from interneurons within a single leech ganglion is little affected by the presence or absence of action potentials (Granzow *et al.*, 1985; unpublished data). Therefore, the output activation of each modeled hidden unit represents its membrane potential rather than its firing frequency.

In order to train the network to produce local bending responses, we constructed a training set of input-output mappings. Inputs to the network consisted of activation of individual or pairs of sensory cells at 0.5 for 'weak' and 1.0 for 'moderate' stimulation. The output values used in the training set were obtained from intracellular recordings of synaptic potentials in motor neurons during activation of sensory neurons. Negative values represented inhibition, positive values represented excitation, and zero was defined to be the resting state. The larger responses of motor neurons to strong input and pairs of stimuli were represented by higher values of excitation and inhibition in the output units, in an approximately linear fashion.

In a typical implementation of the back-propagation routine, an input is presented to the network and activation is allowed to propagate to the output units. The resulting activations of output units are then subtracted from the desired or 'target' activation values, defined by the set of mappings, and the difference or 'error' is used to adjust the synaptic weights of the network. However, since synaptic potentials reflect net *input* to the motor neurons rather than activation, training proceeded with net inputs as targets: the error term was generated by subtracting motor neuron net inputs from target inputs as defined by the training set. Thus motor neuron outputs played a role only in computing the lateral inhibition between pairs of motor neurons. Outputs of inhibitory motor neurons were calculated in the same way as synaptic outputs of interneurons: as a sigmoidal function of net input, biased so that inhibitory connections had no effect in the absence of activation of an inhibitory motor neuron.

The other network, which was capable of both local bending and shortening, was produced in the much the same way, except that the training set was expanded to include input-output mappings which represented shortening responses. Shortening was triggered by 'strong' input activations of 3.0 or 4.0, and resulted in input to motor neurons that was approximately twice as large as the input causing the strongest local bending response.

10.3.2 Simulation of local bending

We examined the performance of networks containing from four to sixteen hidden units. In general, all networks could be trained to criterion (a change in error

(A)

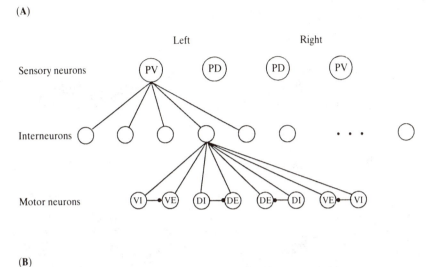

(B)

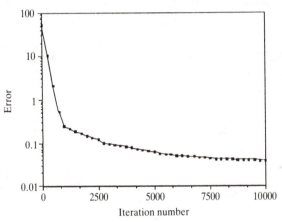

Figure 10.5 Feed-forward modeling of the local bend circuit. **A.** Architecture of the network. A standard three-layered architecture was adapted to conform to constraints derived from behavioral and physiological observations. Four input units correspond to four principal sensory neurons, the two dorsal and two ventral P cells, found in each mid-body segment. Eight output units correspond to eight types of motor neurons. The number of hidden units varied. Each unit was initially connected to every other unit in adjacent layers with activity flowing from top to bottom. Lateral inhibitory connections with fixed weights were inserted between motor neuron pairs in the same quadrant in conformance with actual circuitry. Interneurons were non-linear units (output range: 0 to +1) biased so that the output was 0 with no input, since leech neurons typically do not release transmitter at rest. The network was trained using a back-propagation algorithm to minimize error in net inputs to motor neurons. Motor neurons were therefore viewed as linear output units, except where they made lateral connections. Activation along lateral connections was a biased, non-linear function of net input, as above. Initial random weights were small (0 to +0.3 for sensory to interneuron connections, –0.15 to +0.15 for interneuron to motor neuron connections). **(Cont. overleaf)**

(C)

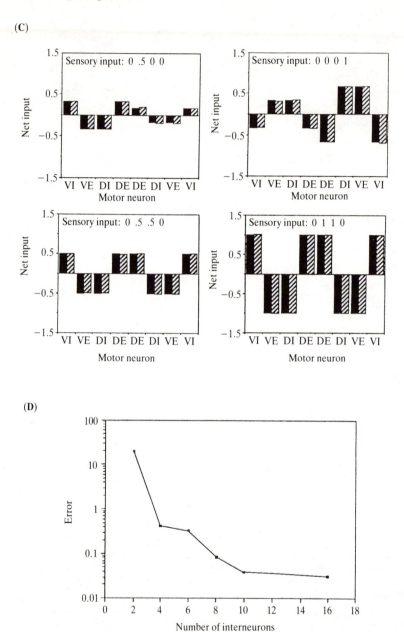

(D)

(Fig. 10.5 cont.) As dictated by physiology, only positive weights were allowed from sensory to interneurons, whereas single interneurons could have positive or negative weights to motor neurons. Abbreviations: V ventral; D dorsal; E excitatory; I inhibitory; P pressure sensory cell. **B.** Error as a function of iteration number for a single network with ten interneurons. Like the one shown, each network was trained on 10 000 cycles (iterations) through the **(cont. opposite)** of less than 0.00002 per iteration) in 10 000 iterations or less (Figure 10.5B). Trained networks could reproduce the target patterns with a high degree of accuracy. Figure 10.5C shows the output of a network with ten hidden units in response to several different input patterns. The similarity of output and target activations suggests that the network found a precise solution to the local bending task. Precision was not substantially improved when the number of hidden units was increased from ten to sixteen (Figure 10.5D). However, the minimum error term was markedly higher when the number of hidden units was decreased, and performance was quite poor with 4 hidden units. This result suggests that a minimum of ten hidden units is required for the task. Thus a complete analysis of the actual local bending circuitry might be expected to yield at least this many local bending interneurons. Of course, we cannot rule out the possibility that a solution exists for a smaller number of hidden units and the back-propagation algorithm has so far been unable to find it.

We analysed the network with ten hidden units in greatest detail. In particular, we were interested in the patterns of connectivity it predicted for the actual local bending interneurons. All the hidden units received connections with significant weights from one, two or three input units, but in no case did a hidden unit have significant connections from all four input units (Figure 10.6). Regardless of the number of inputs to a given hidden unit, most hidden units had substantial weights to every output unit. Interestingly, output weights within a quadrant were always equal and opposite. That is to say, if a particular hidden unit had a strong positive weight onto the left dorsal excitor, the weight onto the left dorsal inhibitor was also strong, but negative. The fact that these weights were equal was caused by the particular values we chose for the connection from inhibitory output units to the excitatory unit in the same quadrant. In the simulations presented here, all lateral inhibitory weights were arbitrarily set to −1 and not adjusted during training. In other simulations, different lateral weights were used. When these weights were set to −3, for example, the inhibitory weights from each hidden unit became smaller, so that its positive and negative influence within a given output quadrant were no longer equal.

Unlike the connections made by a single hidden unit within a quadrant, there did not appear to be a simple correlation between the strength of connections it made between output quadrants. This was true whether one considered the size of the weights or their sign. In addition, running the same training set on a network which

(**Fig. 10.5 cont.**) the set of input and output activation patterns. Learning rate (initially 0.2) was halved every 2500 iterations. C. Performance of the network with ten interneurons after training. Numbers above the graphs represent input activations. The top left graph, for instance, shows the output of the 8 motor neurons when the input pattern consisted of 0.0 input on the left and right PV, and the right PD, and 0.5 input on the left PD. Four of the 9 patterns used to train the network are shown. Ordinate: activation. Abscissa: motor neurons, left to right as in part **A**. Bars are motor neuron (black) and target (grey) activations. **D.** Error as a function of number of hidden units. Each point represents the least error of four different simulations with the indicated number of hidden units. Somewhere between four and ten hidden units are required to produce local bending. Performance does not improve significantly with more than ten hidden units.

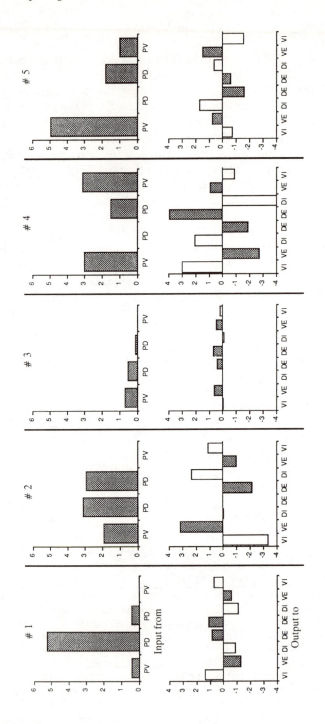

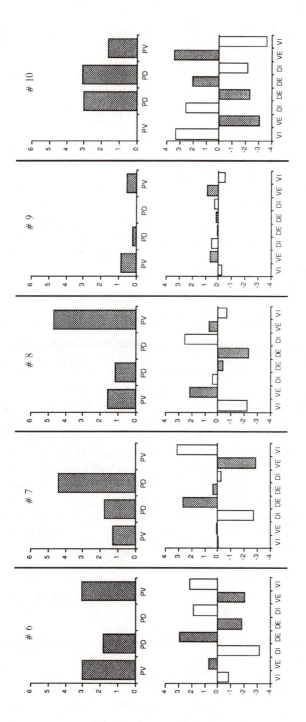

Figure 10.6 Connectivity of hidden units in the network simulating local bending. Each panel (1-10) shows the connections of a hidden unit from the network of Figure 10.5B & C. Ordinate is synaptic weight. Within each panel, upper graphs show connections from sensory cells, left-to-right as in Figure 10.5A, lower graphs show connections to motorneurons, left to right as in Figure 10.5A. In the lower graphs, dark bars indicate connections to excitatory motor neurons, light bars indicate connections to inhibitory motor neurons. Negative weights represent inhibitory connections. Hidden units received connections from 1 to 3 input units, and made connections to most output units.

differed only in its randomly assigned initial connection weights produced variation in the types of hidden units generated. To characterize this variation, we classifiedthe hidden units according to the behavior they would produce if activated individually, as in a typical physiological experiment. We obtained several classes: some units would produce 'lateral' bends (e.g. unit #4 in Figure 10.6), 'dorsal' bends (#1) or 'ventral' bends (#5); others would produce behaviors not in the training set, such as shortening (#3) or diagonal bending (#7). In one study of thirty hidden units from three independently trained networks of ten hidden units each, about a third produced bends in the vertical plane, about a third produced bends in the lateral plane, and a third produced a miscellany of other behaviors. At this point, we are just beginning to seek such patterns. What is clear, however, is that most hidden units are multifunctional rather than committed; i.e. very few of them have both input and output connections appropriate to produce a recognizable leech behavior. Instead, the simulations suggest that all behavioral outputs, including dorsal and ventral bends, are the result of a complex summation of many behavioral acts of different magnitudes.

10.3.3   Simulation of local bending plus shortening

The same three-layered architecture was trained to produce local bending to weak inputs and shortening to strong inputs. This was achieved by adding patterns to the local bending training set so that, in response to stronger input unit activation, all excitatory motor neurons were excited, and all inhibitory motor neurons were inhibited, as physiological and behavioral observations require. We have not yet performed a systematic analysis of the number of hidden units required to solve this problem. However, as Figure 10.7A shows, a network of ten hidden units solved the problem with respectable accuracy. A network with sixteen hidden units had superior performance and required many fewer iterations to train. This suggests that a greater number of hidden units may be required to produce both local bending and shortening than were required to produce local bending alone.

An analysis of the connectivity of hidden units indicated that the addition of shortening produced a new type of hidden unit: one that received substantial weights from all four input units (Figure 10.7B). Hidden units with weights from one, two and three input units were also observed. Connectivity on the output side was unchanged: most hidden units still connected to each output unit. The weights of the connections were equal and opposite within quadrants (e.g. the input connections to the DE and DI motor neurons were nearly equal), and the majority of hidden units were of the lateral-bending sort.

Many accounts of behavioral choice propose that there are subsystems dedicated to the exclusive production of one behavior or another (Davis, 1979; Toates & Halliday, 1980). We therefore examined whether the present network, that was capable of switching from local bending to shortening, was organized in such a way. In particular, we asked whether the network contained hidden units that were reserved for local bending or shortening. This was a simple matter of examining the activation of hidden units during the transition from local bending to

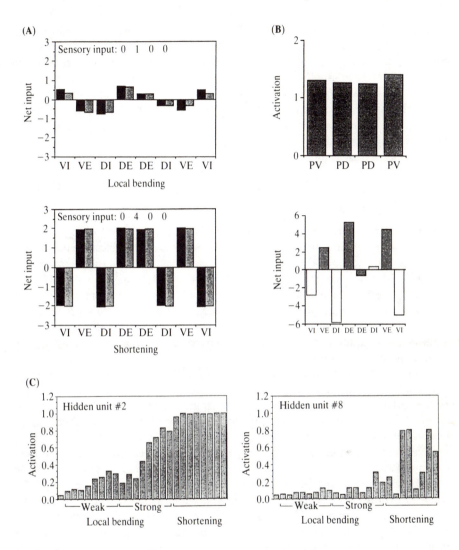

Figure 10.7 Performance of a network trained on local bending plus shortening patterns. The network was initially identical to that shown in Figure 10.5. It was presented with the same input patterns as used to generate Figure 10.5, as well as 8 additional patterns with each iteration, to mimic stronger stimuli. **A.** Examples of training sets used to simulate local bending and shortening. Numbers above the graphs represent input activations. Ordinate: activation. Abscissa: motor neurons, left to right as in Figure 10.5A. Bars are motor neuron (black) and target (grey) activations. These data show that increasing the strength of sensory input activation (from 1 to 4) causes the output to switch from local bending to shortening. **B.** Connectivity of a new type of hidden unit appearing in networks trained to produce both local bending and shortening. Ordinates are synaptic weight. Upper graphs show connections from sensory cells, left to right as in Figure 10.5A; lower graphs show connections to motor neurons, left to right as in **(cont. overleaf)**

shortening. By definition, an exclusive local-bending unit would have high activations in response to local bending input patterns, and low activations to shortening input patterns, whereas an exclusive shortening unit would have the opposite response profile. Such an analysis revealed that, in general, each hidden unit is active in both types of behavior (Figure 10.7C). Some hidden units showed a gradual increase in activation from local bending to shortening, while for others the transition was relatively abrupt. However, even in the case of abrupt transitions, there appeared to be sufficient activation during local bending to rule out interpreting such units as exclusive shortening units.

10.4   Discussion

By recording from interneurons known to be responsible for one behavior while others are taking place, we have shown that some interneurons are committed to a single behavior and some are not. By further characterizing the interneuronal networks and their interconnections, we might find a simple rule by which different kinds of behavioral choice are accomplished. However, experience with other systems shows that there may well not be such simple rules. One reason for this lack of simplicity could be that interneurons are involved in a diverse range of behaviors, so that the strategy for a choice between any two behaviors may depend also on interactions with other behaviors. Another reason might be that selection acts on behavior, not on circuits directly, and that there are a number of different ways to produce a given behavioral output (Dumont & Robertson, 1986); therefore, the particular circuit is more influenced by historical accident than by any 'optimal design'. If this is likely for circuits, it should be even more likely for interactions between circuits.

In some ways, the use of back-propagation to discover possible circuits gives us ways to distinguish between optimal strategies and historical accident. Each run of the back-propagation configuration starts with a different random network. This means that if many different networks can produce the same behaviors, chances are good that the algorithm will find them. By doing many simulations, we can get an idea of the space of possible solutions to the problem. We can then check the connectivity patterns of the hidden units in the model against the interneurons in the animal. If there is some correspondence (i.e. if some interneurons have the same connections as the hidden units in the model), we can investigate other possibilities for why the biological network was selected over other modeled possibilities:

(**Fig. 10.7 cont.**) Figure 10.5A. In the lower graphs, dark bars indicate connections to excitatory motor neurons, light bars indicate connections to inhibitory motor neurons. C. Activation of interneurons during local bending and shortening. Ordinate is activation level. Each bar represents the response of the indicated hidden unit to a single pattern of input to sensory cells. Inputs are arranged along the abscissa in order of increasing strength and number of sensory cells activated. The transitions between weak and strong local bending, and local bending and shortening are indicated at the bottom. In general, all hidden units contributed to both local bending and shortening.

perhaps the selected circuit has a broader functional range than do other possible networks, or perhaps the interneurons have another function that we have not taken into account, such as interganglionic coordination or participation in a third behavior for which the network was not trained.

One should not be too eager to make comparisons between the model network and the neuronal circuitry. One of the biggest limitations of the model is that it uses a gradient descent procedure to minimize error, so that it finds *local* minima in such a surface. The solutions found depend upon the initial parameters (connection strengths) of the network, and the learning parameters chosen. We have tried to circumvent these problems by doing multiple runs, each starting with different conditions, but there is no guarantee that the optimal solution will be found, nor that this has anything to do with the circuit constraints that were operating phylogenetically. Also, as it currently stands, the model is greatly simplified compared to physiological reality. For instance, we have not yet taken into account known lateral (electrical) connections between homologous motor neurons (Ort *et al.*, 1974). In addition, we have yet to impose bilateral symmetry on the hidden layer; i.e. each hidden unit on the left should have a 'mirror image' homolog on the right, a general rule among leech interneurons. A potentially more serious problem is that the model does not incorporate many of the properties of neurons thought to be important for neuronal processing. For instance, all variations in time, from the time-course of synaptic events to the modification of membrane properties, are ignored, and axons are assumed to have no conduction delay. In addition, the units are stateless, in that they do not reflect their history except in terms of learning. Some of these limitations will be corrected by future modifications of the model. Despite even the current limitations, however, the model has made some very provocative predictions. For instance, it predicts that there will be few interneurons committed to a single behavior, and that behavioral choice may be due to differences in the level of activity in many or all of the interneurons rather than to the selection of a particular set of interneurons committed to one behavior. A useful feature of these predictions is that they are testable physiologically.

Acknowledgement

This research was supported by an NIMH research grant, MH43396, to W.B.K.

References

Brodfuehrer P.D. & Friesen W.O. (1986a) Initiation of swimming activity by trigger neurons in the leech subesophageal ganglion; III. Sensory inputs to Tr1 and Tr2. **J. comp. Physiol.** A **159**, pp. 511-519

Brodfuehrer P.D. & Friesen W.O. (1986b) From stimulation to undulation: a neuronal pathway for the control of swimming in the leech. **Science 234**, pp. 1002-1004

Croll R.P., Kovac M.P. & Davis W.J.(1985a). Neural mechanisms of motor pattern switching in the mollusc *Pleurobranchaea*. II. Role of the ventral white cell, anterior ventral and B3 buccal neurons. **J. Neurosci. 5**, pp. 56-63

Croll R.P., Kovac M.P., Matera E.M. & Davis W.J.(1985b) Neural mechanisms of motor pattern switching in the mollusc *Pleurobranchaea*. III. Role of the paracerebral neurons and other identified brain neurons. **J. Neurosci. 5**, pp. 64-71

Davis W.J. (1979) Behavioral hierarchies. **TINS 2**, pp. 5-7

Dumont J.P.C. & Robertson R.M.(1986) Neuronal circuits: an evolutionary perspective. **Science 33**, pp. 849-853

Friesen W.O. (1985) Neuronal control of leech swimming movements: interactions between cell 60 and previously described oscillator neurons. **J. comp. Physiol. A 156**, pp. 231-242

Friesen W.O. (1989) Neuronal control of leech swimming movements. In: **Neuronal and Cellular Oscillators**, J. Jacklet (ed.) pp. 247-294

Friesen W.O., Poon M. & Stent G.S.(1978) Neuronal control of swimming in the medicinal leech IV. Identification of a network of oscillatory interneurones. **J. Exp. Biol. 75**, pp. 25-43

Getting P.A. & Dekin M.S. (1985) *Tritonia* swimming: A model system for integration within rhythmic motor systems. In: **Model Neural Networks and Behavior**. A.I. Selverston (ed.) pp. 3-20

Granzow B., Friesen W.O. & Kristan W.B.Jr. (1985) Physiological and morphological analysis of synaptic transmission between leech motorneurons. **J. Neurosci. 5**, pp. 2035-2050

Kovac M. (1974) Abdominal movements during backward walking in the crayfish. II. The neuronal basis. **J. comp. Physiol. 95**, pp. 71-94

Kovac M.P. & Davis W.J. (1980) Neural mechanism underlying behavioral choice in *Pleurobranchaea* **J. Neurophysiol. 43**, pp. 469-505

Kristan W.B. Jr. (1982) Sensory and motor neurones responsible for the local bending response in leeches. **J. exp. Biol. 96**, pp. 161-180

Kristan W.B. Jr. & Calabrese R.L. (1976) Rhythmic swimming activity in neurones of the isolated nerve cord of the leech. **J. exp. Biol. 65**, pp. 643-668

Kristan W.B. Jr, McGirr S.J. & Simpson G.V. (1982) Behavioural and mechanosensory neurone responses to skin stimulation in leeches. **J. exp. Biol. 96**, pp. 143-160

Kristan W.B. Jr., Stent G.S. & Ort C.A. (1974) Neuronal control of swimming in the medicinal leech; III. Impulse patterns of the motor neurons. **J. comp. Physiol. 94**, pp. 155-176

Kristan W.B. Jr. & Weeks J.C. (1983) Neurons controlling the initiation, generation and modulation of leech swimming. **S.E.B. Symposium XXXVII,** pp. 243-260

Kristan W.B. Jr., Wittenberg G., Nusbaum M.P. & Stern-Tomlinson W. (1988) Multifunctional interneurons in behavioral circuits of the medicinal leech. In: **Invertebrate Neuroethology.** J. Camhi (ed.) **Experientia 44,** pp. 383-389

Lehky S.R. & Sejnowski T.J. (1988) Network model of shape-from-shading: neural function arises from both receptive and projective fields. **Nature 333,** pp. 452-454

Lockery S.R. & Kristan W.B. Jr. (1988) Possible loci for habituation of the leech local bending reflex. **Soc. Neurosci. Abstr.,** in press

Macagno E.R. (1980) Number and distribution of neurons in leech segmental ganglia. **J. comp. Neurol. 190,** pp. 283-302

McClellan A.D. (1982a) Movements and motor patterns of the buccal mass of *Pleurobranchaea* during feeding, regurgitation and rejection. **J. exp. Biol. 98,** pp. 195-211

McClellan A.D. (1982b) Re-examination of presumed feeding motor activity in the isolated nervous system of *Pleurobranchaea* **J. exp. Biol. 98,** pp. 213-228

Muller K.J., Nicholls, J.G. & Stent G.S. (1981) **Neurobiology of the leech.** Cold Spring Harbor Laboratory Press, Cold Spring Harbor, NY.

Nicholls J.G. & Baylor D.A.(1968) Specific modalities and receptive fields of sensory neurons in CNS of the leech. **J. Neurophysiol. 31,** pp. 740-756

Nusbaum M.P., Friesen W.O., Kristan W.B. Jr. & Pearce R.A. (1987) Neural mechanisms generating the leech swimming rhythm: swim-initiator neurons excite the network of swim oscillator neurons. **J. comp. Physiol. 161,** pp. 355-366

Nusbaum M.P. & Kristan W.B. Jr. (1986) Swim initiation in the leech by serotonin-containing interneurones, cells 21 and 61. **J. exp. Biol. 122,** pp. 277-302

Ort C.A., Kristan W.B. Jr., & Stent G.S. (1974) Neuronal control of swimming in the medicinal leech. II. Identification and connections of motor neurons. **J. comp. Physiol. 94,** pp. 155-176

Poon M., Friesen W.O. & Stent G.S. (1978) Neuronal control of swimming in the medicinal leech V. Connexions between the oscillatory interneurones and the motor neurones. **J. exp. Biol. 75,** pp. 45-63

Ramirez J.M. & Pearson K.G. (1988) Generation of motor patterns for walking and flight in motoneurons supplying bifunctional muscles in the locust. **J. Neurobiol. 19,** pp. 257-282

Rumelhart D.E., Hinton G.E. & McClelland J.L. (1986) Learning representations by back-propagating errors. **Nature 323,** pp. 533-536

Selverston A.I. (1985) **Model Neural Networks and Behavior.** Plenum Press, NY.

Stent G.S., Kristan W.B. Jr., Friesen W.O., Ort, C.A., Poon M. & Calabrese R.L. (1978) Neuronal generation of the leech swimming movement. **Science 200**, pp. 1348-1357

Stuart A.E. (1970) Physiological and morphological properties of motoneurones in the central nervous system of the leech. **J. Physiol. 209**, pp. 627-646

Toates F.M. (1980) **Animal behaviour : a systems approach.** Wiley, NY.

Toates F.M. & Halliday T.R. eds. (1980) **Analysis of Motivational Processes** Academic Press, London.

Weeks J.C. (1982a) Synaptic basis of swim initiation in the leech. I. Connections of a swim-initiating neuron (cell 204) with motor neurons and pattern-generating 'oscillator' neurons. **J. comp. Physiol. 148**, pp. 253-263

Weeks J.C. (1982b) Synaptic basis of swim initiation in the leech. II. A pattern-generating neuron (cell 208) which mediates motor effects of swim-initiating neurons. **J. comp. Physiol. 148**, pp. 264-279

Weeks J.C. & Kristan W.B. Jr. (1978) Initiation, maintenance and modulation of swimming in the medicinal leech by the activity of a single neurone. **J. exp. Biol. 77**, pp. 71-88

Wittenberg G. & Kristan W.B. Jr. (1987) Behavioral choice in the isolated leech nervous system: shortening vs. swimming. **Soc. Neurosci. Abstr. 13**, p.388

Wittenberg G. & Kristan W.B. Jr. (1988) Behavioral choice in the leech: characterization of the shortening motor pattern. **Soc. Neurosci. Abstr. 14**, p. 690

Zipser D. & Andersen R.A. (1988) A back-propagation programmed network that simulates response properties of a subset of posterior parietal neurons. **Nature 331**, pp. 679-684

11
Flexibility of Computational Units in Invertebrate CPGs

Allen Selverston & Pietro Mazzoni

11.1 Introduction

The local circuits found in invertebrate central pattern generators (CPGs) are known in greater detail than any other class of neural networks. There are now about 10 CPGs which have been described as virtually complete neuronal circuits (see Roberts & Roberts, 1983; Selverston & Moulins, 1985). The main impetus for analyzing these circuits was persuasive evidence which coalesced in the early 1960s suggesting that virtually all rhythmic motor outputs were centrally generated. New experimental preparations were discovered which could in principle be reduced to their component parts and interconnections (Wilson, 1961; Willows, 1967; Maynard, 1972; Kater, 1974). The idea was that if the central pattern generating circuitry could be determined, then the mechanisms underlying burst and pattern formation would emerge (Kennedy *et al.*, 1967). It has been disappointing therefore, that despite our current knowledge of central pattern generators (CPGs), no formalism for describing their mechanisms exists. More surprisingly, the existing evidence suggests that there can be enormous differences in the way these circuits are arranged even though they produce what are fundamentally very similar rhythmic motor patterns. While many different arrangements of neuronal interconnectivity are present, the basic electrophysiological properties of the individual cells and synapses appear to be very similar.

Except for a few instances (Getting, 1983), attempts at modeling invertebrate CPGs have not provided workers with novel insights which might be helpful in pointing out new experimental directions. Most models have been phenomenological (realistic) in nature, i.e. the model is essentially a replica of the real system in so far as this is possible. Generally such models have no unique computational properties which predict anything other than the results which one observes experimentally (Hartline, 1987).

Despite the fact that current network models are in some ways biologically implausible, they do have computationally interesting properties and offer the possibility of using them to study simple networks in new ways. One hope is that these models may suggest new experimental approaches. It is important to keep in mind that such schemes as the Hopfield (Hopfield & Tank, 1986) or back-propagation algorithms (Zipser & Andersen, 1988), while neurally 'inspired', have no real basis in empirical observations of mammalian or any other 'wet' brain tissue. There is certainly massive connectivity between neurons in the brain which might suggest that neurons in computational circuits are massively interconnected. This makes them similar, but it is a loose similarity. A precise description of neuronal connections in cortex is simply not available. So while these models are computationally interesting, the fact that they have some of the properties of real nervous systems (learn and store 'memories') may only be coincidental. A major problem with the use of theoretical models of the mammalian brain is that they face technical hurdles when it comes to full scale experimental verification. The models are based on specific connectivities, synaptic weights and input-output relationships. This is the kind of data which is most difficult to measure in brain. While computationally interesting in their own right, they are extremely speculative with regard to explaining neuronal function. How much more valuable such models would be if their assumptions were both biologically realistic and experimentally verifiable.

We propose that invertebrate CPG circuits may be helpful in bridging this gap between theory and experiment. Although the invertebrate 'bottom-up' approach has not led to the synthesis that many had hoped for, it has generated a data base with strong links to both behavior and cellular neurophysiology which can be used for modeling studies. The 'top-down' approach favored by some network modelers, will never, by itself, be able to explain mechanisms, and disciplines which build on it (cognitive psychology, for example) may be seriously misled by computationally interesting results without regard to empirical data. The algorithms which have been used in many of the most recent studies depend on limited interactions between large numbers of identical units. We know from invertebrate studies that not only are individual neurons different, but the kinds of synapses which are made between them have enormous plasticity. It is likely that similar differences exist among mammalian CNS neurons. A legitimate question can be raised here however, and that is, are invertebrate central nervous systems relevant to the study of information processing in vertebrate brains?

Certainly at the cellular level the giant axon of the squid provided an enormous amount of empirical data which led to the formulation of one of the most well-known models in neurobiology (Hodgkin & Huxley, 1952). This model describing the action potential was derived from invertebrate data because the large size of single axons made it possible to space clamp an entire region of axon membrane with internal electrodes. Such experiments could not be performed on vertebrate axons. Nevertheless the Hodgkin-Huxley model is still acknowledged to be applicable and useful for the study of action potentials in all vertebrate neurons. If we make the argument that the availability of empirical parametric data was a necessary condition for the development of the axon model, then can we make a similar argument that the favorable features of invertebrate networks can provide the empirical data for modeling neural networks in general? While it is possible that simple networks may compute by methods entirely different from those found in vertebrates, there is no *a priori* reason for thinking this is the case.

While cellular models may indeed be applicable to different phyla, large systems of neurons may not be governed by the same principles as very small systems. At the moment we have no way of knowing. There are microcircuits in the brain which have been studied in neocortex, hippocampus and cerebellum, but very little is known about the actual nature of the connectivity involved. We have been struck by the fact that there appear to be many possible circuit arrangements even for invertebrate CPGs which at a functional level appear to be quite similar.

A major, and as yet unsolvable problem for vertebrate neurophysiology is that there is no reliable way of recording intracellularly from pre- and post-synaptic units in the intact brain and therefore, no way to establish the functional connections between cells even in microcircuits. Arguments that the brain may never be understood in terms of its individual neurons and instead requires a 'higher level' language have been made. The idea is that gas laws or spin glass theories do not have to take into account the details of what each component is doing. But these examples usually derive from physics or chemistry where the particles and their interactions are all alike. These are probably inappropriate systems upon which to base neural models because the available evidence suggests neither individual neurons nor their interconnections are identical. It may be a long time before models incorporating available biologically realistic parameters are integrated into neural network algorithms. It may be even longer before such data from vertebrate brain is available. Meanwhile the data which can be extracted from invertebrate networks, and the ability to use this data for the testing of theoretical models, puts them in a unique position for contributing to this emerging field.

11.2 The study of invertebrate CPGs

The hallmark of an invertebrate CPG is that it can continue to produce a rhythmic pattern when completely isolated from sensory feedback and other forms of rhythmic input (Delcomyn, 1980). The experimental proof for this fact was difficult to obtain and the general acceptance of a totally central origin was not without controversy, some of which has lasted to the present time (Pearson *et al.*, 1983; Wendler, 1983). For the majority of CPGs, some generalized form of non-rhythmic excitatory input is necessary even when sensory feedback is missing.

An isolated CPG preparation is usually not only free of sensory feedback but also of neuroactive substances such as chemical modulators and hormones which can have profound effects on the pattern generating machinery *in vivo*. Due to the fact that invertebrate neural systems contain fewer cells than vertebrate systems and that the cells are large and re-identifiable, the role of each cell in generating a complex motor pattern can be studied. To get at the question of mechanism in these systems we need, at a minimum, an explanation for the source of the bursts and the pattern of firing (the phase relationships) between the different elements of the system. We can also ask about the overall period and the firing frequency within bursts. This information constitutes the 'problem' which must be solved by the circuit. Experimentally, several criteria must be met:

1) All of the neurons which are active during the generation of the rhythm must be identified electrophysiologically and those which are only being driven must be distinguished from those which actually participate in the genesis of the pattern.

2) The functional relationships between the neurons, even in the somewhat artificial experimental situation must be determined, i.e. the monosynaptic connections must be rigorously established.

3) The individual properties of each neuron must be measured and the strength and temporal characteristics of each synapse quantified as well as possible.

11.3   Some examples of invertebrate neural oscillators

Several invertebrate CPGs are particularly illustrative of the heterogeneity present in these small networks. It is not our intention here to go into much detail but merely to point out the general features of these systems for comparative purposes and to illustrate the point that there is considerable variability among CPGs with similar motor outputs. There are three main subdivisions: (1) those which are driven by endogenous or conditional bursters (Selverston & Moulins, 1985), (2) those in which bursting is a result of the cooperative activity between non-bursting neurons, and (3) those in which bursting ensues as a result of both cellular *and* network properties.

The simplest is the heartbeat generator in the cardiac ganglion of lobsters (Tazaki & Cooke, 1983) (Figure 11.1A). Here, a group of endogenously bursting small neurons directly excites a group of large motor neurons. The neurons are all electronically connected and there is some indication that this may contribute to the burst generating mechanism. This is a single phase system so extensive connectivity between neurons is not required.

The leech heartbeat system (Figure 11.1B) makes use of extensive pairs of reciprocal inhibitory synapses forming a closed chain. This form of connectivity is very common in invertebrate systems and has been modeled extensively (Perkel & Mulloney, 1974). The operation of this pattern generator is extremely complex and the diagram does not do justice to the dynamic changes (see Calabrese, 1979) but it is an example of a system which utilizes both endogenously bursting cells and network properties to generate a motor pattern.

The snail feeding oscillator (Figure 11.1C) generates a complex three-phase pattern which controls the buccal mass and radula in snails (Benjamin, 1983). Several of the cells in this network have intrinsic burst generating capabilities. These neurons also show a strong capacity for generating plateau potentials. Some also have extremely strong post-inhibitory rebound properties. The connectivity

(A) Lobster cardiac

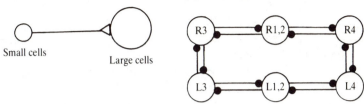

Small cells

Large cells

(B) Leech heart

(C) Snail feeding

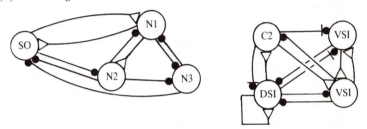

(D) Tritonia swim

(E) Clione swim

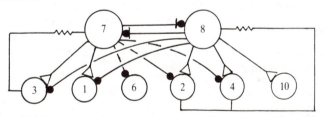

Figure 11.1 Schematic circuits of several invertebrate central pattern generators. Triangles are chemical excitatory synapses and black dots are chemical inhibitory synapses. Lines at the back of some dots signify mixed inhibitory/excitatory synapses. Resistors represent electrotonic junctions.

between all groups of neurons is a mixture of both excitatory and inhibitory synaptic connections.

The *Tritonia* CPG (Figure 11.1D) produces alternating bursts of inputs in the dorsal and ventral swim interneurons. When single cells in the CPG circuit are isolated, none appear to be capable of endogenous bursting and the system as a whole is a network type oscillator (Getting, 1983). A cycle begins with a strong burst in the DSI neuron. C2 is silent because of its high threshold and VSI is silent because it is inhibited by DSI. DSI eventually fires C2 which, after a delay due to an A current, turns on the VSI. When VSI fires it inhibits both DSI and C2. The basis of the swim-generating pattern is reciprocal inhibition paralleled by delayed excitation.

The *Clione* swim CPG is made up of eight groups of neurons connected with both chemical and electrical synapses as shown in Figure 11.1E. Unlike many of the other CPGs, this network is able to generate alternate bursts of motor activity in the absence of tonic excitatory drive suggesting the presence of intrinsic burst generating mechanisms in at least some of the cells. The basic kind of synaptic interaction appears to be reciprocal inhibition between antagonistic groups. One interesting feature of this network is the presence of an additional cell which is active only during periods of intense activity. When active, it interacts with other cells without spiking and has the general effect of increasing the frequency of the swim producing bursts. Like many other CPGs, both network and cellular properties contribute to the generation of the pattern.

For these five examples only the cardiac ganglion is purely endogenously driven; leech, snail and *Clione* are mixed oscillators and *Tritonia* is driven solely by synaptic connectivity. The patterns produced by all of these networks are made up of bursts of impulses in each unit with various phase relationships between them. Despite this similarity in output states, there do not appear to be any generalizable rules or set of first principles which can be extracted from an examination of these particular small systems. What is clear however, is that they do share some fundamental cellular and synaptic properties as well as specific network configurations such as reciprocal inhibition. None of the circuits are connected in a way which links each cell to every other cell. Two additional networks, the lobster gastric and pyloric CPGs are the most well defined and we can use them as examples of how some networks actually operate. We will see that, instead of being rigid 'hard-wired' systems, they are quite flexible and can undergo profound state changes as a result of chemical modulation.

11.4   The stomatogastric central pattern generators

11.4.1   Pyloric rhythm

The pyloric CPG (Figure 11.2B) is composed of 14 neurons in the stomatogastric ganglion and 2 in the commissural ganglia (Figure 11.2A). The two in the commissurals, called P cells (Russell, 1976) provide intermittent excitation to all of the pyloric units except the PD and AB cells. The P cells are phasically inhibited by the AB neuron and this loop must be intact for the ganglion to operate properly. The pyloric pattern, shown in Figure 11.2C, is a three phase pattern with a frequency of about 2 Hz. The PD-AB cells are electrotonically coupled and therefore tend to fire simultaneously which, due to their synaptic connections, strongly inhibits all of the other neurons. When the PD-AB group stop firing, the LP and IC neurons fire, followed by the VD and PY neurons (Figure 11.2C).

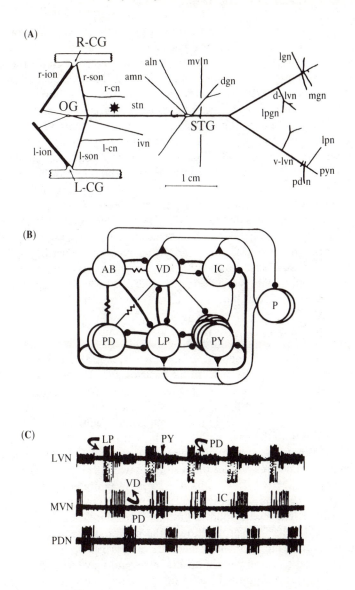

Figure 11.2 The dissected stomatogastric preparation and components of the pyloric rhythm. **A.** Diagrammatic version of the principal nerves of the stomatogastric system. R & L-CG are the right and left commissural ganglia and OG shows the position of the esophageal ganglion. STG, stomatogastric ganglion; stn, the stomatogastric nerve. The star indicates the position where stn can be reversibly blocked. The abbreviations are for the remaining nerves of the system. **B.** Pyloric circuit: black dots represent chemical inhibitions, triangles represent chemical excitation; resistors are electrotonic junctions. **C.** Extracellular recordings of the pyloric motor pattern in a combined preparation (i.e. with commissural ganglia attached). Time bar is 0.5 sec.

The pyloric rhythm was analyzed by reversibly blocking the stomatogastric nerve to remove the influence of the P cells and other neuromodulatory inputs from the commissural ganglia. In addition, neurons were deleted from the pyloric circuit either singly or in groups by means of a dye-sensitized photoinactivation technique (Miller & Selverston, 1979). These procedures allowed us to consider several basic problems such as the relative contribution of each neuron to the overall pattern, and the relative importance of endogenous bursting vs. connectivity to the generation of the output. Using these techniques, it was found that all of the pyloric neurons were intrinsic conditional bursters, i.e. all could fire bursts of action potentials if exposed to the proper chemical environment. The neuromodulators from the commissural ganglia fulfilled this role and also enabled many of the pyloric neurons to express 'plateau potentials' - the holding of depolarized levels for sustained periods. In terms of mechanism, the pyloric system appears to be both a system of coupled oscillators and a resonant network which can oscillate as a result of the connectivity alone. The principal form of connectivity underlying the bursting appears to be reciprocal inhibition, a basic circuit often suggested as underlying alternate bursting. A reduced network of only two pyloric cells (PD and LP) connected in this way has been shown to be capable of bursting (Miller & Selverston, 1982).

11.4.2 *The gastric mill CPG*

The gastric mill is composed of three 'teeth', controlled by striated muscles which receive patterned activity from the gastric CPG. There are two lateral teeth and one medial tooth. A total of 11 neurons comprise the gastric CPG circuit (Figure 11.3), all located in the stomatogastric ganglion. Like the pyloric system, two interneurons (E cells) located in the commissural ganglia provide a generalized excitatory feedback to the gastric CPG via the stomatogastric nerve. The bursts of impulses in the motor nerves are arranged antagonistically. The LG and MG units fire at about the same time and, *in situ*, cause the two lateral teeth to come together. Their antagonists, the two LPG units, are strongly inhibited by LG and MG and when activity in these units ceases, the LPGs fire strong bursts which act to pull the lateral teeth apart. The medial tooth is protracted by four GM units and retracted by the DG and AM units. The protraction is the power stroke and normally occurs during the time that the two lateral teeth are closely opposed. The neural circuit which generates the gastric pattern differs in several ways from the circuit which generates the pyloric rhythm. Instead of all of the neurons in the CPG being intrinsic oscillators, there is only one, the DG neuron. As a result, both the burst generating and the pattern forming mechanisms arise from the connections within the network. When the medial tooth neurons are removed from the circuit the lateral teeth pattern is hardly affected which suggests that the intrinsic bursting of the DG acts in parallel with network burst forming properties found in the lateral teeth network, i.e. int 1, LG and MG. The evidence points to the fact that the medial tooth neurons are driven by the lateral teeth units but the mechanism by which these neurons actually generate the pattern remains uncertain.

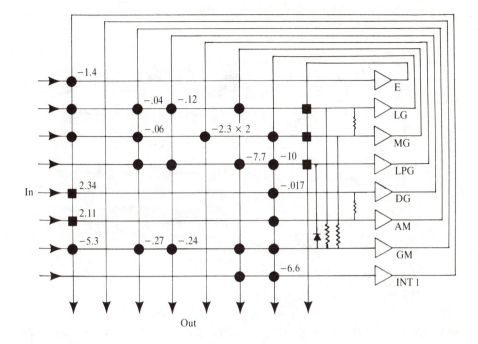

Figure 11.3 Connectivity matrix for neurons making up the gastric CPG. Circles are chemical inhibitory synapses and squares are chemical excitatory synapses. Resistors represent electrical connections with the diode symbol representing a rectifying electrotonic junction. Relative synaptic strengths are indicated.

11.4.3   *Neuromodulator induced flexibility*

The lobster contains a large number of putative neuromodulatory substances as shown by both immunohistochemistry (Marder, 1987) and radioimmunoassay (Vigna, 1985). These substances differ from conventional neurotransmitters in two main ways. Instead of being released directly onto post-synaptic sites where they bind quickly with receptor molecules and are then rapidly destroyed by enzymes, they are released either into the general vicinity of the neurons or into the bloodstream in much the same way as hormones are released. A second difference is that their mode of action is via second messenger systems which induce major changes in cellular properties as a result of intracellular phosphorylations. Many of these modulators are peptides or amines which can be shown to be contained in cell bodies 'upstream' from the stomatogastric ganglion. These neurons send axons into the ganglion via the stomatogastric nerve. In the ganglion, they branch into a diffuse neuropil. Immunostaining of this region reveals extensive staining over the entire neuropilar region but cell bodies are not observed. This arrangement suggests these particular neurons act like neurosecretory cells which integrate information converging onto the commissurals and whose firing elicits the release of neuromodulators into the CPG architecture of the ganglion. Once released, the

(A)

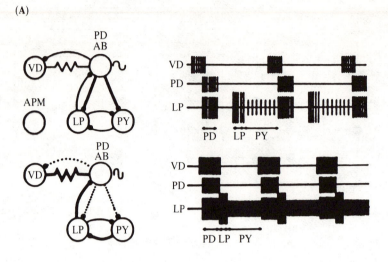

(B)

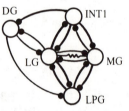
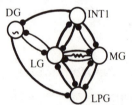

Control

Proctolin 10^{-5} M

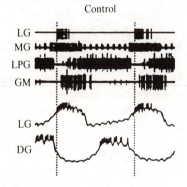
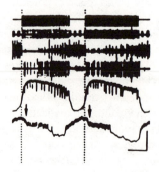

modulators can either act on an ongoing rhythm or start up a quiescent system (Harris-Warrick, 1988).

While it is well known that hormones and other neuromodulatory substances can affect nervous systems, very little is known about the mechanisms involved at the cell and circuit level. The CPG circuits in the stomatogastric ganglion are excellent systems with which to study such interactions since they respond to a large number of intrinsic substances. The first demonstration of the usefulness of this system for such investigations was shown by Nagy & Dickinson (1983). A cell in the small esophageal ganglion (Figure 11.2A) was found which released acetylcholine into the stomatogastric ganglion and caused extensive changes in the pyloric motor output pattern (Figure 11.4A). When the physiological basis for these changes was examined, these workers found that profound alterations in synaptic strengths had occurred and that in effect a new functional circuit had been 'sculpted' out of the old one. Since this groundbreaking study, a large number of substances have been found which can alter the function of both the gastric and pyloric circuits (for reviews see Marder, 1987, and Harris-Warrick, 1988). The overall rationale is to demonstrate that a particular substance exists naturally in the animal and if possible to localize it by immunocytochemical or radioimmunoassay. When cells containing these substances are found, their direct stimulation should lead to measurable release of the modulator and to physiological changes which are identical to those produced by bath application. When these criteria are met, it then becomes possible to describe exactly how both the gastric and pyloric patterns can be modified and what the cellular and possibly subcellular mechanisms are. More explicitly, this means how does the binding of a particular neuromodulator to certain cells eventually lead to the changes in conductance or transmitter release, which might account for the overall change in the output state of the network?

The action of neuromodulators may be a useful tool for studying a network's computational properties. Neuromodulator induced changes in cellular properties and synaptic strengths may be incorporated into models. Additionally, combined use of neuromodulators and the dye-sensitized photoinactivation of neurons permits studying their effects on reduced circuits of one or two cells. It has been shown that single isolated cells respond differently to particular modulators (Harris-Warrick, 1988). It would be useful to try and resynthesize these single cell responses with models to see if taken together they could account for the global changes in the pattern (adding, of course, the changes which occur in synaptic weights as well).

Two substances can be used to illustrate the general action of peptides on the gastric mill CPG - proctolin and cholecystokinin (CCK). Proctolin is a pentapeptide which can interact with both the pyloric and gastric systems. Using polyclonal antibodies, immunohistochemical studies have shown that proctolin containing neurons exist throughout the stomatogastric nervous system (Marder *et al.*, 1986).

Figure 11.4 (opposite) A. Modification of the pyloric pattern by the muscarinic action of the APM neuron. Functional changes in the circuit are shown on the left with three synapses becoming very weak and three becoming very strong. Changes in the firing pattern are shown on the right. (Modified from Nagy & Dickinson, 1983). **B.** Changes in the *in vitro* combined gastric pattern as a result of the bath application of proctolin. See text for details.

Cell bodies were found in the commissural ganglia and fibers were found in the nerves leading to the stomatogastric ganglion. There was widespread staining of the stomatogastric ganglion neuropile, but the microstructural distribution of the proctolinergic terminals could not be ascertained. The effects of proctolin on the gastric pattern could be studied both intra- and extracellularly (Heinzel & Selverston, 1988) by bath application (Figure 11.4B). In addition, the actual behavioral changes induced by proctolin could be studied by visual observation of the teeth with an endoscope. Direct perfusion of the stomatogastric ganglion *in vitro* with dosages well within physiological ranges suggested the action of proctolin was directly on the neurons of the gastric oscillator. Specifically, there were large increases in burst duration as well as increases in frequency for all neurons except the LPGs. The strongest effects were on the DG and LG neurons and were accompanied by a phase change in the DG burst so that instead of terminating at the onset of the LG burst, it continued on into the time of the LG and GM bursts. Behaviorally this would correlate with the observation of a different chewing pattern.

A peptide, immunologically crossreactive with mammalian CCK, has been found in the stomatogastric system (Turrigiano & Selverston, 1987); however, its effects on the gastric pattern, while clear, require very high doses to work. This suggests the mammalian material is not the same as the intrinsic compound. A CCK-like material isolated from the stomach of the shrimp (Favrel, 1988) has been shown to have physiological activity more potent than commercially available CCK. It remains to be seen exactly how the change in the pattern is caused by cellular and synaptic responses to both forms of CCK.

The work on the lobster system has shown that both CPGs can switch into different stable states depending on the chemical environment and these cellular changes may provide a useful database for computational studies on neural networks. Although the basic network is probably anatomically stable, the functional properties appear to be flexible. We do not know as yet whether or not all of the different output states seen by bath application *in vitro* have true behavioral significance, but the means are available to find this out. The point here is that chemical modulators have the effect of functionally rewiring a circuit for as long as they are present. This means that these circuits are not rigid 'hard-wired' entities and most are probably multifunctional. Circuits can change not only by altering their synaptic weights but also by modifying many physiological parameters. Whether or not such flexibility extends to mammalian cortical circuits remains an intriguing question.

11.5   A preliminary network model

A neural system such as the stomatogastric ganglion presents the investigator with a myriad of phenomenological details. The stomatogastric ganglion, for example, contains such disparate variables as intracellular potential, transmitter release kinetics and synaptic strengths. As we have seen, the character of these variables can be temporarily modified. Each cell in the ganglion has its own membrane time constant, neuropil length constant, and a set of individual conductance channels, from slow to fast, from passive to active. Unlike physics, which has summarized classical electromagnetism into four equations, neurobiology is far from having synthesized the diversity of phenomena it studies into a few sets of simple laws that predict and explain them. Although the existence of such first principles is not assured in neurobiology, the simplification which their discovery would produce amply justifies a search for them. It is in the search for these biological first principles that modeling plays an important role. A model allows the investigator to postulate basic laws governing the behavior of a biological system, and to test whether these laws can produce the behavior observed and predict the system's response to external perturbations.

We have begun an analysis of a three-cell subnetwork of the pyloric system. This subnetwork is a central pattern generator (CPG), as it produces a steady oscillatory output when synaptically isolated from the rest of the cells in the ganglion. As mentioned earlier, there are two major contributions to this oscillatory behavior. One is the endogenous bursting ability of each cell in the network. The other is the reciprocally inhibitory connectivity among the cells, together with adaptation characteristics of their output. We studied the latter contribution by building a model network of three cells connected as in the biological system, possessing an adaptive input-output (I-O) function and a few passive membrane properties, i.e. units similar to those described in Hopfield models. From this very simplified model we obtained oscillations that are strikingly similar to those observed experimentally.

11.5.1   The biological system

The three cells studied are shown with their connections in Figure 11.5A. LP has reciprocal inhibitory synaptic connections with PD and VD, and the latter are electrically coupled by a gap junction. In addition, the VD and LP normally receive phasic excitatory input from neurons in the commissural ganglia. Simultaneous recordings of each cell's intracellular potential *in vitro* show the oscillation pattern of the CPG (Figure 11.5B). The oscillations have 10 - 15 mV amplitudes and 1 - 2.5 Hz frequencies. As each cell's potential rises above the cell's threshold for action potentials, it produces a burst of spikes that travel down the axon to the muscle. The bursts have definite phase relationships (LPs in opposite phase to PDs and VDs, and PDs slightly delayed after VDs) that are important in driving antagonistic movements of the pyloric muscles (Figure 11.5C). But the spikes appear to be of little consequence in the actual burst-generating and phase-producing mechanisms (Graubard, 1978; Raper, 1979).

11.5.2   The model

The model we developed is a neural network derived from the type created by Hopfield (Hopfield & Tank, 1986). Hopfield's network simulates cells as simple operational amplifiers (Figure 11.6A) with an input voltage *u* (corresponding to the

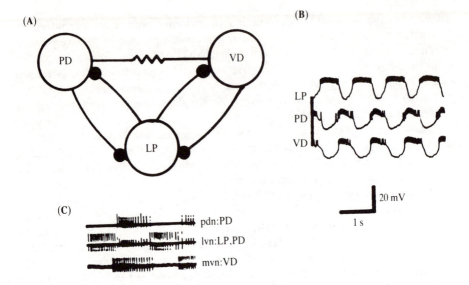

Figure 11.5 Production of patterned activity by a subset of the pyloric network. **A.** The three-cell central pattern generator. Large circles represent single cells. Filled circles are inhibitory chemical synapses. The resistor indicates a gap junction. PD, pyloric dilator; LP, lateral pyloric; VD, ventricular dilator. **B.** Simultaneous recordings of the intracellular potentials of the cells in **A**. This is the pattern that we attempted to model. **C.** Simultaneous extracellular recordings from nerves carrying the motor axons of the neurons in **A**. Note the definite phase relationships of this motor pattern. pdn, pyloric dilator nerve; lvn, lateral ventral nerve; mvn, medial ventral nerve. (Figure reprinted from Miller & Selverston, 1982, by authors' permission.)

intracellular potential), a set of input currents (synaptic, electrotonic and external inputs), and an output V (synaptic activity). The sum of the input currents determines the value of u, and u in turn determines V according to the input-output (I-O) function $V(u)$. Each cell's input is connected to ground through a resistor and a capacitor that simulate the passive resistance and capacitance of the cell membrane. A cell's output is connected to the inputs of other cells through conductances reproducing chemical synapses. The output is inverted for inhibitory synapses. The

Figure 11.6 (opposite) Elements of the model. **A.** Model neuron. The operational amplifier has an input voltage u representing the intracellular potential; a resistor and a capacitor to ground representing the passive cell membrane; a voltage $V(u)$ simulating graded synaptic output; and a set of input currents. I_{syn}, synaptic input from other cells in the network; I_{ext}, steady input from the commissural ganglia; I_{gj}, current from gap junctions. **B.** A schematic diagram of the complete model network, reproducing the connections of the three cells in Figure 11.5A. The operational amplifiers have inverted outputs because all the chemical synapses in the biological network are inhibitory. Filled squares and diamonds are resistors representing chemical and electrical synapses, respectively, with conductances (synaptic strengths) T_{ij} and S_{ij}. u represents intracellular potential and I, the external input from the commissurals. **C.** The sigmoid monotonic input-output relation used for the model neurons. At the half-maximum potential (u_{hm}), the neuron's synaptic activity is half of its maximum value.

(A)

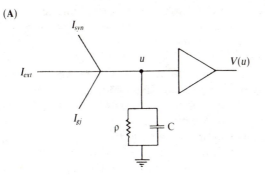

(B)

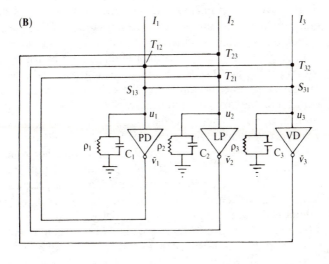

(C)

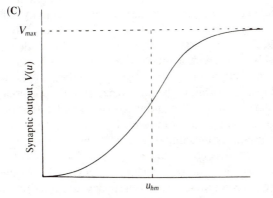

multiple connections of each unit's output to the other cells' inputs makes the ensemble of units into a neural network with positive and/or negative feedback.

We connected three such units into a network (Figure 11.6B) according to the empirically determined circuitry of the pyloric PD-LP-VD central pattern generator (Figure 11.5A), each unit representing a cell. Our network differs from Hopfield's original network by having gap junctions (simulated by resistors between input voltages) and a non-linearly adapting I-O function (discussed below).

The main variables of our model are intracellular potential, u, and transmitter release, $V(u)$. V depends on u according to the sigmoidal curve of Figure 11.6C, increasing from 0 to a maximum value V_{max} as the potential increases from 0 to large positive values. Note that u is the intracellular potential relative to the cell's resting potential (RP), so that RP corresponds to $u = 0$, and positive values of u are depolarizations above RP. As in Hopfield's network, this function is sigmoidal, but we added some modifications suggested by the physiology of these cells.

First of all, our sigmoid is centered around a finite positive value of u (u_{hm}, half-maximal potential) at which transmitter is released at half its maximum rate. The value of u_{hm} is set at 10 - 20 mV above resting potential, so that, with the sigmoid's steepness adjusted accordingly, the cell is almost silent at its lowest potential value, i.e. the trough of the slow wave, which corresponds to the physiological behavior of the pyloric cells.

The other major characteristic peculiar to our I-O relation is its ability to simulate adaptation properties of synaptic activity by shifting horizontally along the u axis in response to changes in the intracellular potential. Suppose a cell's potential is stable at some finite positive value - for example, by steady depolarization from the commissural inputs. Then, as a pulse of depolarizing current is injected into the cell, its potential shifts to the right and $V(u)$ initially increases too. After a delay, however, the value of the half-maximum potential (the sigmoid's center) also shifts to the right, moving the whole sigmoid toward the new value of u and reducing transmitter release. The adaptation is less than linear in the sense that, within physiological ranges, the sigmoid's shift is smaller than the change in potential. Thus, a depolarization produces a net increase in synaptic activity, but with an initial peak followed by a decay to a steady-state value. The effect observed in the post-synaptic cell is a PSP with an initial peak (negative in this case, due to the inhibitory synapse) followed by a decay to a smaller-magnitude steady value (Figure 11.7). The response is symmetrically opposite for hyperpolarizations. In Figure 11.7, there is another downward peak in the post-synaptic cell's potential, which occurs at the end of the depolarizing pulse and is smaller than the first peak. This is not observed in the biological system (Figure 11.7, inset). At this point, we cannot fully explain the presence or meaning of this extra peak. It may be an artefact of the step repolarization which has no bearing on the behavior of the network as a whole, a behavior that consists of continuous changes in potentials. On the other hand, it may be indicative of a more serious discrepancy between our model and the biological system. In any case, we hope to be able to use this discrepancy, as well as others (see Section 11.5.4), to assess more fully the limitations of our model.

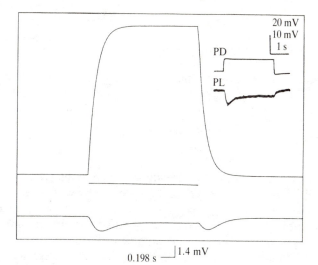

Figure 11.7 Two-cell current pulse experiments. All synapses in the network are suppressed except for the one from PD to LP. Post-synaptic cell's (LP) response to depolarization of pre-synaptic cell (PD) is shown to illustrate the time course of synaptic activity. The shape of the PSP in LP reflects the synaptic output (graded synaptic transmission) of PD. Note the initial downward peak of the response, followed by a higher steady-state value, and the similarity between modified and real responses (inset).

These adaptive properties of the I-O curve were built into the model to simulate analogous properties exhibited by neurons of the stomatogastric ganglion. In two-cell current-pulse experiments in the biological system, the PSP elicited in the post-synaptic cell has a peak-and-steady-value shape similar to that of Figure 11.7, indicating that synaptic activity indeed adapts or fatigues in a similar manner. The presence of an observable decrease in action potential frequencies within bursts (Figure 11.5B) also suggests the presence of an adaptation mechanism. The phenomenon of post-inhibitory rebound, by which a cell's ability to fire at a given potential increases following a steady hyperpolarization, suggests an opposite adaptation behavior for negative potential changes.

The variable that plays the leading role in our model is u_i, the electric potential at the input of unit i. It represents the intracellular potential of the cell which the unit stands for, and it is this variable that we monitor in computer runs of our model as well as in physiological experiments.

Because each unit in our model is represented by an ideal operational amplifier (Figure 11.6A), its input potential u is determined by the simple relationship

current out = current in

or, in our case,

$$I(membrane) = I(syn) + I(gj) + I(ext).$$

Using mathematical expressions for these currents, we get

$$C_i \frac{du_i}{dt} + \frac{u_i}{R_i} = \sum_{j=0}^{2} [T_{ij} V_j(u_j)] + \sum [S_{ij} u_j] + I_i \tag{11.1}$$

which is a first-order non-linear differential equation in the variable u_i. The left-hand side terms are the capacitative and resistive currents between the ith unit's input and ground, representing the currents through the cell membrane due to its passive properties. On the right-hand side, the first term is the sum of synaptic inputs, which are currents given by the product of the neighboring cells' outputs ($V_j(u_j)$) and the strength of the synaptic connections they make with cell i (T_{ij}). Similarly, the second term is the sum of the gap junction currents, with S_{ij} representing the coupling strength between units i and j. Note that both T_{ij} and S_{ij} are 0 when $i = j$, since none of our units makes any synaptic or electrotonic connections with itself. Finally, I_i, the last term on the right, represents the external input from the commissural ganglia.

As one can see from Equation 11.1, the output voltage V (representing rate of transmitter release) of each unit affects the input potential of other units in the network. For each unit with an input potential u, this output is given by

$$V(u) = \frac{Vmax}{2} [1 + tanh\{s(u - u_{hm})\}], \tag{11.2}$$

which gives the sigmoid in Figure 11.6C. s is a parameter providing the steepness of the sigmoid, while u_{hm} (described above) is the potential for half-maximum output.

Since the differential Equation 11.1, governing the behavior of the input potential u of unit i, contains terms (the two sums on the right-hand side) which depend on the value of u for other units, our network as a whole is described by a system of differential equations in the form of Equation 11.1. In our case, there are three such equations, and the computer implementation of our model consisted of a program integrating this system of equations over time by numerical methods.

11.5.3   Results

The model as described produces oscillations (Figure 11.8A) qualitatively similar to those of the biological system. The amplitudes and frequencies are within a factor or two of the corresponding physiological values, and the phase relationships are correct. No action potentials 'ride' the oscillating voltages as they do in the real system, since we excluded action potentials from our model. Graubard *et al.*

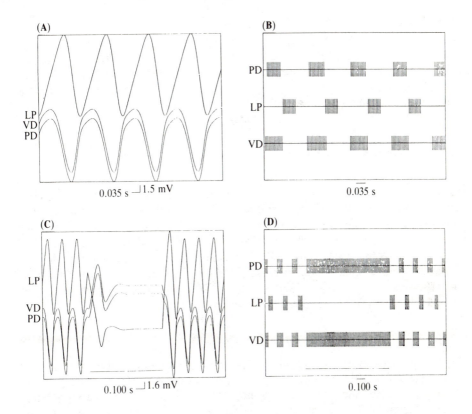

Figure 11.8 Behavior of the model network. **A.** Patterned activity produced by the model network of Figure 11.5B. This record is a simulation of simultaneous intracellular potential recordings in the PD-LP-VD network. Compare with Figure 11.5B. **B.** Simulation of extracellular recordings from the model network. This record was obtained from the intracellular simulation of Figure 11.5A by setting threshold levels for action potential production at each cell's average potential. This type of display was used only as an aid in visualizing the pattern's periods, phase relationships, and responses to current pulses. The action potentials play no role in the model network's activity. **C.** Response of the model network to an external perturbation, in this case, a hyperpolarization of LP. The change in activity of each cell is as expected from the connectivity and as observed in the animal. Also as observed experimentally, the model network returns to its original pattern of activity after the perturbation is over. **D.** Simulated extracellular record of the perturbation experiment of part **C**, obtained from the record in **C** as described in **B**. As observed experimentally, the strong hyperpolarization of LP makes this cell silent, while the release of inhibition on PD and VD induces them to fire tonically.

(1983) have shown that graded transmitter release is sufficient to produce oscillations even in the absence of spikes. The latter seem a consequence rather than a cause of the oscillations, and their importance lies in the production of motor impulses to the muscles.

We did use spikes as a visual aid in the study and comparison of the model's oscillations, however. A threshold for action potentials was set near the average value of each cell's oscillating voltage, and spikes were displayed for potentials above threshold. We thus obtained displays of action potential bursts such as Figure 11.8B, which aid in the quick visualization of period, phase relationships, and the effects of current injections, which can be directly compared to extracellular recordings from the nerves (Figure 11.5C).

11.5.4   Response of the model to perturbations

A model is particularly useful if it can predict the real system's response to external perturbations. In this respect our model has not yet reached the status of a reliably predictive simulation. We perturbed the model by injecting square current pulses into individual cells. The changes observed in the oscillation pattern are similar to those obtained in experiments and expected from the pattern of connections. A hyperpolarization of LP should release its inhibition of the other two cells, whose potentials should increase, hyperpolarizing LP even more. This effect is observed in the model (Figures 11.8C, D), and so is the converse effect (depolarization of LP producing a hyperpolarization of PD and VD).

11.5.5   A word about parameters

Our model belongs to the class of parameter-measured models, that is, it uses parameters obtained from physiological experiments and not arbitrarily adjusted to give the desired behavior (see Hartline, 1987). The parameters we used are all within factors of 2 - 3 of physiological values, which we obtained from our own experiments and from searches through the literature. The physiological values themselves vary by factors of 2 or 3 as well, thus setting a limit on the accuracy of the model. For example, measured values for PD's membrane resistance varied from 7 to 30 megohms, and our model used 10 megohms. Details of the I-O function (its steepness and maximum value) and of its adaptation mechanism could not be measured directly, but were adjusted to reproduce the physiological results of two cell experiments. In other words, we imposed a 2 - 3 factor agreement between model and physiology for the PSP's amplitude, shape, and adaptation time constant, which are together determined by $V(u)$, its adaptation properties, and synaptic strengths. Our model, therefore, is not one in which parameters are adjusted to give one particular fit with an observed behavior, but rather one that reproduces pyloric oscillations using independently measured parameters.

This simple model of a pyloric CPG produces oscillations remarkably similar to the biological CPG's. We have demonstrated that an adaptive synaptic activity function, reciprocal inhibitory connectivity and passive membrane properties are sufficient for the production of physiologically plausible oscillations. Perkel & Mulloney (1974) had shown previously that two cells connected by reciprocal inhibitory and fatiguing synapses can produce alternating bursts of action potentials. Their model, however, required the arbitrary adjustment of a large number of parameters, such as conductances and time delays, for the production of an acceptable pattern. We used a very small number of parameters with physiological values which independently produced an interesting pattern.

We treated the neuron as a computational unit, in the sense of having properties which allow it to interact with other cells to produce behaviors not intuitively predictable from the behavior of the cell alone. These properties are the passive membrane characteristics, an adaptive transmitter release function, and an inhibitory output. They allowed three cells to oscillate steadily when connected according to the anatomy of a biological CPG. Without this or some other adaptive parameter the model would reach a steady non-oscillatory state.

It is important to note that our model network produces oscillations without having any endogenous oscillator built into it. The oscillations appear to be an emergent property of the network as a whole. It was a point of the modeling study to exclude the pyloric cells' endogenous bursting properties, and our demonstration that these are not necessary for generating the basic pattern raises the question of their function in the biological system. In this regard, we must point out that the frequency of our network's oscillations is fixed by the membrane time constant of the simulated neurons. No change in the parameters expected to vary most readily (commissural inputs, synaptic strengths) can change the network's oscillation period. In the biological system, on the other hand, the period changes easily by factors of 3 - 4. The endogenous bursting properties may play a role in these changes by coupling to the oscillations emerging from the network.

Finally, we have obtained oscillations from a modified Hopfield-type neural network. This opens many new computational possibilities. Oscillations involve more variables than the steady outputs of Hopfield's original network, such as period, phase, amplitude and frequency composition, and could thus handle more information in even more interesting ways. For example, different levels of external inputs to our network produce oscillation patterns differing in amplitudes and average levels of potentials. Such possibilities are worth exploring both for the sake of new computational theories for artificial networks of neuron-like units, and for a better understanding of how information is encoded in biological neural networks.

Acknowledgements

This research was supported by ONR award No. N00014-88-K-0328. We thank Lynn Ogden and Iteh Hsieh for technical assistance.

References

Benjamin P.R. (1983) Gastropod feeding: Behavioral and neural analysis of a complex multicomponent system. In: **Neural Origin of Rhythmic Movements**. pp. 159-183, A. Roberts & B.L. Roberts (eds.) Cambridge University Press, Cambridge.

Calabrese R.L. (1979) The role of endogenous membrane properties and synaptic interactions in generating the heartbeat rhythm of the leech *Hirudo medicinalis*. **J. exp. Biol. 82**, pp. 163-176

Delcomyn F. (1980) Neural basis for rhythmic behavior in animals. **Science 210**, pp. 492-498

Favrel P. (1988) Purification et caracterisation biochimique de peptides immunologiquement apparentes aux gastrines/cholecystokinines chez quelques crustaces decapodes: Recherche d'un role biologique. Ph.D. Dissertation, University of Rennes, Concarneau, France.

Getting P.A. (1983) Mechanisms of pattern generation underlying swimming in *Tritonia*. II. Network reconstruction. **J. Neurophysiol. 49**, pp. 1017-1035

Graubard K. (1978) Synaptic transmission without action potentials: Input-output properties of a nonspiking presynaptic neuron. **J. Neurophysiol. 41**, pp. 1014-1025

Graubard K., Raper J.A. & Hartline D.H. (1983) Graded synaptic transmission between identified spiking neurons. **J. Neurophysiol. 50**, pp. 508-521

Harris-Warrick R.M. (1988) Chemical modulation of central pattern generators. In **Neural Control of Rhythmic Movements in Vertebrates**, pp. 285-292, A. Cohen, S. Rossignol & S. Grillner (eds.) John Wiley & Sons, NY.

Hartline D. (1987) Modeling stomatogastric ganglion. In **The Stomatogastric Ganglion**. A.I. Selverston & M. Moulins (eds.) Springer-Verlag, NY.

Heinzel H.G. & Selverston A.I. (1988) Gastric mill activity in the lobster. III. Effects of proctolin on the isolated central pattern generator. **J. Neurophysiol. 59**, pp. 566-585

Hodgkin A.L. & Huxley A.F. (1952) A quantitative description of membrane current and its application to conduction and excitation in nerve. **J. Physiol. (Lond.) 117**, pp. 500-544

Hopfield J.J. & Tank D.H. (1986) Computing with neural circuits: A model. **Science 233**, pp. 625-633

Kater S.B. (1974) Feeding in *Helisoma trivolvis*: The morphological and physiological basis of a fixed action pattern. **Amer. Zool. 14**, pp. 1017-1036

Kennedy D., Selverston A. & Remler M.P. (1967) Analysis of restricted neural networks. **Science 164**, pp. 1488-1496

Marder E. (1987) Neurotransmitters and modulators. In **The Crustacean Stomatogastric System**. pp. 263-306, A.I. Selverston & M. Moulins (eds.) Springer-Verlag, NY.

Marder E., Hooper S.L. & Siwicki K.K. (1986) Modulatory action and distribution of the neuropeptide proctolin in the crustacean stomatogastric nervous system. **J. comp. Neurol. 243**, pp. 454-467

Maynard D.M. (1972) Simpler networks. **Ann. New York Acad. Sci. 193**, pp. 59-72

Miller J.P. & Selverston A.I. (1979) Rapid killing of single cells by irradiation of intracellularly injected dye. **Science 206**, pp. 702-704

Miller J.P. & Selverston A.I. (1982) Mechanisms underlying pattern generation in lobster stomatogastric ganglion. **J. Neurophysiol. 48**, pp. 1416-1432

Nagy F. & Dickinson P. (1983) Control of a central pattern generator by an identified interneurone in Crustacea. I. Modulation of the pyloric output. **J. exp. Biol. 105**, pp. 33-58

Pearson K.G., Reye D.N. & Robertson R.M. (1983) Phase-dependent influences of wing stretch receptors on flight rhythm in the locust. **J. Neurophysiol. 49**, pp. 1168-1181

Perkel D. & Mulloney B. (1974) Motor pattern production in reciprocally inhibitory neurons exhibiting post-inhibitory rebound. **Science 185**, pp. 181-183

Raper J.A. (1979) Non-impulse-mediated synaptic transmission during the generation of a cyclic motor program. **Science 205**, pp. 304-306

Roberts A. & Roberts B.L. (1983) In: **Neural Origin of Rhythmic Movements**. SEB Symposia, Cambridge University Press, Cambridge.

Russell D.F. (1976) Rhythmic excitatory inputs to the lobster stomatogastric ganglion. **Brain Res. 101**, pp. 582-588

Selverston A.I. & Moulins M. (1985) Oscillatory neural networks. **Ann. Rev. Physiol. 47**, pp. 29-48

Tazaki K. & Cooke I.M. (1983) Neuronal mechanisms underlying rhythmic bursts in crustacean cardiac ganglia. In **Neural Origin of Rhythmic Movements**. pp. 129-157, A. Roberts & B.L. Roberts (eds.) Cambridge University Press, Cambridge.

Turrigiano G. & Selverston A.I. (1987) Presence and release of a CCK/gastrin-like molecule in the lobster stomatogastric ganglion. **Soc. Neurosci. Abstr. 13**, p. 1257

Vigna S. (1985) Cholecystokinin and its receptors in vertebrates and invertebrates. **Peptides 6**, pp. 283-287

Wendler G. (1983) The influence of proprioceptive feedback on insect flight coordination. **J. comp. Physiol. 88**, pp. 173-200

Willows A.O.D. (1967) Behavioral acts elicited by stimulation of single, identifiable brain cells. **Science 157**, pp. 570-574

Wilson D.M. (1961) The central nervous control of flight in a locust. **J. exp. Biol. 38**, pp. 471-490

Zipser D. & Andersen R.A. (1988) A back-propagation programmed network that simulates response properties of a subset of posterior parietal neurons. **Nature 331**, pp. 679-684

12

A Mechanism for Switching in the Nervous System: Turning ON Swimming in a Frog Tadpole

Alan Roberts

Summary

In many cases a brief stimulus can lead to a prolonged change in behaviour but it is not clear how the nervous system can switch ON and sustain a prolonged change in motorneuron discharge. An analysis of the anatomy and physiology of neurons in the spinal cord of frog embryos has led to a simple hypothesis to explain how these embryos turn ON and sustain their swimming activity. Reflexes are not required. Sustained rhythm generation depends on short reciprocal inhibition between neurons on either side of the cord, and long, mutual re-excitation among excitatory neurons within each side. The evidence leading to the mutual re-excitation hypothesis is outlined and simulations to test its plausibility are presented. The simulations and experiments make it clear that particular membrane and synaptic properties are critical to the operation of the spinal network underlying swimming.

12.1 Introduction

A common logical function in electronic computation is switching, where a brief command leads to a permanent change of state, from OFF to ON or from ON to OFF. Neurons and the behaviour they control also need to be turned ON and OFF by brief commands. Such sustained responses to brief stimuli are ubiquitous - the eyes move from one fixation point to another, a limb adopts a new posture, an insect flies off when disturbed. Yet in no case is it clear how the brief stimulus leads to a maintained change in motorneuron discharge frequency which far outlasts the stimulus. Typically, neurons are good at continuously converting input into output. As individuals they do not generally show changes of state which continue after the stimulus and yet this is what whole behaving animals do all the time. This may sometimes depend on reflexes, but sustained responses can also occur without them. My aim here is to consider one such case where, in the absence of reflexes, an animal's response far outlasts the stimulus which initiates it. This allows us to ask how an OFF-ON-OFF switching function can be achieved by neurons when they are connected in a simple network.

Young clawed toad tadpoles (*Xenopus laevis*) will swim when touched on the flank. They can then continue swimming for many seconds but usually stop when they bump into something. A motor discharge pattern closely paralleling this behaviour can be recorded in immobilized embryos. This 'fictive' swimming is initiated by a brief touch and can be stopped by pressure on the head skin or cement gland (Kahn *et al.*, 1982; Roberts & Blight, 1975). The animal does not move, so movement related feedback reflexes cannot be involved. Our analysis of the anatomical and physiological basis of this sustained fictive swimming has led to a mutual re-excitation hypothesis to explain how brief stimuli can turn locomotion ON. In this hypothesis, swimming is sustained from cycle to cycle by a mutual synaptic re-excitation within the population of spinal interneurons which drive motorneurons. A form of positive feedback is involved. My aim here is to outline the evidence which led to the hypothesis and to illustrate computer simulations designed to test its plausibility (see also Roberts *et al.*, 1986 for a fuller review of the physiological evidence).

12.2   The physiological evidence: turning ON swimming

Swimming and 'fictive' swimming can be initiated by touching the skin. This excites sensory Rohon-Beard neurons (Clarke *et al.*, 1984) which in turn excite spinal sensory interneurons (Clarke & Roberts, 1984; Sillar & Roberts, 1988 a,b). The excitation is distributed to both sides of the spinal cord producing a long excitatory potential in motorneurons (about 200-300 ms in duration). If large enough this usually leads to impulse firing, beginning with the side opposite the stimulus, while on the same side firing is prevented by a brief inhibition (Figure 12.1) (Clarke & Roberts, 1984; Roberts *et al.*, 1985; Sillar & Roberts, in prep.). There is no evidence for any prolonged firing in the sensory pathways. (After an electrical stimulus to the skin, firing is over within 30 ms.) When stronger stimuli initiate swimming there is therefore no possibility that it continues as a result of continued activity in the sensory pathways.

During 'fictive' swimming we now have substantial evidence that three principal classes of spinal neuron are active: motorneurons (MNs), 'commissural' (C) interneurons, and 'descending' (D) interneurons are all depolarized by 10-20 mV, excited phasically to fire one impulse per swimming cycle, and receive mid-cycle inhibition when their counterparts on the opposite side are active (Figure 12.1) (Roberts & Kahn, 1982; Soffe & Roberts, 1982a,b; Soffe *et al.*, 1984; Roberts *et al.*, 1986). This pattern of motorneuron discharge is suitable to produce the alternating contractions of the trunk muscles which result in swimming. By recording from each cell type we have shown that they all have: rather negative resting potentials (near –75 mV), a non-overshooting impulse, an inability to fire repeatedly when depolarized, an ability to fire on rebound if hyperpolarized during such depolarization, and a common synaptic input during swimming (Figures

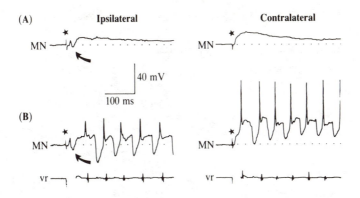

Figure 12.1 Initiation of 'fictive' swimming by stimulation of the trunk skin (at stars) with a 0.5 ms current pulse. Intracellular recordings from a rhythmic neuron (probably a motorneuron, MN) and below a motor root record (vr) from the same side. The top two records show how a stimulus subthreshold for swimming produces a fast rising long excitation on the opposite side to the stimulus (B) and on the same side (A) a similar excitation whose peak is delayed by an early inhibition (at arrow). The lower records show how stronger stimuli lead to 'fictive' swimming where the first impulse usually occurs on the side opposite to the stimulus. In 'fictive' swimming (B) the neuron is depolarized from the resting potential (dots), fires one impulse per cycle (compare with motor root record, vr), and is inhibited with strong hyperpolarization mid-cycle when rhythmic neurons on the opposite side fire. Note: in **A**, depolarizing current was passed into the neuron to accentuate inhibitory potentials. Recordings provided by Dr. K. T. Sillar.

12.2A & B). By recording from pairs of neurons we have examined synaptic connections. 'Commissural' (C) interneurons have glycine-like immunoreactivity (Dale *et al.*, 1986; Roberts *et al.*, 1988) and produce strychnine-sensitive inhibition of neurons on the opposite side of the cord and occasionally also on the same side (Figure 12.2C) (Dale, 1985). 'Descending' (D) interneurons are very likely to be the excitatory interneurons which produce dual-component excitatory post-synaptic potentials (EPSPs) in more caudal neurons on the same side by activating both kainate-quisqualate and NMDA receptors (Figure 12.2D) (Dale & Roberts, 1985). The slow component of these EPSPs is NMDA dependent and longer (200 ms) than the swimming cycle period. The long EPSPs will therefore sum to produce a steady depolarization when repeated at swimming frequencies (10-20 Hz, Figure 12.2E). Motorneurons do not appear to make any strong central connections. In our earlier papers we had assumed that some of the synaptic input needed to produce the rhythmic activity of spinal neurons during 'fictive' swimming would come from hindbrain motor centres (e.g. Kahn & Roberts, 1982). In particular we thought that higher centres would provide a 'tonic drive' to control rhythm production (cf. Brown, 1911). However, recordings showed that all the synaptic inputs seen in intact embryos were still present in spinal preparations (Roberts *et al.*, 1985). We therefore asked whether this could be achieved on the basis of the synaptic connections of 'C' and 'D' interneurons. The simplest proposal was that 'C'

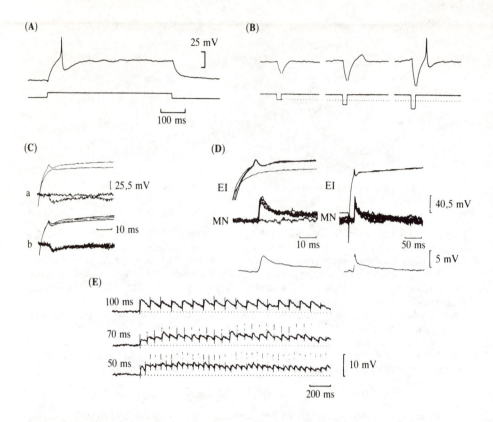

Figure 12.2 Properties and synaptic inputs to rhythmic spinal neurons including motorneurons. **A.** Most spinal rhythmic neurons respond to depolarizing injected current (lower trace) with a single non-overshooting impulse and do not fire repetitively. **B.** Hyperpolarization from the resting potential (near −75 mV) does not lead to rebound firing (not shown), but brief hyperpolarization of a depolarized neuron can lead to a single rebound impulse. (Traces and calibration as A). **Ca,b.** A short, hyperpolarizing inhibitory potential in a rhythmic neuron (lower traces) is produced when an impulse is evoked by current injection into a 'commissural' interneuron (upper traces). This inhibition is blocked by strychnine. **D.** A fast rise, long duration excitatory potential in a motorneuron (MN) is produced when an impulse is evoked in an excitatory interneuron (EI). The records are displayed at two time scales and the bottom traces are averages of 32 synaptic potentials. **E.** When excitatory synaptic potentials in rhythmic neurons are evoked repetitively at intervals similar to the swimming cycle period they can sum to produce a maintained depolarization. This depends on the slow NMDA component of these dual-component potentials. **A & B** from Roberts *et al.* (1986). **C** from Dale (1985). **D & E** from Dale & Roberts (1985).

interneurons inhibited all rhythmically active neurons on the opposite side while 'D' interneurons excited all rhythmically active neurons on the same side. Figure 12.3 summarizes the anatomy and these major connections and shows that 'C' and 'D' interneurons synapse onto members of their own neuron class. 'C' interneurons therefore produce mid-cycle, short duration, reciprocal inhibition across the cord while 'D' interneurons produce cycle-by-cycle, long duration re-excitation of neurons on the same side. If 'D' interneurons could in this way keep neurons on either side depolarized by a summation of the long NMDA component of the EPSPs that they produce (Figure 12.2D & E), then mid-cycle inhibitory post-synaptic potentials from 'C' interneurons could lead to delayed rebound excitation (Figure 12.2B) and keep activity going following stimulation. This simple network could therefore be turned ON by a brief stimulus and, once ON, stay ON until some later stimulus turned it OFF.

The important new proposal in this spinal cord network is the mutual re-excitation among the excitatory 'D' interneurons on each side. This positive feedback within the population of 'D' interneurons eliminates the need for any external source of 'tonic' excitation from higher centres. Since direct experiments based on recordings from pairs of 'D' interneurons have not so far proved possible, how can we evaluate these proposals and test their plausibility? We have used three approaches: pharmacology, lesions and computer simulations. To eliminate the voltage dependent conductance of NMDA receptor channels (Mayer *et al.*, 1984) most of our experiments have been done in Mg^{2+}-free saline. 'Fictive' swimming still occurs but can be prevented by strychnine which blocks glycinergic inhibition, PDA which blocks all three excitatory amino acid receptors, and APV which specifically blocks NMDA receptors (Dale & Roberts, 1984; Roberts *et al.* 1985). We have concluded that inhibition and the long, NMDA component of excitation are both needed for sustained rhythm generation in Mg^{2+}-free saline. Lesions can also interfere with excitation and inhibition. The presumed excitatory 'D' interneurons have mainly descending projections and lie in the rostral cord and caudal hindbrain (Roberts & Clarke, 1982; Roberts and Alford, 1986). Cutting across one half of the spinal cord removes this descending excitation and blocks rhythmic activity on the cut side caudal to the cut (Soffe & Roberts, 1982b). Cutting completely across the hindbrain at progressively more caudal levels removes more and more 'D' interneurons and leads to reduction in both the frequency and episode length of 'fictive' swimming (Roberts & Alford, 1986). The inhibitory 'C' interneurons project mainly to the opposite side, so dividing the nervous system along the midline will cut these axons. When this is done, a single isolated side of the spinal cord with some hindbrain attached can still produce rhythm but in Mg^{2+}-free saline this ability is blocked by strychnine (Kahn & Roberts, 1982; Soffe, in prep.). This evidence indicates that rhythm generation can depend on glycinergic inhibition and can occur within each side of the spinal cord (Figure 12.3) (Dale, 1985). However, recent experiments indicate that in the presence of 1mM Mg^{2+} other forms of rhythmicity exist which are not dependent on inhibition (Soffe, in prep.). The main evidence from pharmacology and lesions is therefore compatible with the connection scheme of Figure 12.3C and with the proposal that in zero Mg^{2+}, rhythm generation depends on rebound from inhibition from 'C' interneurons and is sustained by feedback re-excitation from the population of excitatory 'D' neurons.

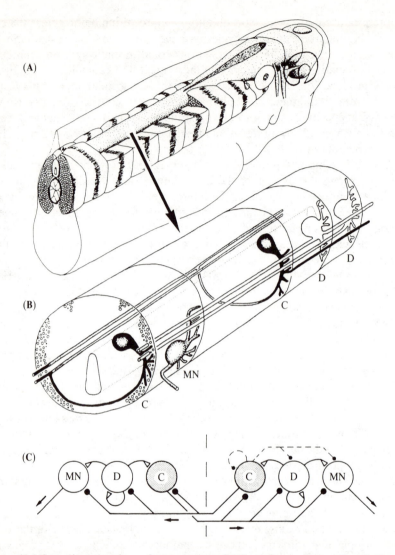

Figure 12.3 Synaptic connections of motorneurons (MN), excitatory 'descending' interneurons (D) and inhibitory 'commissural' interneurons (C) in the spinal cord. **A.** A view of the *Xenopus* embryo at stage 37/38 showing the rostral part with the spinal cord lying between the myotomes or swimming muscles (partly removed). **B.** A diagram of a short length of spinal cord (about 100 μm in diameter) showing examples of the three principal rhythmic neuron classes each with dendrites in the marginal zone of longitudinal axons at the lateral edges of the cord. 'MN' project from the cord to innervate the swimming muscles. 'D' project caudally and rostrally along the cord to excite other rhythmic neurons via axo-dendritic synapses. 'C' project to the opposite side, via the ventral commissure, then branch to run along the cord and make axo-dendritic or -somatic synapses on the opposite side. A few 'C' axons also project along the same side to inhibit rhythmic neurons (and sensory interneurons (Sillar & Roberts, 1988a)). **C.** Diagrammatic scheme to show the main excitatory (open triangles) and inhibitory (closed circles) synaptic contacts **(cont. opposite)**

12.3 Simulating the OFF/ON switch for swimming

The final way in which we have evaluated our proposals is by using the physiological and anatomical evidence to build simple networks representing those in the spinal cord. We have used the 'Manuel' programs designed by D. H. Perkel (late of Department of Psychobiology, University of California, Irvine, California, USA). These allow physiologically realistic modelling of membrane, cell morphological and synaptic properties. We can therefore ask: if we incorporate the properties and connections derived from our experiments on the *Xenopus* spinal cord neurons, will the resulting network be able to generate the 'fictive' swimming pattern and sustain its production after a brief initiating stimulus? [This approach was attempted using a system of programs which did not allow such physiological accuracy and while the resulting network with mutual re-excitation could generate sustained responses these were not the stable alternations seen during 'fictive' swimming (Roberts *et al.*, 1984)]. The first step in the simulation process was to produce 'neurons' with appropriate membrane properties. We have done this by using a three compartment model. This has an axon with properties like the squid giant axon (Hodgkin & Huxley, 1952) with a soma and dendrite which are similar but with reduced Na+ and K+ conductances (Figure 12.4B). If depolarizing current is injected into the soma of this 'neuron' a non-overshooting impulse is evoked when threshold is exceeded. There is no repetitive firing during depolarization, but short hyperpolarizations can evoke single impulses on rebound (Roberts *et al.*, 1986). Synapses are made onto the soma or dendrite. Inhibitory synapses activate a brief conductance increase with a Nernst potential at –80 mV, 5 mV more negative than the –75 mV resting potential (Soffe, 1987). Excitatory synapses activate a fast rising but slowly falling conductance with a Nernst potential at 0 mV. This models the dual-component excitatory potentials seen in Mg^{2+}-free saline which have a prolonged NMDA component (Dale & Roberts, 1985). The synaptic potentials (PSPs) resulting from these conductances are similar in time course to unitary PSPs (Figure 12.2) but were increased in amplitude to correspond to the sizes of compound PSPs seen during swimming or its initiation (Figure 12.4E).

Once the cell and synapse properties showed a good match with the evidence from the spinal cord, model neurons were connected following the scheme of Figure 12.3, but amalgamating inhibitory and excitatory neurons and omitting the motorneurons (Figure 12.5A). The network was stimulated, as it would be normally, by the sensory pathways - one side received a synaptic excitation and the other side received the same excitation after a delay of 25 ms (cf. Figures 12.1 and 12.5). If the initiating excitation was large enough an impulse was evoked on each side. As a result, first, reciprocal inhibition was produced and, second, the neurons excited themselves (Figure 12.5B). If the feedback excitation or the reciprocal

(**Fig. 12.3 cont.**) between populations of neurons in the spinal cord. Each large circle represents the whole population (longitudinal column) of each neuron class on one side of the spinal cord. Compare with anatomy in B and see text. The weak dashed lines indicate contacts made by a minority of 'C' neurons onto neurons on the same side. A is based on a drawing by Dr. S. R. Soffe.

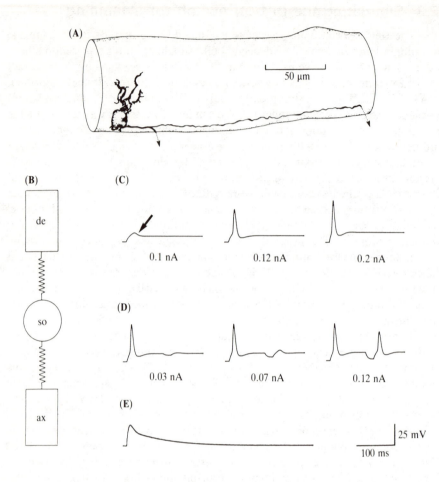

Figure 12.4 Simulating the responses and synaptic input to rhythmic neurons. **A.** A typical large motorneuron drawn after backfilling with horseradish peroxidase and viewed from the side. It has dorsal dendrites, a ventral soma and a caudally directed axon which exits in two places (arrowheads) to innervate the swimming muscles. **B.** The simulated neuron has 3 resistively coupled compartments representing the dendrites (de), soma (so) and axon (ax). Further details in text. **C.** When depolarizing current is injected into the soma a single non-overshooting impulse can be evoked in the soma (see Figure 12.2A). There is no repetitive firing because soma and dendrite membrane is relatively inexcitable and has a voltage dependent K+ channel, apparent from the drop in voltage response at 0.1 nA (arrow). **D.** If brief hyperpolarizing current is injected into the soma during depolarization single impulses can be evoked on rebound (see Figure 12.2B). **E.** When a single excitatory synaptic potential occurs in the dendrite, the response in the soma is as shown. A from Roberts & Clarke, 1982. **B to D** Roberts & Tunstall, unpublished.

(A)

(B)

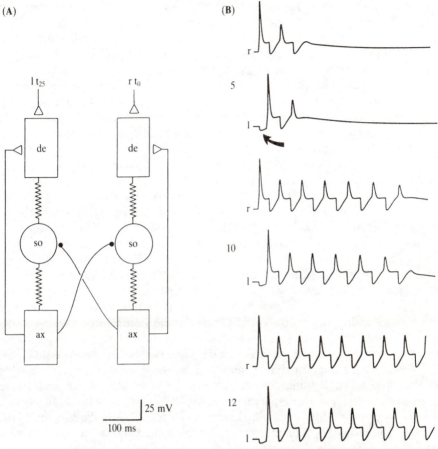

Figure 12.5 Simulating neuron activity during 'fictive' swimming. **A.** The reduced 2 'neuron' network with short duration reciprocal inhibition (closed circles), and long duration self-excitation (open triangles). Each 'neuron' represents the population of excitatory *and* inhibitory (D and C) neurons on one side of the spinal cord. Activity is initiated by a single long excitation (200 ms) of the form in Figure 12.4E, given at 0 ms to the right side (r_t0) and 25 ms later to the left side (l_{t25}). **B.** Shows simulated activity in the soma (so) on left (l) and right (r) sides when a stimulus is given to the left side. The strength of self re-excitation (arbitrary units) was increased from 5 (top) to 12 (bottom) when it was sufficient to produce self-sustaining swimming activity (compare Figure 12.1B). When self re-excitation is weaker the excitation at right side (0 ms) leads to an impulse. This produces reciprocal inhibition on the left (arrow, see Figure 12.1A), and self re-excitation to hold the right neuron depolarized. When the left neuron is excited at 25 ms its impulse produces inhibition of the right neuron. The form and short duration of the inhibitory potential are clear and lead to a rebound impulse which completes one cycle of activity. The second cycle is not completed because the self re-excitation is insufficient. As this is increased (to 10 units) the number of cycles increases to become self-sustaining at values over 12 (lowest 2 records). From Roberts & Tunstall, unpublished.

inhibition was too weak then no further impulses occurred. However, when both were sufficient, a single impulse occurred on rebound from each inhibition and the activity became self sustaining (Figure 12.5B). This form of network will generate alternating impulse discharge over a wide range of inhibitory and excitatory synaptic strengths, even if excitation and inhibition are asymmetric on the two sides.

A more complete network with separate excitatory and inhibitory neurons on each side showed similarly robust rhythm generation after a brief initiating excitation. The simulations therefore show that the mechanisms proposed could provide a sufficient basis for rhythmic pattern generation underlying swimming in the *Xenopus* embryo spinal cord. In particular, although a number of simplifications are made, the network with only two neuron types can show a switching function and be turned from OFF to ON by a simple, brief command.

In the simulations some major simplifications have been made. The most important is that single neurons have been used to represent populations. Variation in the swimming cycle period would normally depend on the number of excitatory 'D' interneurons firing on each cycle (Roberts & Alford, 1986). The number firing will depend on the amount of excitation and the range of firing thresholds within the population. However, as the number of excitatory 'D' neurons firing is increased, the number of inhibitory 'C' neurons firing is likely to rise as well. Unfortunately it is not at all clear how one can experimentally treat these possibilities except through more large scale simulations, or with rather crude lesion techniques. Another simplification is the omission of some known synaptic connections such as those that inhibitory 'C' interneurons make on the same side of the spinal cord (Figure 12.3C). These are implicated in the ability of one single side of the spinal cord to generate prolonged rhythmic activity (Soffe, in prep.). Finally, all the work I have described is directed to preparations in Mg^{2+}-free saline where the voltage dependency of the NMDA activated channels is blocked. As in the lamprey spinal cord, it is now very likely that rhythm production in the *Xenopus* embryo also has a contribution from the voltage dependent properties of these synaptic channels (Wallén & Grillner, 1987; Soffe, in prep.).

12.4 Conclusion: the operation of an OFF/ON switch

The physiological and anatomical evidence from the *Xenopus* embryo spinal cord has suggested a mechanism for the operation of a neuronal switch which controls swimming behaviour. The simulations show that this mechanism could work on the basis of the membrane properties and synaptic connections of spinal cord neurons. In essence the mutual-re-excitation hypothesis replaces the 'tonic drive', which is a common feature of many other locomotor generator proposals from Brown (1911) onwards (see Grillner, 1975), with a cycle-by-cycle self re-excitation. This positive feedback is controlled by neuron membrane properties which limit repeated firing, and by inhibition which also provides a mechanism of delayed excitation. The OFF/ON switch for *Xenopus* swimming therefore depends on two classes of neurons, excitatory and inhibitory.

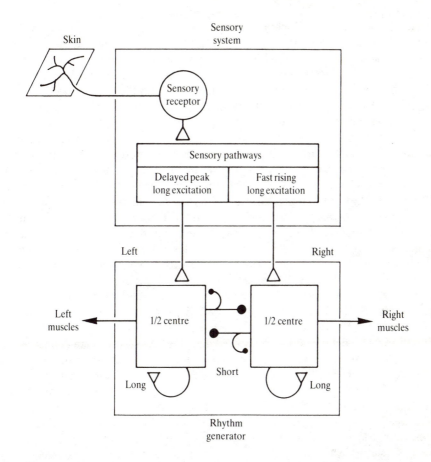

Figure 12.6 Diagram to summarize the spinal cord circuitry which turns ON swimming activity. The sensory receptors respond to touch. The sensory pathways deliver a long (200 ms) excitation to both sides. The rhythmic spinal neurons in each half centre (side of the cord) excite neurons in their own half centre and inhibit neurons in the other half centre. (There is also some inhibition within each half centre indicated by smaller filled circles.) As a result of self re-excitation and delayed excitation following rebound from inhibition, activity in the rhythm generator can be self-sustaining once started. Open triangles: synapses producing long NMDA-dependent excitation. Closed circles: synapses producing short glycinergic inhibition.

The switch operates as follows (see Figure 12.6). A touch to the skin excites a small number of sensory neurons which then excite many sensory pathway interneurons along the same side of the spinal cord. These amplify the signal and produce a fast rising long excitation (200 ms) on the opposite side and a similar excitation with a delayed peak on the same side (Figure 12.1). Rhythmic neurons are excited and all of them will only fire once when depolarized. On each side the rhythmic cells form a half centre and fire together (but with a slight rostro-caudal delay). When the excitatory 'D' neurons fire they produce a long (200 ms) excitation of all types of rhythmic neuron on the same side of the spinal cord (C, D and MN), so all neurons are excited just after they fire. However, they do not fire again because firing is limited by their particular membrane properties. When inhibitory 'C' neurons fire, they produce a short (25 to 50 ms) inhibition of all rhythmic neurons (C, D and MN) in the half centre on the opposite side. If these neurons are still depolarized by the long re-excitation, the inhibition will result in delayed, rebound excitation and firing (Figures 12.2, 12.4 and 12.5).

The spinal cord network, based on interconnections between longitudinal columns of the excitatory (D) and inhibitory (C) neurons, will generate self-sustaining activity following a single brief input. It therefore acts as an OFF/ON switch. The embryo normally stops swimming when its head bumps into something (Roberts & Blight, 1975) and evidence is now available to suggest that normally this activates GABA-ergic (gamma-aminobutyric acid) inhibition which turns OFF the switch (Boothby & Roberts, 1988). Even if the full mechanism for rhythm generation involves other additional mechanisms, for example a membrane based rhythmicity involving voltage dependent NMDA receptor activated channels (Soffe, in prep.) our evidence still suggests that activity is maintained by mutual re-excitation. This re-excitation always involves an NMDA-dependent slow component (Dale & Roberts, 1984, 1985). This type of re-excitation was not present in another related proposal made by Perkel and Mulloney (1974). In a hypothetical model network they showed that when two neurons are connected by reciprocal inhibition they will produce self-sustaining alternating discharge, provided that inhibition (hyperpolarization) leads to rebound firing *from the resting potential*. This is not the case for *Xenopus* embryo neurons. More recently, the continuous swimming of a small pelagic marine mollusc, *Clione*, has been shown to depend on this principle (Arshavsky *et al.*, 1985; Satterlie, 1985). However, in this animal swimming is permanently turned ON, and can only be temporarily stopped by certain stimuli.

I have described a simple switching mechanism to turn ON swimming in the *Xenopus* embryo. The spinal cord circuitry for swimming rhythm generation appears to be able to sustain its own activity by a form of positive feedback within a population of neurons which I have called mutual re-excitation. Brief sensory stimuli can therefore easily affect this 'swimming machine' to turn it ON or OFF or adjust its operation. It is I think surprising, firstly, how simple the basic network is, and secondly, how difficult it has been to obtain direct evidence on the mechanisms, even in such a simple system. It is clear that the embryo is an extreme case. Its pattern of activity during 'fictive' swimming is faster than in most larger animals. During its 'fictive' swimming sensory feedback has so far not been demonstrated. However, in nearly all studied cases of more complex animals, sensory feedback is a central feature of all movements. This, again, makes the unravelling of basic mechanisms even more difficult. However, I suspect that we will find that mutual re-excitation will be a basic mechanism for behavioural switching, and maintaining responses *after* stimulation. It relates broadly to the rather discredited ideas of reverberatory circuits first raised in motor systems (Ranson & Hinsey, 1930), championed by Lorente de Nó (1935) and then made a part of learning theory by

Hebb (1949). However, evidence is now emerging from hippocampal slices which suggests that mutual re-excitation mechanisms exist (e.g. Miles & Wong, 1986). Regardless of where neuronal activity needs to be maintained, some form of positive feedback seems the most obvious suggestion. In general, people have been afraid of it, but our simple spinal network simulations, based on careful physiological modelling, show sensible, robust behaviour. Similar principles may well underlie many other cases where OFF/ON switching or maintained changes in firing frequency are required.

Acknowledgements

I would like to acknowledge the role that the late D.H. Perkel played in making the simulations reported here possible, and to thank Dave Rogers, Mike Oram and Mark Tunstall for extensive help with computation in Bristol. Thanks are also due to my colleagues Drs Steve Soffe and Keith Sillar for advice, and to the SERC, MRC, Nuffield Foundation and Wellcome Trust for financial support.

References

Arshavsky Y.I., Beloozerova I.N., Orlovsky G.N., Panchin Y.N. & Pavlova G.A. (1985) Control of locomotion in marine mollusc *Clione limacina* III. On the origin of locomotory rhythm. **Exp. Brain Res. 58**, pp. 273-284

Boothby K.M. & Roberts A. (1988) Descending GABA neurones inhibit swimming in the amphibian embryo, *Xenopus laevis*. **J. Physiol. (Lond.) 401**, p. 38P

Brown T.G. (1911) The intrinsic factor in the progression of the mammal. **Proc. R. Soc. Lond. B 84**, pp. 308-319

Clarke J.D.W., Hayes B.P., Hunt S.P. & Roberts A. (1984) Sensory physiology anatomy and immunohistochemistry of Rohon Beard neurones in embryos of *Xenopus laevis*. **J. Physiol. (Lond.) 348**, pp. 511-525

Clarke J.D.W. & Roberts A. (1984) Interneurones in the *Xenopus* embryo spinal cord: Sensory excitation and activity during swimming. **J. Physiol. (Lond.) 354**, pp. 345-362

Dale N. (1985) Reciprocal inhibitory interneurones in the *Xenopus* embryo spinal cord. **J. Physiol. (Lond.) 363**, pp. 61-70

Dale N. & Roberts A. (1984) Excitatory amino acid receptors in *Xenopus* embryo spinal cord and their role in the activation of swimming. **J. Physiol. (Lond.) 348**, pp. 527-543

Dale N & Roberts A. (1985) Dual-component amino acid-mediated synaptic potentials: Excitatory drive for swimming in *Xenopus* embryos. **J. Physiol. (Lond.) 363**, pp. 35-59

Dale N., Ottersen O.P., Roberts A. & Storm-Mathiesen J. (1986) Inhibitory neurones of a motor pattern generator in *Xenopus* revealed by antibodies to glycine. **Nature 324**, pp. 255-257

Grillner S. (1975) Locomotion in vertebrates: central mechanisms and reflex interaction. **Physiol. Revs. 35**, pp. 247-304

Hebb D.O. (1949) **The Organisation of Behaviour.** Chapman and Hall, London.

Hodgkin A.L. & Huxley A.F. (1952) A quantitative description of membrane current and its application to conduction and excitation in nerve. **J. Physiol. (Lond.) 117**, pp. 500-544

Kahn J.A. & Roberts A. (1982) Experiments on the central pattern generator for swimming in amphibian embryos. **Phil. Trans. R. Soc. B 296**, pp. 229-243

Kahn J.A., Roberts A. & Kashin S.M. (1982) The neuromuscular basis of swimming movements in embryos of the amphibian *Xenopus laevis*. **J. exp. Biol. 99**, pp. 175-184

Lorente de Nó, R. (1935) Facilitation of motoneurons. **Amer. J. Physiol. 113**, pp. 505-523

Mayer M.L., Westbrook G.L. & Guthrie P.B. (1984) Voltage-dependent block by Mg^{2+} of NMDA responses in spinal cord neurones. **Nature 309**, pp. 261-263

Miles R. & Wong R.K.S. (1986) Excitatory synaptic interactions between CA3 neurons in the guinea-pig hippocampus. **J. Physiol. (Lond.) 373**, pp. 397-418

Perkel D.H. & Mulloney B. (1974) Motor pattern production in reciprocally inhibitory neurons exhibiting post-inhibitory rebound. **Science 185**, pp. 181-183

Ranson S.W. & Hinsey J.C. (1930) Reflexes in the hind limbs of cats after transection of the spinal cord at various levels. **Amer. J. Physiol. 94**, pp. 471-495

Roberts A. & Alford S.T. (1986) Descending projections and excitation during fictive swimming in *Xenopus* embryos: neuroanatomy and lesion experiments. **J. comp. Neurol. 250**, pp. 253-261

Roberts A. & Blight A.R. (1975) Anatomy, physiology and behavioural role of sensory nerve endings in the cement gland of embryonic *Xenopus*. **Proc. R. Soc. Lond. B 192**, pp. 111-127

Roberts A. & Clarke J.D.W. (1982) The neuroanatomy of an amphibian embryo spinal cord. **Phil. Trans. R. Soc. B 296**, pp. 195-212

Roberts A., Dale N., Ottersen O-P. & Storm-Mathison J. (1988) Development and characterization of commissural interneurons in the spinal cord of *Xenopus laevis* revealed by antibodies to glycine. **Development 103**, pp. 447-461

Roberts A., Dale N., Evoy W.H. & Soffe S.R. (1985) Synaptic potentials in motoneurons during fictive swimming in spinal *Xenopus* embryos. **J. Neurophysiol. 54**, pp. 1-10

Roberts A., Dale N. & Soffe S.R. (1984) Sustained responses to brief stimuli: swimming in *Xenopus* embryos. **J. exp. Biol. 112**, pp. 321-335

Roberts A. & Kahn J.A. (1982) Intracellular recordings from spinal neurons during 'swimming' in paralysed amphibian embryos. **Phil. Trans. R. Soc. B 296**, pp. 229-243

Roberts A., Soffe S.R. & Dale N. (1986) Spinal interneurons and swimming in frog embryos. In: **Neurobiology of vertebrate locomotion**. S. Grillner, R. Herman, P.S.G. Stein & D. Stuart (eds.) Macmillan, London.

Satterlie R.A. (1985) Reciprocal inhibition and postinhibitory rebound produce reverberation in a locomotor pattern generator. **Science 229**, pp. 402-404

Sillar K.T. & Roberts A. (1988a) A neuronal mechanism for sensory gating during locomotion in a vertebrate. **Nature 331**, pp. 262-265

Sillar K.T. & Roberts A. (1988b) Unmyelinated cutaneous afferent neurons activate two types of excitatory amino acid receptor in the spinal cord of *Xenopus laevis* embryos. **J. Neurosci. 8**, pp. 1350-1360

Soffe S.R. (1987) Ionic and pharmacological properties of reciprocal inhibition in *Xenopus* embryo motoneurons. **J. Physiol. (Lond.) 382**, pp. 463-473

Soffe S.R., Clarke J.D.W. & Roberts A. (1984) Activity of commissural interneurons in spinal cord of *Xenopus* embryos. **J. Neurophysiol. 51**, pp. 1257-1267

Soffe S.R. & Roberts A. (1982a) Tonic and phasic synaptic inputs to spinal cord motoneurons active during fictive locomotion in frog embryos. **J. Neurophysiol. 48**, pp. 1279-1288

Soffe S.R. & Roberts A. (1982b) The activity of myotomal motoneurons during fictive swimming in frog embryos. **J. Neurophysiol. 48**, pp. 1274-1278

Wallén P. & Grillner S. (1987) N-methyl-D-aspartate receptor induced, inherent oscillatory activity in neurons active during fictive locomotion in the lamprey. **J. Neurosci. 7**, 2745-2755

13
Reflex Circuits and the Control of Movement

Malcolm Burrows & Giles Laurent

13.1 Introduction

The problem to be addressed in this chapter is how the sensory signals generated by mechanoreceptors on one leg of the locust are processed in the central nervous system so that an appropriate adjustment of posture or locomotion is produced. We will first show how these pathways are designed to allow local adjustments of one leg, and then how the movements of this leg are integrated with those of the other legs so that an adaptive behaviour of the whole animal is possible. Finally we will show that these problems are of general importance in the design and functioning of circuits that must produce a patterned output capable of change. The design solutions will be illustrated by reference to the properties of known interneurones and the ways that they are connected to form reflex pathways that are responsible for the modification of movements by a locust hindleg. The emerging principles of information flow in local networks will then be summarized.

13.1.1 The integrative problem

Some 10 000 sensory axons from each of the 2 hindlegs of a locust converge onto the metathoracic ganglion which is the segmental ganglion for the last thoracic segment. Many of these afferents are from different types of mechanoreceptors that provide information about touch, strain in the cuticle and about movement of the joints. In sharp contrast, no more than about 100 motor neurones are responsible for generating the complex patterns of muscular contractions required in locomotion and in adjusting posture of one leg. Considerable convergence and integration is therefore indicated and much of this must be carried out locally in the segmental ganglion. Each half of the metathoracic ganglion contains no more than 1000 interneurones and of these, more than half have no axons and have branches (neurites) restricted entirely to this ganglion. These local interneurones are of two physiological types: those which normally produce action potentials, *spiking* local interneurones, and those which do not normally produce action potentials, *nonspiking* local interneurones. Other types of interneurone have axons that project to adjacent ganglia in the segmental chain and are called intersegmental or projection interneurones. They receive sensory stimuli from the front and middle legs or other parts of the body, and project to the metathoracic ganglion. These local and intersegmental neurones provide the basic framework within which motor actions must be organized on a short time scale, but the many neurosecretory cells that are present must be expected to exert longer term 'modulatory' influences.

Specific local reflexes can be evoked by stimulation of specific arrays of receptors indicating that the spatial information provided by the mechanoreceptors on a leg is preserved (Siegler & Burrows, 1986). For example, touching hairs on the dorsal surface of the tibia causes the trochanter to levate and move the femur forwards, the tibia to flex and the tarsus to levate (Figure 13.1A). Touching hairs a few millimetres away on the ventral tibia causes the opposite sequence of movements (Figure 13.1B). These reflexes are organized locally by the segmental ganglion but can normally only take place in the context of the movements of the other legs. Two layers of organization must therefore be considered: the local circuits within a ganglion and the intersegmental influences which place the effects of these local circuits in a broader context. To understand these different levels of organization, answers must be sought to the following questions:

1) How are the local reflex pathways organized so that spatial information is preserved and the small number of motor neurones controlled to produce movements that are precise, delicate and adaptive?

2) How is the gain of these reflex pathways adjusted so that the movements are appropriate for different circumstances?

3) How are the local reflex pathways modified so that the movements of one leg are appropriate in the context of the movements of the other legs?

Finally from this analysis of circuit connections and interneuronal properties we can ask whether any general principles emerge about the organization of the pathways or about the integrative action of individual neurones.

13.2 Analysis of the neural networks

13.2.1 *Processing of afferent signals*

Afferents diverge to connect both with several members of a particular class of neurone and with members of different classes of neurone. Considerable parallel processing therefore occurs. Spiking local interneurones play a prominent initial role in this processing (Figure 13.1C-E). Moving a hair evokes a burst of spikes in its only afferent neurone, which is followed by a depolarization and sometimes a spike in a spiking local interneurone belonging to a ventral midline population (Figure 13.1C) (Siegler & Burrows, 1983, 1984). Each afferent spike is followed, after a short and constant latency, by an excitatory post-synaptic potential (EPSP) in the interneurone (Figure 13.1D). The connection would appear to be direct and

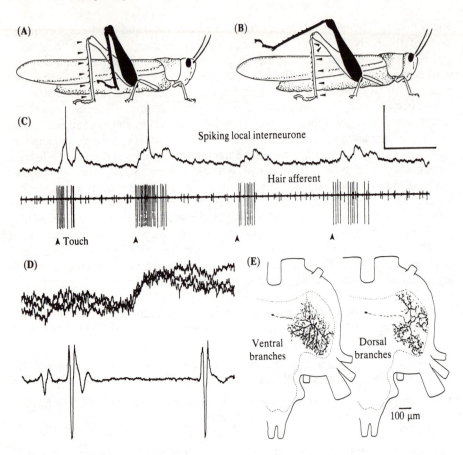

Figure 13.1 Spiking local interneurones preserve spatial information from exteroceptors. A,B. Local reflexes elicited by touching hairs on a hindleg. The arrows show the hairs that are touched, and the silhouettes the resulting reflex movement of the hindleg. C. The spikes of a single hair afferent are associated with depolarizations of a spiking local interneurone. D. Each afferent spike is followed at a constant latency by an EPSP in the interneurone. The upper trace shows 3 superimposed EPSPs, the lower trace a single sweep of the afferent spikes. The sweeps are triggered from the first, large afferent spike (arrow). E. A drawing to show the morphology of a spiking local interneurone stained by the intracellular injection of cobalt. Half of the metathoracic ganglion is shown. The ventral branches of the interneurone are on the left and its more dorsal branches on the right. Calibration: horizontal C 500 ms, D 12.5 ms; vertical C 10 mV, D 2.5 mV.

chemically mediated. All the interneurones in this group have cell bodies at the ventral midline, primary neurites in a particular ventral commissure and extensive branches in the most ventral regions of neuropil to which hair afferents also project. These ventral branches are linked by a thin process to a sparser array of branches in more dorsal regions where motor neurones also project (Figure 13.1E). An

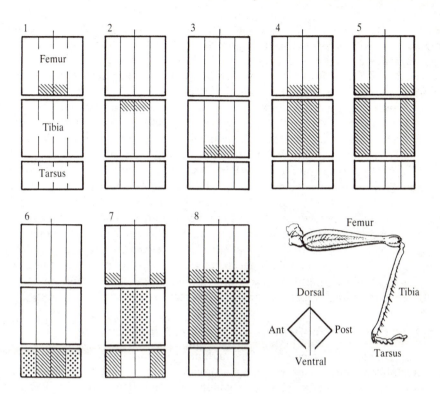

Figure 13.2 The receptive fields of 8 spiking local interneurones. All receive inputs from exteroceptors on one hindleg which is shown as if opened by a ventral midline incision and then laid flat. The femur, tibia and tarsus are each divided into four quadrants. Regions of the leg providing excitation are hatched and those providing inhibition are stippled.

individual interneurone has a distinctive shape that is an elaboration of this basic ground plan. Electron microscopy of these interneurones, intracellularly labelled with horseradish peroxidase, shows the ventral branches to have predominantly input synapses, and the dorsal branches to have mostly output synapses (Watson & Burrows, 1985). Some polarization of function within these neurones is therefore indicated, but the juxtaposition of some input and output synapses suggests that local modification of either the input or output signals can still occur.

A particular interneurone receives inputs only from specific arrays of receptors (Burrows, 1985; Burrows & Siegler, 1985). The distribution of these receptors therefore defines the receptive field of an interneurone (Figure 13.2). A receptive field can be small, often associated with an area of cuticle near a joint, or can be more extensive, sometimes encompassing one surface of the leg. Some receptive fields contain inhibitory regions that result from interactions in the central nervous system and not from direct, inhibitory afferent inputs. A result of this organization is that one region of the leg will be represented in the receptive fields of several interneurones, so that parallel and distributed processing within this class of interneurone will occur. For example, touching the distal, dorsal tibia will affect interneurones 3, 4, 7 and 8 (Figure 13.2). Moreover, the spatial information provided by the receptors will be preserved by this arrangement. For example, information from receptors on the dorsal tibia that is required for the execution of the local reflex in Figure 13.1A, is preserved by interneurone 4 (Figure 13.2).

In addition to the connections made with spiking local interneurones, mechanoreceptive afferents also make parallel connections with other classes of neurone. In particular, widespread direct connections are made with non-spiking local interneurones (Figure 13.3A) (Burrows *et al.*, 1988; Laurent & Burrows, 1988b). A few afferents also connect directly with motor neurones in some larval (Weeks & Jacobs, 1987) and adult (Laurent & Hustert, 1988) insects (Figure 13.3B). Finally, afferents connect directly with intersegmental interneurones so that information about events in one leg is conveyed to ganglia controlling other legs (Figure 13.3C) (Laurent, 1988; Laurent & Burrows, 1988a). A single afferent may thus make divergent and direct connections with at least four classes of neurone (Figure 13.3D). The question now is how the integrated sensory information is delivered to the motor neurones to produce a coordinated movement of the leg.

13.2.2 *Output connections of the local interneurones*

Spiking local interneurones of the midline group make a restricted number of direct inhibitory connections with motor neurones that innervate leg muscles (Figure 13.4) (Burrows & Siegler, 1982). Touching a single hair evokes spikes in a particular spiking local interneurone and inhibitory post-synaptic potentials (IPSPs) in a specific motor neurone (Figure 13.4A). Each spike is followed after a short and constant latency by an IPSP, indicating that the connection is direct and chemically mediated (Figure 13.4B). Only the spike is able to produce a measurable voltage change in the post-synaptic motor neurone so that there is no evidence for graded release of transmitter. A more widespread series of inhibitory connections is made with non-spiking interneurones (Burrows, 1987) and with intersegmental interneurones (Laurent, 1987b) (Figure 13.4C). These spiking local interneurones therefore:

1) collate afferent information from arrays of receptors while preserving spatial information (Siegler & Burrows, 1986).

2) reverse the sign of the afferent signal from excitatory to inhibitory (Burrows & Siegler, 1982; Burrows, 1987).

3) delimit and enhance the borders of the receptive fields of non-spiking and intersegmental interneurones through lateral inhibition (Burrows, 1987; Laurent, 1987b).

4) exclude the action of non-spiking interneurones whose motor effects would be inappropriate for a particular motor response, and disinhibit those whose action would be appropriate (Burrows, 1987).

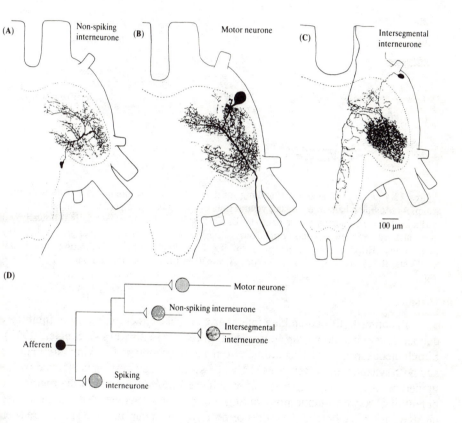

Figure 13.3 Divergent connections of afferents from exteroceptors with different classes of neurones. **A-C.** Drawings of representatives of 3 of these classes of neurone: **A**. non-spiking interneurone: **B**. flexor tibiae motor neurone: **C**. intersegmental interneurone with an ascending axon. **D**. Diagram of the excitatory connections (triangles) made by mechanosensory afferents. Each of the connections has been established by electrophysiological analysis, but an individual afferent may not connect with all the types of neurone shown. The same constraints apply to flow diagrams shown in subsequent figures.

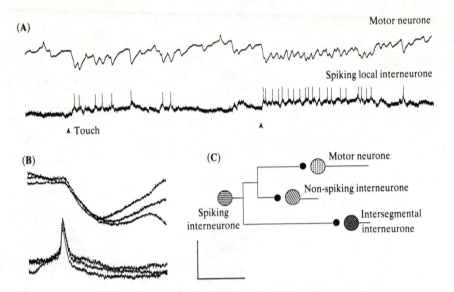

Figure 13.4 Output connections of spiking local interneurones belonging to a ventral midline group. A. Moving a hair on the distal, ventral tibia evokes spikes in a particular interneurone and IPSPs in the levator tarsus motor neurone. B. Each spike in the interneurone is followed by a short latency IPSP in the motor neurone. C. Flow diagram of the divergent, inhibitory connections (filled circles) made by a spiking local interneurone. Calibration: horizontal A 500 ms, B 7.5 ms; vertical, interneurone A 5 mV, B 1.6 mV, motor neurone A 25 mV, B 6 mV.

In contrast, the non-spiking interneurones make either excitatory or inhibitory connections with the motor neurones (Figure 13.5) (Burrows & Siegler, 1978). Simultaneous intracellular recordings from a pre-synaptic non-spiking interneurone and post-synaptic motor neurones show that synaptic transmission is effected by the graded release of chemical transmitter (Figure 13.5A). Changes in the membrane potential of a pre-synaptic non-spiking interneurone cause graded and sustained changes in the membrane potentials of post-synaptic neurones. No spikes are seen in the pre-synaptic interneurone and signals of only a few millivolts are required to effect release of transmitter so that small sustained shifts of its membrane potential will result in tonic release. The outputs of these interneurones converge on groups of motor neurones and each motor neurone in turn is driven by several interneurones (Figure 13.5B) (Burrows, 1980). Electron microscopy shows that the input and output synapses of a non-spiking interneurone can be closely apposed on the same neurite (Watson & Burrows, 1988). The action of these non-spiking interneurones is to organize the motor neurones into sets whose combined action would be a component of a normal movement. By virtue of its pattern of connections each interneurone controls a particular set of motor neurones, though there is considerable overlap between these sets. Furthermore, some of the non

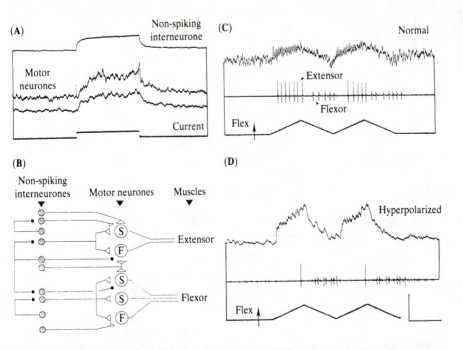

Figure 13.5 The role of non-spiking interneurones in local reflexes. **A**. Depolarizing a non-spiking interneurone with a pulse of current causes a depolarization of two post-synaptic motor neurones. **B**. Some of the connections made by non-spiking interneurones with flexor and extensor tibiae motor neurones of a hindleg. Only 3 flexor motor neurones are shown. S = Slow, F = Fast motor neurone. Note the one-way, lateral inhibitory connections between some of the non-spiking interneurones. **C,D**. A local reflex is changed when the membrane potential of a non-spiking interneurone is altered. **C**. At normal membrane potential, movement of the tibia (3rd trace) evokes a depolarization of the interneurone (1st trace) and strong resistance reflexes in muscles that move the tibia (myograms on the 2nd trace). **D**. Hyperpolarizing the interneurone reduces the frequency of extensor spikes during the imposed movement. Calibration: horizontal A 330 ms, C, D 500 ms; vertical, A motor neurone 4 mV, interneurone 40 mV, current 35 nA, C,D 4 mV.

spiking interneurones make inhibitory connections with other non-spiking interneurones (Burrows, 1979) which can have two effects:

1) they inhibit interneurones that excite certain motor neurones, whose contribution to the movement will thereby be excluded;

2) they excite some motor neurones by disinhibiting a tonic inhibitory input from a second non-spiking interneurone thereby allowing them to contribute to a movement.

We have not found excitatory connections amongst non-spiking interneurones or any output connections with intersegmental or spiking local interneurones.

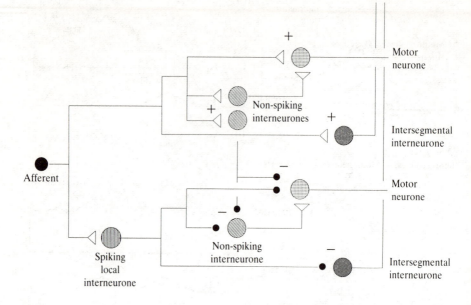

Figure 13.6 Flow diagram of the pathways involved in a local reflex of a hindleg initiated by exteroceptive inputs. Excitatory synapses are shown as open triangles, inhibitory synapses as filled circles.

13.2.3   Reflex pathways

From these experimentally determined features of connectivity, it is possible to summarize the general properties of the pathways underlying a local reflex (Figure 13.6).

1) Afferents make divergent, excitatory connections with several classes of neurone. Parallel processing abounds.

2) Spiking local interneurones make divergent, inhibitory connections with several classes of neurones.

3) Lateral inhibitory interactions occur between the local interneurones.

4) The outputs of the afferents and the local interneurones then converge onto sets of motor neurones.

5) Outputs from a local circuit are then conveyed by intersegmental interneurones to ganglia controlling adjacent legs.

13.2.4   Gain control of local reflexes

If these are the pathways responsible for local reflexes, then which elements can be modified to permit a response to be adapted to the differing behaviour of the locust? Non-spiking interneurones, by virtue of their connections with pools of motor neurones, their inputs from afferents and from spiking local interneurones, appear as crucial elements. An electrode in one of these neurones can be used to manipulate its membrane potential and test the effect on a local reflex (Burrows, Laurent & Field, 1988; Siegler, 1981). The interneurone shown in Figures 13.5C and D receives direct inputs from afferents that are excited when the tibia is forcibly flexed. The result of this input is a resistance reflex in which an extensor motor neurone is made to spike and would cause a contraction of the extensor muscle opposing the imposed movement (Figure 13.5C). A pulse of current injected into this interneurone shows that it makes a direct excitatory connection with the extensor motor neurone. If the interneurone is now hyperpolarized with a steady current and the same sensory stimulus is delivered, the resulting resistance reflex in the extensor motor neurone is much reduced (Figure 13.5D). This result indicates that the interneurone is directly involved in the reflex and that, despite the parallel processing, a single interneurone can change the gain of a reflex pathway. Any synaptic inputs to the non-spiking interneurone can therefore be expected to change the gain of the reflex because the release of transmitter from it is graded. Does this result suggest a more widespread mechanism by which local reflexes are fitted appropriately into the behaviour of the animal as the result of information from the other legs?

13.2.5 *Intersegmental influences on local circuits*

The local reflexes of one leg can only occur if the positions and movements of the other legs are appropriate at that time. How is sensory information from another leg transmitted, and how is it integrated into the local circuits controlling a particular leg so that local reflexes can be appropriately adjusted? Consider the signals received by a middle leg on the same side of the body as the hindleg we have been describing. Members of a population of intersegmental interneurones with cell bodies in the mesothoracic ganglion receive inputs from a middle leg and have axons that project to the metathoracic ganglion (Laurent, 1987a). The receptive fields of these interneurones are shaped by direct excitation from afferents and by inhibition from spiking local interneurones (Laurent, 1987b; 1988) in the same way as the metathoracic neurones. These intersegmental interneurones make direct excitatory (Figure 13.7A,B) or inhibitory connections with motor neurones and with non-spiking interneurones in the metathoracic ganglion (Laurent & Burrows, 1989a). The connections are specific and are related to the receptive field of the intersegmental interneurone and to the output connections of the non-spiking interneurone.

The connections do not seem to be designed to produce a stereotyped intersegmental reflex, but instead appear to act by altering local metathoracic reflexes. This possibility can be tested by recording from a non-spiking interneurone and a motor neurone and simulating the effect of an input from an intersegmental interneurone by the application of current to the non-spiking interneurone. A local reflex elicited by touching exteroceptors on the metathoracic

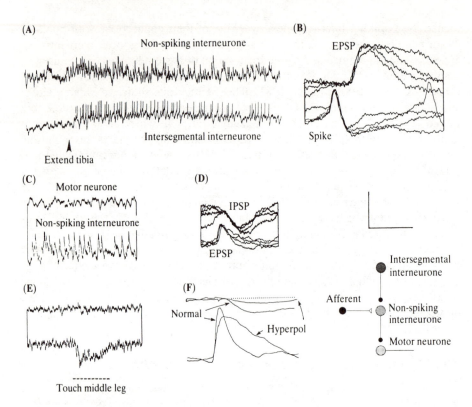

Figure 13.7 Intersegmental influences on a local reflex. **A,B**. Spikes in an intersegmental interneurone excited by extension of the tibia of the ipsilateral middle leg evoke EPSPs in a metathoracic non-spiking interneurone. **B**. Each spike in the intersegmental interneurone is followed by an EPSP in the non-spiking interneurone. **C-F**. Inhibitory inputs from an intersegmental interneurone can alter the effectiveness of a non-spiking interneurone in controlling a motor neurone. **C**. An afferent input from the hindleg evokes EPSPs in a non-spiking interneurone and IPSPs in a flexor tibiae motor neurone. **D**. Each EPSP is followed after a constant latency by an IPSP in the motor neurone. **E**. Touching the middle leg evokes a hyperpolarization of the non-spiking interneurone but has no effect on the motor neurone. **F**. Hyperpolarizing the non-spiking interneurone with an applied current reduces the size of the IPSP in the motor neurone that is caused by the EPSP in the interneurone. The inset shows the pathways involved. Calibration: vertical, **A** 4 mV, **B** 2 mV, **C,E** 7.1 mV, **D** non-spiking interneurone 7.1 mV, motor neurone 3.5 mV: horizontal **A** 500 ms, **B** 6.3 ms, **C,E** 700 ms, **D** 11.6 ms, **F** 10 ms.

tibia evokes EPSPs in the non-spiking interneurone and IPSPs in a leg motor neurone (Figure 13.7C). The IPSPs in the motor neurone consistently follow the EPSPs in the interneurone (Figure 13.7D), and injecting depolarizing current into the interneurone reveals a direct inhibitory connection with the motor neurone (Burrows, 1979). Touching the mesothoracic leg evokes a hyperpolarization of the interneurone but has no effect on the motor neurone (Figure 13.7E). If the

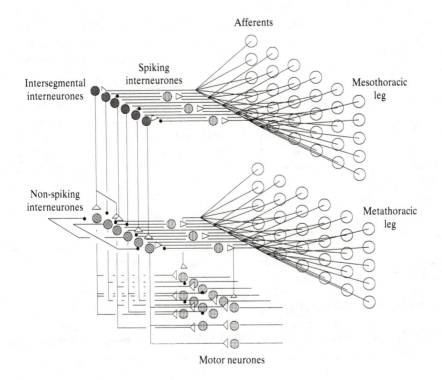

Afferents

Spiking
interneurones

Intersegmental
interneurones

Mesothoracic
leg

Non-spiking
interneurones

Metathoracic
leg

Motor neurones

Figure 13.8 Diagram of the pathways by which afferent inputs to a middle leg influence the motor output to the ipsilateral hindleg. The conventions are the same as in Figure 13.6.

mesothoracic effect is simulated by hyperpolarizing the non-spiking interneurone with injected current, touching the metathoracic leg now produces smaller IPSPs in the motor neurone (Figure 13.7F) and consequently a reduction in the efficacy of the reflex inhibition. An intersegmental neurone can therefore gate a local reflex by its effects on a non-spiking interneurone (Figure 13.8).

13.3 Emerging principles of organization in neural networks

13.3.1 Information flow in the networks

The interconnections between the afferents, the local interneurones and the motor neurones make up the local networks which underlie postural adjustments and adaptive reflexes. Afferents from mechanosensory receptors can affect local motor output either directly (1 synapse) or more generally, after processing by 1 or 2 layers of interposed interneurones (2 or 3 synapses). Furthermore, these networks can be modified by sensory inputs received by another leg which are no more than an additional 2 synapses from the output motor neurones. The effective pathways can thus involve as few as 2 to 3 successive layers of interneurones or stages of input transformation (Figure 13.8).

The ratio of afferents to interneurones varies between 10 or 100 to 1 depending on the class of interneurone. The afferents also diverge to several classes of interneurones, and to several individuals within a class, so that each sensory signal is systematically distributed over many parallel channels. The 'image' of a sensory stimulus conveyed to an output element is thus not derived from one specific interneuronal pathway or labelled line, but from the parallel activation of many interneurones whose receptive fields overlap at the site of stimulation and whose outputs ultimately converge on the active motor pool.

Not all the interneurones, however, are activated by a particular sensory input, and no interneurone is connected with all the output units (motor neurones). This contrasts with the patterns of connections made by the 'hidden' or 'internal representation' units in most associative, multilayered networks, as defined by Hopfield (1982) or as used, for example, by Rumelhart *et al.* (1986a) to solve specific tasks (see, however, Rumelhart *et al.*, 1986b). Furthermore, although lateral inhibitory connections between the local interneurones are common, reciprocal inhibitory connections have not been found. The flow of information always appears to be unidirectional, and shows no symmetry or back-coupling equivalent to that in Hopfield nets.

13.3.2 *Interdependence of receptive and projective fields*

Interneurones may have complex and composite receptive fields comprising excitatory and inhibitory regions. Some of these receptive fields are readily understood from a functional point of view: for example, a tactile excitatory region of a receptive field that is bordered by an inhibitory region would serve as an edge-sharpening device to specify better the location of a stimulus. For other interneurones the excitatory and inhibitory regions of their receptive fields may not be contiguous (see Burrows, 1985; Laurent, 1987b) and may even involve different types of mechanosensory stimuli. These arrangements are easily understandable only if the two fields are likely to be stimulated at the same time, when the interneurone would become a 'feature detector' - the excitatory input is only detected when the inhibitory input is absent. The functional relevance of other composite receptive fields is difficult to grasp if only the inputs are known. Knowledge of the output properties ('projective fields', Lehky & Sejnowski, 1988) may, however, be helpful. Consider an example where two interneurones A and B converge on a third interneurone C (Laurent & Burrows, 1989a). A and B each have excitatory regions of their receptive fields which do not overlap, but A has an inhibitory region identical to the excitatory region of B. Therefore, when B is excited, A is inhibited. Interneurone A has an excitatory and B an inhibitory connection with C. The result of this organization is that the inhibitory action of B on C cannot be opposed by the excitatory action of A. Understanding the receptive field of such a neurone as interneurone A, even in a very simple network of this type, may thus require the knowledge of its output connections and the output of all the neurones sharing the same target. This is similar to the conclusion reached by Lehky & Sejnowski (1988) in their study of a neural network model with one layer of hidden units: 'understanding the function of a neurone within a network appears to require not only knowledge of the pattern of input connections forming its receptive field but also knowledge of the pattern of output connections, which form its projective field. Indeed, the same neurone may have a number of different functions if it projects to several regions'.

13.3.3   Formation of receptive fields

How are the precise connections that must underlie a receptive field formed? For model neural networks with hidden units, several supervised or unsupervised 'learning' algorithms exist (Hopfield nets: Hopfield, 1982; back-propagation in Boltzmann machines: Hinton & Sejnowski, 1986; Rumelhart *et al.*, 1986; Lehky & Sejnowski, 1988; recirculation: North, 1987) that allow the network to reach a dynamically stable configuration or 'ultrastability' (Ashby, 1950) after a given number of trials. In neural networks of the locust, the same problems exist, but must be posed in terms of the development and maturation of the complex wiring patterns. Does the wiring of 10 000 afferent neurones undergo remodelling, as the precise receptive fields of the interneurones or 'hidden units' are refined during post-embryonic development, perhaps in an activity-dependent manner? Three questions for future experiments are thus posed.

1) What are the basic receptive fields of the local interneurones at birth? In other words, what is the basic genetic framework for the representation of sensory space?

2) Are there equivalents of the 'learning rules', or the algorithms for 'back-propagation' or 'recirculation' in a maturing animal, that could adjust synaptic weights until each receptive field is adapted to its task(s)?

3) How, in a population of interneurones involved in many different tasks (behaviours), is the 'desired' output defined? The receptive fields of individual interneurones seem to be the same from one adult locust to another. Consequently, either the synaptic weights in the network are adjusted in the same way in every animal to reach the same stable configuration, or few post-embryonic changes occur.

13.3.4   Interneurones, hidden units, and neuronal function

What is the specific function of an interneurone in a class of homologues, or of a hidden unit in a layer? Both neurophysiological experiments and computational theory agree on the ambiguity of the term 'neuronal function'. Function cannot be deduced without invoking the other homologue interneurones in the class, or the other hidden units in the layer. The co-operative action of the interneurones, or the units, in transforming incoming data is also reflected in the cooperativity of their function. We believe that it is at worst wrong, or at best inadequate, to speak of specific interneuronal function. An interneurone has several output targets, themselves often involved in different tasks, and it may therefore participate in several circuits working independently in certain circumstances.

13.3.5   *Non-linear interactions*

Many models of network functioning attach little importance to the precision of the circuit wiring. For example, Hillis (1988) invokes the Gestalt of a thinking machine: 'The notion of emergence would suggest that such a network, once it reached some critical mass, would spontaneously begin to think'. For Hopfield (1982), 'it becomes relevant to ask whether the ability of a large collection of neurones to perform "computational" tasks may in part be due to a spontaneous collective consequence of having a large number of interacting simple neurones'. Moreover, computation with coarsely tuned units can be made accurate and reliable if the information is distributed among members of a population (von Neumann, 1956; Ballard *et al.*, 1983; Cowan & Sharp, 1988).

In the central nervous system of the locust, two facts argue against coarse coding as a mechanism of integration. First, the number of available interneurones is restricted. For example, no more than 100 spiking local interneurones in the midline group may be present (Siegler & Burrows, 1984). Second, the receptive field of an individual interneurone is usually precisely defined and consistent from locust to locust. In addition, some ideas from artificial network theory contrast with the experimental observations of possible non-linear interactions on dendritic branches of neurones (e.g. Laurent & Burrows, 1989b). Conductance changes on the branches of certain non-spiking local interneurones appear to alter the ability of these neurones to integrate other inputs. Since these interactions occur without spikes, a neurone might well be able to perform several computations at the same time. This mode of computation adds a further word to the 'vocabulary of computational operations' (Shepherd, 1979) and for us, strongly argues in favour of great specificity of synaptic wiring, against a loose anatomical ground plan.

Acknowledgement

This work was supported by NIH grant 16058 and by a grant from the SERC (UK). Gilles Laurent is a Locke Research Fellow of the Royal Society of London.

References

Ashby W.R. (1950) The stability of a randomly assembled nerve-network. **EEG Clinical Neurophysiol. 2**, p. 471

Ballard D.H., Hinton G.E. & Sejnowski T.J. (1983) Parallel visual computation. **Nature 306**, pp. 21-26

Burrows M. (1979) Graded synaptic transmission between local pre-motor interneurons of the locust. **J. Neurophysiol. 42**, pp. 1108-1123

Burrows M. (1980) The control of sets of motoneurones by local interneurones in the locust. **J. Physiol. 298**, pp. 213-233

Burrows M. (1985) The processing of mechanosensory information by spiking local interneurones in the locust. **J. Neurophysiol. 54**, pp. 463-478

Burrows M. (1987) Inhibitory interactions between spiking and nonspiking local interneurones in the locust. **J. Neurosci. 7**, pp. 3282-3292

Burrows M. & Siegler M.V.S. (1978) Graded synaptic transmission between local interneurones and motoneurones in the metathoracic ganglion of the locust. **J. Physiol. 285**, pp. 231-255

Burrows M. & Siegler M.V.S. (1982) Spiking local interneurons mediate local reflexes. **Science (NY) 217**, pp. 650-652

Burrows M. & Siegler M.V.S. (1985) The organization of receptive fields of spiking local interneurones in the locust with inputs from hair afferents. **J. Neurophysiol. 53**, pp. 1147-1157

Burrows M., Laurent G.J. & Field L.H. (1988) Nonspiking local interneurones receive direct inputs from a proprioceptor and contribute to local reflexes of a locust hindleg. **J. Neurosci. 8**, pp. 3085-3093

Cowan J.D. & Sharp D.H. (1988) Neural nets and artificial intelligence. **Proc. Am. Acad. Arts & Sci. 117**, pp. 85-121

Hillis W.D. (1988) Intelligence as an emergent behavior; or, the songs of Eden. **Proc. Am. Acad. Arts & Sci. 117**, pp. 175-190

Hinton G.E. & Sejnowski T.J. (1986) Learning and relearning in Boltzmann Radiuses, In: **Parallel distributed processing. Explorations of the microstructure of cognition.** Vol. I., pp. 282-314, D.E. Rumelhart, J.L. McClelland & the PDP research group (eds.) MIT Press, Cambridge MA & London.

Hopfield J.J. (1982) Neural networks and physical systems with emergent collective computational abilities. **Proc. Natl. Acad. Sci. USA 79**, pp. 2554-2558

Laurent G. (1987a) The morphology of a population of thoracic intersegmental interneurones in the locust. **J. comp. Neurol. 256**, pp. 412-429

Laurent G. (1987b) The role of spiking local interneurones in shaping the receptive fields of intersegmental interneurones in the locust. **J. Neurosci. 7**, pp. 2977-2989

Laurent G. (1988) Local circuits underlying excitation and inhibition of intersegmental interneurones in the locust. **J. comp. Physiol. 162**, pp. 145-157

Laurent G.J. & Burrows M. (1988a) Direct excitation of nonspiking local interneurones by exteroceptors underlies tactile reflexes in the locust. **J. comp. Physiol. 162**, pp. 563-572

Laurent G. & Burrows M. (1988b) A population of ascending intersegmental interneurones in the locust with mechanosensory inputs from a hind leg. **J. comp. Neurol. 275**, pp. 1-12

Laurent G. & Burrows M. (1989a) Distribution of intersegmental inputs to nonspiking local interneurones and motor neurones in the locust. **J. Neurosci.**, In press.

Laurent G. & Burrows M. (1989b) Intersegmental interneurones can control the gain of reflexes in adjacent segments by their action on nonspiking local interneurones. **J. Neurosci.**, In press.

Laurent G.J. & Hustert R. (1988) Motor neuronal receptive fields delimit patterns of motor activity during locomotion of the locust. **J. Neurosci.** in press

Lehky S.R. & Sejnowski T.J. (1988) Network model of shape-form-shading: neural function arises from both receptive and projective fields. **Nature 333**, pp. 452-454

North G. (1987) A celebration of connectionism. **Nature 328**, p. 107

Rumelhart D.E., Hinton G.E. & Williams R.J. (1986a) Learning internal representations by error propagation. In: **Parallel distributed processing. Explorations of the microstructure of cognition.** Vol. I, pp. 318-362, D.E. Rumelhart, J.L. McClelland & the PDP research group (eds.) MIT Press, Cambridge MA & London.

Rumelhart D.E., Hinton G.E. & Williams R.J. (1986b) Learning representations by back-propagating errors. **Nature 323**, pp. 533-536

Shepherd G.M. (1979) **The synaptic organization of the brain.** Oxford University Press, NY.

Siegler M.V.S. (1981) Postural changes alter synaptic interactions between nonspiking interneurons and motor neurons of the locust. **J. Neurophysiol. 46**, pp. 310-323

Siegler M.V.S. & Burrows M. (1983) Spiking local interneurons as primary integrators of mechanosensory information in the locust. **J. Neurophysiol. 50**, pp. 1281-1295

Siegler M.V.S. & Burrows M. (1984) The morphology of two groups of spiking local interneurones in the metathoracic ganglion of the locust. **J. comp. Neurol. 224**, pp. 463-482

Siegler M.V.S. & Burrows M. (1986) Receptive fields of motor neurones underlying local tactile reflexes in the locust. **J. Neurosci. 6**, pp. 507-513

von Neumann J. (1956) Probabilistic logics and the synthesis of reliable organisms from unreliable components. In: **Automata Studies.** C.E. Shannon & J. McCarthy (eds.) Princeton University Press, Princeton, NJ.

Watson A.H.D. & Burrows M. (1985) The distribution of synapses on the two fields of neurites of spiking local interneurones in the locust. **J. comp. Neurol. 240**, pp. 219-232

Watson A.H.D. & Burrows M. (1988) The distribution and morphology of synapses on nonspiking local interneurones in the thoracic nervous system of the locust. **J. comp. Neurol. 272**, pp. 605-616

Weeks J.C. & Jacobs G.A. (1987) A reflex behavior mediated by monosynaptic connections between hair afferents and motoneurons in the larval tobacco hornworm. **J. comp. Physiol. 160**, pp. 315-329

14
Idiosyncratic Computational Units Generating Innate Motor Patterns: Neurones and Circuits in the Locust Flight System

Meldrum Robertson

Summary

To what extent do general models of neural networks reflect the operation of real circuits of neurones? A consideration of the central neuronal circuitry underlying the generation of the deafferented flight rhythm in the locust reveals that, in this system, the individual computational units (identified neurones) and the ways in which they are organized and interact are highly idiosyncratic. The unique character of this system results from its evolutionary and developmental history as well as from pure, functionally adaptive constraints. Many details of operation may be suboptimal and/or baroque and these may simply be the unavoidable burden of an individual history. This implies that detailed models of systems with different histories, while very important for generating and testing hypotheses specific to the particular systems, are likely not to be transferrable to other systems. Circuits that are unique in their organization and operation demand unique models if such models are to be useful. Nevertheless, assuming that general principles of network operation exist, generalized modelling with idealized units is a valid approach as a means of determining such principles. However, most of the general network models which are currently available do not address the issue of innate motor patterning. The principle of operation in the locust flight system is likely to be largely independent of many of the fine details of the way in which the system actually operates.

14.1 Introduction

Can the essence of the computing neurone, the neurone as a computational unit, be distilled? That is to say, is it possible to define those characteristics that are necessary and sufficient to enable neuronal networks to perform similar computations? Neurones exist in an almost infinite variety of shapes and sizes within an organism and between species. This variability in morphology alone is able to affect physiology, but neurones also possess, in different proportions, a plethora of intrinsic biochemical and membrane properties to increase still further the diversity in the ways that they operate (Bullock, 1980). In addition, there is a variety of ways in which neurones can interact to form operating circuits. Finally, the situation is complicated when one recognizes that the current make-up of nervous systems, like that of other biological systems, reflects their evolutionary and developmental histories and thus not all of the features and characteristics of a neuronal circuit are necessarily adaptive for the particular function under investigation (Dumont & Robertson, 1986). One result of all this variety is that any definable output of a circuit, i.e. the end result of the 'computation' of the neuronal assemblage, might be produced by any of a number of different theoretical systems (i.e. the hardware), and the algorithms might be different. In order to recognize general computational strategies that could be used by biological neural networks it is therefore necessary to document the different characteristics of specific networks and try to determine the relevance, if any, of these differences to network function and computing ability.

One class of neuronal circuit which has been comparatively well studied in recent years includes the circuits that are responsible for patterning the motor activity underlying simple behaviours in invertebrates (see e.g. Kristan *et al.*, Chapter 10; Selverston & Mazzoni, Chapter 11). The motor patterns are generated and controlled by central (Delcomyn, 1980) and peripheral (Pearson, 1985b) nervous mechanisms. Whatever the relative contribution of the two to the final motor output in different systems, it is indisputable that circuits of interneurones in central nervous systems repeatably produce measurable patterns of output. The central circuits controlling simple invertebrate behaviours are composed of relatively few neurones most of which can be uniquely identified on the basis of an idiosyncratic set of morphological and physiological characteristics (e.g. Hoyle, 1977; Bullock, 1980). These systems are highly represented in the literature because of the persuasive argument that such systems are inherently more tractable due to the ability to characterize the individual components. However, in spite of impressive advances in the knowledge of the cellular and network processes underlying specific systems, few general principles of organization and function have emerged (Burrows, 1984; Pearson, 1985a; Dumont & Robertson, 1986). Such systems are characterized by much complexity within them and diversity between them. This is in sharp contrast to the computational 'neural' networks which are the subject of other chapters in this volume. In these artificial systems the neurone-like units are simple, the operational rules are straightforward and there is much general similarity between different systems. Modification of such networks according to certain learning rules during a training period can greatly diversify the interactions between the units (e.g. Rumelhart *et al.*, 1986). Furthermore, the systems are clearly very powerful and they can perform the same sorts of tasks as nervous tissue. However the question remains whether the artificial systems are true models of neuronal systems, operating on the same principles, or simply very good mimics. It is only with a detailed knowledge of the functional organization and mode of operation of different biological systems that it will be possible to answer this question.

14.2   The locust flight system

Locust flight is a behaviour which has received a lot of attention in the past and much is known about many aspects of its control. Much of this need not concern us here and I will concentrate on the neural mechanisms underlying the rhythmical beating of the wings. There are two pairs of wings and two homologous sets of wing muscles and their motoneurones. The motor pattern during straight and steady flight is simply described (Wilson & Weis-Fogh, 1962). There is currently some controversy over the role of peripheral sense organs in generating the motor pattern (Pearson, 1985b; Pearson & Wolf, 1987; Stevenson & Kutsch, 1987; Wolf & Pearson, 1987a), however this is not an issue I wish to pursue here. Suffice it to say that the deafferented thoracic nervous system produces a rhythmical motor output which is obviously related to flight (Wilson, 1961) and which indicates the existence of an important central component of the control mechanism, comprising circuits of interneurones and motoneurones. Many flight interneurones have now been described (Robertson & Pearson, 1983; Pearson & Robertson, 1987; Reye & Pearson, 1987; Ramirez & Pearson, 1988) and the individual and network properties of many of these neurones have been described (Robertson & Pearson, 1985a; Robertson & Reye, 1988; Robertson & Wisniowski, 1988). My intention is to review the properties of locust flight interneurones and their circuits in order to illustrate the general point that features of organization and operation contributing to the complexity in the system are not necessarily related to adaptive function. A negative consequence of this observation is that systems of this sort are likely to be composed of idiosyncratic computational units, to be unique in the details of their operation, and to be generally unpredictable. A positive consequence is that for the formulation of general models many of the fine details could be ignored as they are likely to have little functional relevance.

14.3   General properties of flight interneurones and circuits

Fixing functional labels to particular interneurones is a dangerous business, first because of the fact that in the majority of cases the data on the interneurone have been accumulated under experimental rather than natural conditions, and second because of the possibility that an interneurone is involved in more than one behaviour. The term 'flight interneurone' indicates at the very least that the membrane potential of the interneurone shows pronounced oscillations in phase with the flight motor pattern, but it does not preclude the interneurone having another, possibly more important, functional role. For most of the interneurones that have been described as being involved in flight the evidence is more substantial (Figure 14.1). These neurones show sharply-defined bursts of spikes at a high intraburst frequency (200 - 400 impulses per second) riding upon large (15 - 25 mV) membrane potential oscillations; depolarizing stimulation of some of these neurones is capable of inducing rhythmical activity in the system at rest. Short

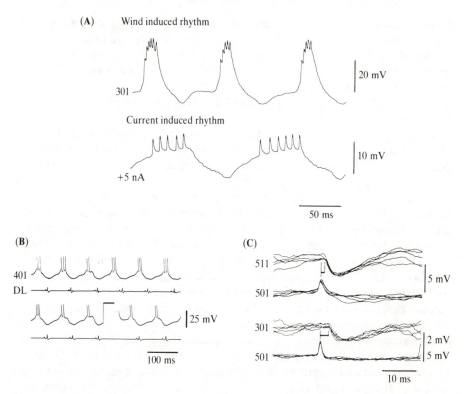

Figure 14.1 Criteria to determine the participation of interneurones in the generation of the flight rhythm. Intracellular recordings are taken from the neuropil segments of selected interneurones in the thoracic ganglia using glass microelectrodes. A. Ability to generate rhythmical activity related to flight. Interneurone 301 fires bursts during the elevator phase of the flight rhythm induced by a wind stimulus to the preparation (upper trace). Moderate depolarization of this interneurone with +5 nA of tonic current injection induces rhythmical activity in the system (lower trace). Note the rhythmical synaptic input evident in the membrane potential waveform indicating that other interneurones are rhythmically active. This stimulus also induces rhythmical activity of wing muscle motoneurones and flight-like phase relationships are maintained (not shown). B. Ability to reset the flight rhythm. Interneurone 401 fires bursts during the elevator phase (upper pair of traces). The time of depression is indicated by the electromyographic monitor of the activity of a dorsal longitudinal (DL) wing depressor muscle. Stimulation of this interneurone with a short duration pulse of depolarizing current (indicated by bar above lower pair of traces) resets the flight rhythm by increasing the duration of the cycle (indicated by successive bursts of DL activity) in which the stimulus occurs. C. Direct synaptic connections to wing muscle motoneurones (not shown) or with other flight interneurones. Successive sweeps of the oscilloscope triggered off the rising phase of the spike recorded from 501 show that each 501 spike is followed after a short and constant latency by an IPSP in interneurone 511 (upper pair of traces), and in interneurone 301 (lower pair of traces). The shortness and constancy of the latencies (indicated by bars) show that the connections are probably monosynaptic. 501 and 511 are in the same ganglion (metathoracic) and the latency is around 1 ms. 301 is in the next anterior ganglion (mesothoracic) and the increase in latency (of around 1.3 ms) is consistent with it simply being due to an increase in conduction path length of the 501 spike. (Robertson & Pearson, 1985a; Robertson, unpublished)

pulses of current delivered to some of these neurones during the expression of the flight rhythm can reset the timing of the rhythm by delaying or advancing the occurrence of the subsequent cycle; and some can be shown to be important in generating the wingbeat by virtue of their synaptic connections either directly or indirectly to the motoneurones of the wing muscles.

The flight interneurones that have been described to date are, for the most part, large intersegmental interneurones in the meso- and metathoracic ganglia. This raises the question of whether there is a sampling bias such that smaller local interneurones have been neglected due to technical limitations. This is certainly possible but, in my opinion, it is unlikely that we have missed a large population of small, important neurones. Stable recordings can be made from small local interneurones. Moreover, all of the intracellular recordings are taken from the branches of the interneurones in the neuropil rather than from the neuronal somata, and at this level the disparity in size between intersegmental and local interneurones is much reduced. A more likely possibility is that, for one reason or another, particular regions of the thoracic ganglia have not been submitted to detailed scrutiny. Almost invariably the dendritic and axonal branching is confined to the most dorsal layer of the neuropil just under the ganglionic sheath. Interneurones that can be segregated according to the motor pattern with which they are active, can also be segregated according to the location of their branching in the neuropil with the branching of flight interneurones occupying the dorsal rind of neuropil (Ramirez & Pearson, 1988). Excluding serial homologues (see below) and the contralateral partner of a bilaterally symmetrical pair, most flight interneurones are strikingly unique in their structure (Figure 14.2). Each has an idiosyncratic morphology which suggests an idiosyncratic set of input and output connections.

Undoubtedly as a consequence of its idiosyncratic set of input connections, each interneurone has unique membrane potential waveforms during expression of the flight rhythm. It is usually possible to identify individual interneurones solely on the basis of their physiology (rate and extent of depolarization and hyperpolarization, number and magnitude of different phases of synaptic input, number and frequency of spikes/burst). To date there is no evidence for endogenous membrane properties contributing to membrane potential oscillations - the rhythm is generated via synaptic interactions in a network of interneurones. Three types of synaptic interaction have been described: chemically-mediated excitatory connections which result in excitatory post-synaptic potentials (EPSPs) of 2 - 5 mV following each pre-synaptic spike; similar inhibitory connections to give inhibitory post-synaptic potentials (IPSPs) which are likely to be the result of a gamma-aminobutyric acid (GABA) mediated increase in conductance to chloride ions; and a delayed excitatory connection which is probably the result of disynaptic disinhibition with tonic release of inhibitory transmitter at least at the second synapse (Robertson & Pearson, 1985a). A local, subthreshold interaction between flight interneurones has been described (Robertson & Reye, 1988) but the functional relevance of this is still unclear (see below). Each functional synaptic connection is likely to be the summed effect of several hundred ultrastructurally

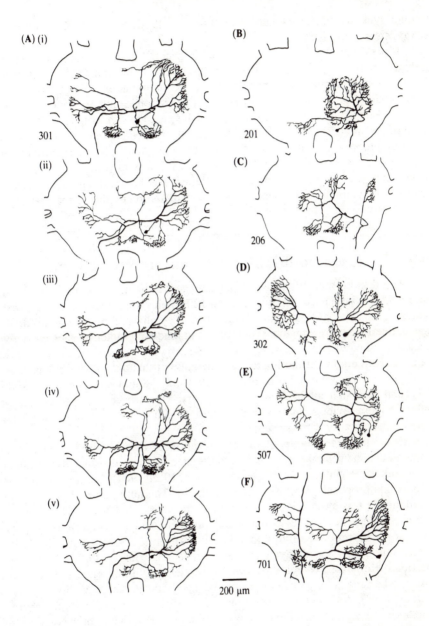

Figure 14.2 Idiosyncratic morphology of flight interneurones. **A (i-v).** Drawings of the right 301 in the mesothoracic ganglion of five different individuals to illustrate the range within which the morphology of an identified neurone can vary. **B-F.** Drawings of five different identified flight interneurones with cell somata in the right mesothoracic hemiganglion to illustrate the idiosyncratic nature of an identified neurone's morphology. (Robertson & Pearson, 1983; Robertson, unpublished)

distinct synaptic contacts (Watson & Burrows, 1983; Killmann & Schurmann, 1985; Peters *et al.*, 1985).

It is evident that most units involved in generating the output pattern in this system have unique, characteristic sets of properties. In the course of investigating the system it has not yet been possible to predict neuronal or circuit properties by extrapolation from an emerging pattern of organization. Some prediction has been possible (Pearson & Robertson, 1987) but in this case the similarity is likely to be a result of common developmental origins rather than reflecting functional adaptation. An early proposal that it may be possible to segregate flight interneurones into functional classes (Robertson & Pearson, 1983) was proved to be premature (Robertson & Pearson, 1985a). Nevertheless it has been possible to determine some of the interneuronal circuitry in the system and relate this to features of the output pattern.

14.4   Features contributing to the output pattern

The deafferented flight motor pattern can be characterized as follows: the pattern repeats with a frequency of around 12 Hz; elevator motoneurones alternate their activity with that of depressor motoneurones; equivalent motoneurones on the right and left sides are active in synchrony; and hindwing motoneurones are active in advance of equivalent forewing motoneurones by 5 - 10 ms. Different aspects of the central circuitry contributing to the generation of this output pattern have been relatively recently reviewed (Robertson & Pearson, 1985b; Robertson, 1985, 1986, 1987) and to do so again in detail is unnecessary. My purpose here is to provide an update to these reviews based on recent findings and to comment in more general terms on the circuitry in the system.

Based on observations of the organization of flight interneurones it was proposed that the central pattern generating system is a unit distributed throughout the pterothoracic ganglia (Robertson & Pearson, 1983, 1984). Recent experiments support this proposal (Wolf & Pearson, 1987b). The neuronal basis for rhythm generation in this system is unknown. Certain elements of the known circuitry would certainly contribute to burst generation and under conditions of tonic excitation can produce rhythmical output. Circuits of reciprocal inhibition (Robertson, 1987) and delayed excitation with feedback inhibition have been described (Robertson & Pearson, 1985a). Models of similar circuits have been shown to be capable of generating rhythmical activity (Perkel & Mulloney, 1974; Getting, 1983). Although it is possible to identify candidate circuits for rhythm generation it is unlikely that it will be possible to identify a single source or a unique mechanism for the underlying oscillation. Stimulation of different single interneurones produces rhythms with different characteristics and with a different active subset of the flight interneurone population (Robertson, 1987). It seems that to generate alternating activity is a trivial problem for nervous tissue whereas the crucial task is co-ordinating the activity of rudimentary oscillators and organizing the appropriate timing of such activity.

Elements of the described circuitry do contribute to the co-ordination of the timing of different components of the output. A relatively constant latency from elevator motoneurone activation to depressor motoneurone activation in deafferented preparations has been described as occurring either usually (Hedwig & Pearson, 1984; Pearson & Wolf, 1987) or occasionally (Stevenson & Kutsch, 1987). A circuit which could underlie this observation has been described (Robertson & Pearson, 1985a). Separate synaptic pathways exist from a single interneurone to both elevator motoneurones and depressor motoneurones. The pathway to the elevator motoneurones is direct, whereas that to the depressor motoneurones is indirect through a cascade of synapses. In this instance the mechanism controlling the timing of alternate activation of elevator and depressor motoneurones is that of an increased delay to the depressor motoneurones via a greater number of synapses in the pathway. Interestingly, a proposal for the mechanism controlling the timing of the lag between activation of the hindwing and forewing depressor motoneurones is that of an increased conduction delay, because of a greater path length to the forewing motoneurones, even though the number of synapses in the pathway to the depressor motoneurones is the same (Robertson & Pearson, 1985b). Finally there is a high degree of synchronous firing of the two members of pairs of bilaterally symmetrical interneurones (Robertson, in preparation). In some cases the synchrony is such that single spikes occur within 1 ms of each other in the two interneurones (Figure 14.3). To date, any direct excitatory interaction between the interneurones has been found to be small (<1 mV) and unable to account for the synchrony. Rather, it appears that synchronous firing of bilateral homologues is a result of a large amount of common synaptic input and that it is dependent upon activation of a sufficient proportion of the flight circuitry - rhythmical activity can be obtained by partial activation of the system but the activity shows inappropriate timing.

The point of this section is to demonstrate that circuit analysis in this system is possible and that functional roles can be assigned to many features of the circuit. However, and in spite of this ability, it has not been possible to recognize any coherent pattern to the organization of the circuit. Individual components of the system resemble components of other invertebrate pattern generating networks, but the selection and assembly of these components appear idiosyncratic to the locust flight system and seem almost arbitrary when viewed from a functional perspective.

14.5 Features apparently unrelated to the output pattern

The hypothesis that a feature of organization and operation in a neuronal circuit is sub-optimal or not adaptive is hazardous to make. The counter claim, that we have merely not provided the system with the appropriate context to reveal the importance of the feature, is irrefutable. The original hypothesis is therefore justifiable only with the existence of a convincing, non-adaptive explanation for the presence of the feature. Moreover the hypothesis does not imply that the feature is

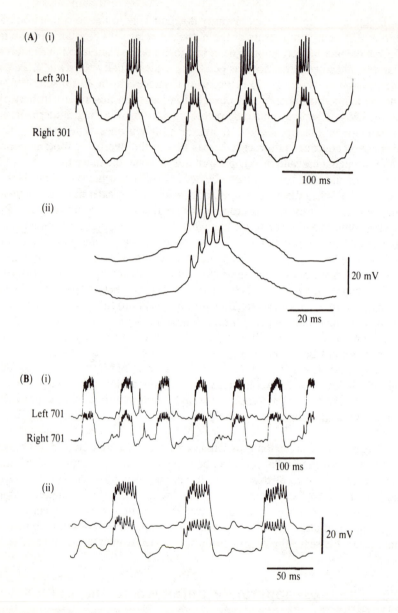

Figure 14.3 Synchronous activity of bilaterally symmetrical interneurones during expression of the flight rhythm. **A (i)**. Simultaneous intracellular recordings from the left 301 and from the right 301 show highly synchronous bursts. **(ii)**. A single burst from a flight sequence demonstrates that spikes in one neurone occur within 1 ms of spikes in the other. **B (i)**, **(ii)**. Other flight interneurones (e.g. 701) show highly synchronous bursts but without intraburst synchrony of single spikes. (Robertson, unpublished)

non-functional, or unnecessary, but it does follow that the system in which it occurs is unpredictable from purely functional principles.

The effect of evolution on neuronal interactions is obvious at a gross level. Different taxa use differents sets of components to construct their circuits. For example electrical connections are rare in insects (Robertson, 1987) but more common in molluscs and crustacea; the multi-component synapses of the *Tritonia* escape circuit (Getting, 1981), which figure prominently in an associative neural network model for pattern generation (Kleinfeld & Sompolinsky, 1988), have not yet been reported in other biological pattern generating systems. More subtle effects of evolution can be observed. An early finding in the investigation of the locust flight system was of sets of serially homologous interneurones in the four fused neuromeres of the metathoracic ganglionic mass (Robertson *et al.*, 1982). Each interneurone in a set has similar morphological features and, as far as has been determined, similar physiology. Furthermore they all have important roles to play in generating the rhythm and driving wing muscle motoneurones. This peculiar arrangement has no obvious adaptive benefit for the control of flight and it has been argued in detail elsewhere (Robertson *et al.*, 1982; Dumont & Robertson, 1986) that this organizational feature reflects a prior stage in the evolution of the flight system and is sub-optimal in its design as flight circuitry. A similar lack of optimal design is evident in the escape circuitry of the crayfish (Dumont & Wine, 1987) and in the characteristics of certain midbrain neurones of electric fish (Rose *et al.*, 1987).

A further point is that the evolution of biological systems is a continuing, dynamic process. It would therefore be expected that our investigations at one particular stage in this process will reveal features that are in the process of being eradicated by selection, and other features which are the substrate of future elaborations or at least have not reached their full potential. Many of the weak synaptic connections whose effects on the spiking activity of post-synaptic neurones are negligible, could be considered candidates for such features. Thus the evolutionary histories of different systems have constrained their current organizations with the result that their organizations are not predictable from general modelling principles.

The developmental history of the system may also result in features which increase its complexity in ways not adapted to its function. As illustrated in the example above, serially homologous interneurones with similar morphology and physiology can be recognized. By observing the embryonic development of interneurones in the segmental ganglia it is possible to identify serial homologues which have diverged during evolution (Pearson *et al.*, 1985). In spite of differing in certain aspects of their phenotype such homologous interneurones retain a common ground plan of organization which reflects their common developmental origins (Bastiani *et al.*, 1984). Moreover, as the large intersegmental interneurones enlarge and extend their processes during development they become transiently dye-coupled both to neurones originating from the same neuroblast and to unrelated neurones in their early environment (Raper & Goodman, 1982; Raper *et al.*, 1983). Such dye-coupling suggests the existence of gap junctions and electrical interaction, i.e. the existence of electrical synapses between the neurons. These interactions are thus related to pathfinding rather than to the generation of appropriate patterns of nervous activity. It has been suggested that some ultrastructurally defined gap junctions in adult locusts may be relics of developmental history (Killmann & Schurmann, 1985). Indeed, the only example of an electrical connection in the locust thoracic nervous system is that between a leg muscle motoneurone and its supernumerary partner (Siegler, 1982) - a developmental anomaly rather than a functional necessity. A further example can be seen in the transmitter type of inhibitory flight interneurones. GABA is often assumed to be the central inhibitory transmitter in invertebrates. Indeed most of the inhibitory flight interneurones that have been examined show a positive GABA-like immunoreactivity indicating that these neurones are probably GABA-ergic (Robertson & Wisniowski, 1988). However at least one inhibitory interneurone does not show GABA-like immunoreactivity. This particular interneurone is different in other ways (Pearson & Robertson, 1987) and it is a reasonable assumption that it is different as a result of its different developmental history. There are two ways to view this observation: either the use of a different inhibitory transmitter is necessary to allow the interneurone to fulfil the detailed requirements of its functional role; or the nature of the transmitter is not germane to a consideration of its functional role. Given that the known physiological characteristics of the IPSPs caused by activity in this interneurone do not seem measurably different to the IPSPs from GABA-ergic interneurones, and in the continuing absence of contradictory evidence, then the conclusion that the identity of the inhibitory transmitter of this interneurone is not crucial to the operation of the system is valid. It is clear from the above examples that the full complement of adult characteristics of interneurones and circuits contains traces which link neurones with their origins and with the developmental pathways from those origins.

Finally, a problem arises in consideration of the reductionist way in which most circuits are investigated. How much of the detailed information that can be experimentally determined about a system ought to be incorporated into any model? It is an unavoidable consequence of physical, pharmacological, or other dissection of a system that many features will be altered in ways that are difficult to determine. Thus it is more than likely that the dissected system has features which are either relics, or transformations, of the real phenomena underlying the operation of the system. Another danger is that phenomena which can be characterized are reified and assume a significance that they do not really warrant. For example, Figure 14.4 shows a plateau-like potential recorded in a flight interneurone as a result of a short duration pulse of current elsewhere in the neurone. The basis for this is thought to be a disynaptic, disinhibitory, feedback circuit from the neurone to itself operating beneath the threshold for spike generation (Robertson & Reye, 1988). The important point is that the findings indicate a role for subthreshold and local interactions in the operation of the flight system. It is quite possible that the plateau-like potential has limited significance, as a phenomenon in its own right, for the generation of the flight rhythm. Much apparent complexity and diversity in different

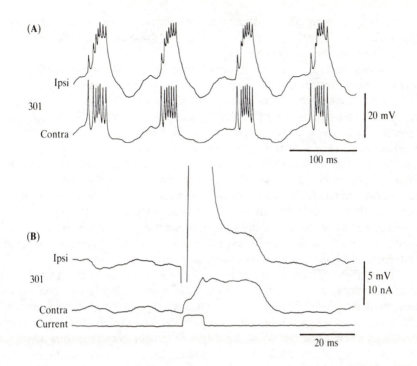

Figure 14.4 Subthreshold activation of a membrane potential event whose duration exceeds that of the stimulus. **A.** Simultaneous intracellular recordings from two sites in a single 301. Ipsi and contra indicate electrode positions in the neuropil segment on either side of the midline ipsilateral and contralateral to the cell soma respectively. The relative sizes of the spikes and membrane potential oscillations alter as a consequence of the relative electrotonic distance from the sites of action potential generation and synaptic input. **B.** A short pulse of subthreshold depolarizing current delivered to the neurone through the ipsilateral electrode induces a depolarizing potential which is maintained longer than the stimulus. This, with other evidence (not shown), is evidence for the subthreshold activation of local synaptic circuitry in the flight system. (Robertson & Reye, 1988)

systems may arise as the result of restricted viewpoints, and thus may be irrelevant for modelling these systems.

Conclusions

A picture is emerging of the locust flight system as a complex and idiosyncratic mix of different neuronal processes. Its unique character results from a combination of adaptive and non-adaptive constraints in the course of its evolution. Similar systems, i.e. small networks of identified neurones controlling innate behaviours, are likely to be similarly idiosyncratic. It is conceivable that the allure of the identified neurone has focussed interest on idiosyncratic systems and hindered the discovery of more general strategies for control. In my concluding remarks I should like to consider briefly the implications of these ideas in the context of this volume - neuronal network modelling.

Models of neurones and networks exist in at least two general classes - models of how systems actually work, and models of the principles by which they work. The first class includes models that are very specific to particular systems and these provide a useful means of generating and testing hypotheses relevant to those systems. These models necessarily have to be very detailed and include all the described features of a system, whatever their origins, in order to be as realistic as possible. Several of the ideas of how different components of the locust flight circuitry operate, could and should be tested more rigorously with such specific models. Unfortunately, if circuits are unique in the details of their organization and operation then models of this sort have little value as exemplars of general solutions. For the same reason any general network model incorporating simplified neurone-like elements is unlikely to be able to serve as an accurate, or even useful, representation of, for example, how the locust flight system operates.

Nevertheless, if there is any hope of extracting some general principles of functional organization which are applicable to different neuronal systems throughout the phyla, then general computational modelling, to produce models within the second class mentioned above, is a valid and worthwhile approach. The operating principles of the locust flight system remain to be determined but, when discovered, they will undoubtedly be formulated without reference to the mass of detail actually present in the system. Much of the detail simply represents the burden of the flight system's history. Examining the current collection of network and associative models there is little that I find particularly relevant to locust flight, or systems like it. Possibly the computational unit of these models should not be mapped to the neurone in systems comprised of few, identified neurones, but to some other definable unit. The models are arguably more relevant to the large arrays of similar neurones in vertebrate brains (e.g. Rolls, Chapter 8). In these cases the features that seem to have been selected include the general ones of increased computational potential, capacity and flexibility, and ability to make associations, rather than any specific computational task. In addition, many of the motor patterns tend to be constructed by association with sensory feedback and learned post-embryonically rather than being innate. It is not surprising therefore if network models applicable to such systems are much less applicable to the locust flight system, which is innate and which has been selected for one specific computational task - the generation of the flight motor pattern. I look forward to future generations of network models with the hope that they have more to say about neuronal computation in invertebrate motor systems.

References

Bastiani M., Pearson K.G. & Goodman C.S. (1984) From embryonic fascicles to adult tracts: organization of neuropile from a developmental perspective. **J. exp. Biol. 112**, pp. 45-64

Bullock T.H. (1980) Reassessment of neural connectivity and its specification. In: **Information processing in the nervous system.** pp. 199-220, H.M. Pinsker & W.D. Willis Jr. (eds.) Raven Press, NY.

Burrows M. (1984) The search for principles of neuronal organization. **J. exp. Biol. 112**, pp. 1-4

Delcomyn F. (1980) Neural basis for rhythmic behavior in animals. **Science 210**, pp. 492-498

Dumont J.P.C. & Robertson R.M. (1986) Neuronal circuits: an evolutionary perspective. **Science 233**, pp. 849-853

Dumont J.P.C. & Wine J.J. (1987) The telson flexor neuromuscular system of the crayfish. III. The role of feedforward inhibition in shaping a stereotyped behaviour pattern. **J. exp. Biol. 127**, pp. 295-311

Getting P.A. (1981) Mechanisms of pattern generation underlying swimming in *Tritonia*. I. Neuronal network formed by monosynaptic connections. **J. Neurophysiol. 46**, pp. 65-79

Getting P.A. (1983) Mechanisms of pattern generation underlying swimming in *Tritonia*. II. Network reconstruction. **J. Neurophysiol. 49**, pp. 1017-1035

Hedwig B. & Pearson K.G. (1984) Patterns of synaptic input to identified flight motoneurons in the locust. **J. comp. Physiol. 154**, pp. 745-760

Hoyle G. (ed.) (1977) **Identified neurons and behavior of Arthropods.** Plenum Press, NY.

Killmann F. & Schurmann F.W. (1985) Both electrical and chemical transmission between the 'lobula giant movement detector' and the 'descending contralateral movement detector' neurons of the locust are supported by electron microscopy. **J. Neurocytol. 14**, pp. 637-652

Kleinfeld D. & Sompolinsky H. (1988) Associative neural network model for the generation of temporal patterns: theory and application to central pattern generators. **Biophys. J.** (in press)

Pearson K.G. (1985a) Neuronal circuits for patterning motor activity in invertebrates. In: **Comparative Neurobiology: modes of communication in the nervous system.** pp. 225-244, M.J. Cohen & F. Strumwasser (eds.) John Wiley & Sons, NY.

Pearson K.G. (1985b) Are there central pattern generators for walking and flight in insects? In: **Feedback and motor control in invertebrates and** vertebrates. pp. 307-315, W.J.P. Barnes & M.H. Gladden (eds.) Croom Helm, London.

Pearson K.G., Boyan G.S., Bastiani M. & Goodman C.S. (1985) Heterogeneous properties of segmentally homologous interneurons in the ventral nerve cord of locusts. **J. comp. Neurol. 233**, pp. 133-145

Pearson K.G. & Robertson R.M. (1987) Structure predicts synaptic function of two classes of interactions in the thoracic ganglia of *Locusta migratoria*. **Cell Tissue Res. 250**, pp. 105-114

Pearson K.G. & Wolf H. (1987) Comparison of motor patterns in the intact and deafferented flight system of the locust. I. Electromyographic analysis. **J. comp. Physiol. 160**, pp. 259-268

Perkel D.H. & Mulloney B. (1974) Motor pattern production in reciprocally inhibitory neurons exhibiting postinhibitory rebound. **Science 185**, pp. 181-183

Peters B.H., Altman J.S. & Tyrer N.M. (1985) Synaptic connections between the hindwing stretch receptor and flight motor neurones in the locust revealed by double cobalt labelling for electron microscopy. **J. comp. Neurol. 233**, pp. 269-284

Ramirez J.M. & Pearson K.G. (1988) Generation of motor patterns for walking and flight in motoneurons supplying bifunctional muscles in the locust. **J. Neurobiol. 19**, pp. 257-282

Raper J.A. & Goodman C.S. (1982) Transient dye-coupling between developing neurons reveals patterns of intracellular communication during embryogenesis. In: **Cell communication during ocular development**. pp. 85-96, J. Sheffield & S.R. Hilfer (eds.) Springer-Verlag, NY.

Raper J.A., Bastiani M. & Goodman C.S. (1983) Pathfinding by neuronal growth cones in grasshopper embryos. II. Selective fasciculation onto specific axonal pathways. **J. Neurosci. 3**, pp. 31-41

Reye D.N. & Pearson K.G. (1987) Projections of the wing stretch receptors to central flight neurons in the locust. **J. Neurosci. 7**, pp. 2476-2487

Robertson R.M. (1985) Central neuronal interactions in the flight system of the locust. In: **Insect locomotion**. pp. 183-194, M. Gewecke & G. Wendler (eds.) Paul Parey Verlag, Hamburg.

Robertson R.M. (1986) Neuronal circuits controlling flight in the locust: central generation of the rhythm. **TINS 9**, pp. 278-280

Robertson R.M. (1987) Insect neurons: synaptic interactions, circuits and the control of behavior. In: **Nervous systems of invertebrates**. pp. 393-442, M.A. Ali (ed.) Plenum Press, NY.

Robertson R.M. & Pearson K.G. (1983) Interneurons in the flight system of the locust: distribution, connections and resetting properties. **J. comp. Neurol. 215**, pp. 33-50

Robertson R.M. & Pearson K.G. (1984) Interneuronal organization in the flight system of the locust. **J. Insect Physiol. 30**, pp. 95-101

Robertson R.M. & Pearson K.G. (1985a) Neural circuits in the flight system of the locust. **J. Neurophysiol. 53**, pp. 110-128

Robertson R.M. & Pearson K.G. (1985b) Neural networks controlling locomotion in locusts. In: **Model neural networks and behavior**. pp. 21-35, A.I. Selverston (ed.) Plenum Press, NY.

Robertson R.M., Pearson K.G. & Reichert H. (1982) Flight interneurons in the locust and the origin of insect wings. **Science 217**, pp. 177-179

Robertson R.M. & Reye D.N. (1988) A local circuit interaction in the flight system of the locust. **J. Neurosci. 8**, pp. 3929-3936

Robertson R.M. & Wisniowski L. (1988) GABA-like immunoreactivity of identified interneurons in the flight system of the locust, *Locusta migratoria*. **Cell Tissue Res. 254**, pp. 331-340

Rose G., Keller C. & Heiligenberg W. (1987) 'Ancestral' neural mechanisms of electrolocation suggest a substrate for the evolution of the jamming avoidance response. **J. comp. Physiol.**, pp. 491-500

Rumelhart D.E., Hinton G.E. & Williams R.J. (1986) Learning representations by back-propagating errors. **Nature 323**, pp. 533-536

Siegler M.V.S. (1982) Electrical coupling between supernumerary motor neurones in the locust. **J. exp. Biol. 101**, pp. 105-119

Stevenson P.A. & Kutsch W. (1987) A reconsideration of the central pattern generator concept for locust flight. **J. comp. Physiol. 161**, pp. 115-129

Watson A.H.D. & Burrows M. (1983) The morphology, ultrastructure and distribution of synapses on an intersegmental interneurone of the locust. **J. comp. Neurol. 214**, pp. 154-169

Wilson D.M. (1961) The central control of flight in a locust. **J. exp. Biol. 38**, pp. 471-490

Wilson D.M. & Weis-Fogh T. (1962) Patterned activity of co-ordinated motor units, studied in flying locusts. **J. exp. Biol. 39**, pp. 643-667

Wolf H. & Pearson K.G. (1987a) Comparison of motor patterns in the intact and deafferented flight system of the locust. 2. Intracellular recordings from flight motoneurons. **J. comp. Physiol. 160**, pp. 269-279

Wolf H. & Pearson K.G. (1987b) Flight motor patterns recorded in surgically isolated sections of the ventral nerve cord of *Locusta migratoria*. **J. comp. Physiol. 161**, pp. 103-114

15
Neuronal Computation in the Mammalian Spinal Cord

Dimitri Kullmann

Summary

The stretch reflex studied in extensor muscles of the decerebrate cat offers a window on the low-level organization of the mammalian motor system. A striking feature of this system is that shifts in motor output can be achieved without any change in the slope of the length-tension curve. In other words, the steady state stiffness of the stretch reflex appears to be regulated by the nervous system. In this chapter it is argued that stiffness regulation cannot be accounted for by the linearizing action of feedback arcs (cf. Houk, 1979). Instead, changes in motor output can be achieved without altering stiffness if motor unit firing rate and recruitment modulation are linked in a precise relationship.

The model presented here successfully accounts for motor unit behaviour in the stretch reflex on the basis of the distribution of synaptic inputs across the alpha motoneurone pool. This implies that stiffness regulation is achieved by differentially tailoring synaptic inputs to motoneurones, depending on their biophysical properties.

15.1 Introduction

Of all areas of the mammalian central nervous system, the spinal cord is perhaps the most thoroughly studied from the point of view of the biophysics, organization and behaviour of the constituent neurones. It has however been relatively neglected in the recent expansion of interest in computational models of neural processing. This can to some extent be explained by the lack of consensus about the precise functions of the lowest levels of the motor system. Not only is there disagreement about the nature of the controlled or regulated variables (Stein, 1982), but also about the roles of individual receptor types (Hasan & Stuart, 1988). Two possible reasons for this state of affairs spring to mind. First, it may reflect a profound ignorance of the mechanical regularities which underlie limb movements. Indeed, if no regularities exist, then it may not even be possible to identify any rules governing the relationships between inputs and outputs of the spinal cord: all pathways would then be tailored to local idiosyncrasies, rather than reflecting some general principles of motor organization. Second, the lack of consensus may result from the application of inappropriate tools to study the organization of the spinal circuitry. So far, all control systems modelling has been carried out in the context of single-channel linear operators (e.g. Houk, 1979; Windhorst, 1988). These are quite at variance with the manifestly non-linear behaviour of receptors, effectors and interneurones, all wired up in parallel, which perform the neuronal computations.

In this chapter it will be argued that some rules do govern the lowest levels of motor behaviour, at least in extensor muscles of the decerebrate cat. It will also be shown that this behaviour cannot be accounted for by the action of linear feedback loops operating at the segmental level. It can however be explained by a model which makes use of the parallel organization of the nervous system, and relies on the distribution of biophysical properties across the population of alpha motoneurones supplying a muscle. The implications of this model will be examined in the light of recent evidence on the control of synaptic strength.

15.2 Regularities of motor behaviour

The stretch reflex measured in extensor muscles of the decerebrate or mesencephalic cat has provided some of the strongest evidence that at least one parameter of motor output may be held constant by the nervous system. As a muscle is slowly stretched to different lengths, its contractile tension is found, above a threshold, to vary roughly linearly with length. The slope, or stiffness, of this length-tension curve is then found to be remarkably stable in the face of perturbations which alter the amount of extensor tone, such as afferent or supraspinal stimulation. The length-tension curve is simply shifted to longer or shorter lengths, without any major change in shape (Matthews, 1959; Feldman & Orlovsky, 1972).

The importance of this observation is that stiffness is *regulated* by the nervous system; that is, it appears to vary less than the behaviour of individual components of the circuitry. For instance, if muscles are isolated from the central nervous system and the nerves supplying them are stimulated electrically, then length-tension curves are obtained whose slopes vary with the stimulation frequency (Rack & Westbury, 1969). A similar principle emerges if the transient change in tension is measured when a muscle is subjected to a small rapid change in length: the instantaneous stiffness varies less with motor output if the reflex arc is intact than if the muscle is deafferented by cutting the dorsal roots (Nichols & Houk, 1976). This is not to say that stiffness is necessarily held constant at all times in these animals (e.g. Hoffer & Andreassen, 1981; Nichols & Steeves, 1986). The observations simply indicate that in some well-defined circumstances changes in motor output can be achieved without a major effect on stiffness.

Stiffness regulation has important advantages for the coordination of motor commands. Since a given length change elicits similar tension changes at different levels of contraction, the postural muscles can be treated as shock-absorbers which

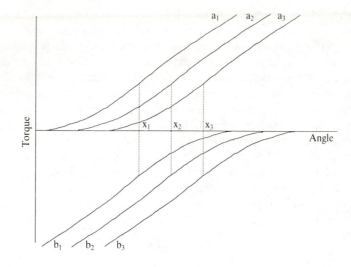

Figure 15.1 A simplified model of joint position control. The torque-angle curves a_1, a_2, a_3 and b_1, b_2, b_3 correspond to length-tension curves for agonist and antagonist muscles respectively, at different levels of motor output. Over small deviations, the non-linearities introduced by relating muscle force to joint angle, instead of length, can be ignored. Neglecting the effects of external loads, the joint angle is at equilibrium when the torques generated by agonist and antagonist muscles balance one another. Thus, position x_1 can be maintained by the higher centres by choosing the torque-angle curves a_1 and b_1. Another angle, x_2, can be specified by relaxing the agonist to obtain a_2, and further contracting the antagonist to obtain b_2. Motor planning is greatly simplified if changes in motor output are achieved without altering the stiffness of each muscle, that is, without altering the slope of the torque-angle curve.

have constant impedance, but whose length can be altered. A change in load distribution, as might occur during a change in stance, should then cause predictable displacements along the length-tension curves of every contracting muscle. These can then be taken into account in planning changes in descending signals. If stiffness were variable, it might still be possible to predict the effect of a perturbation, but at a greater computational cost because the dependence of stiffness on motor output would have to be known. On a more speculative level, stiffness regulation may simplify the computation of motor signals required for a limb to reach a given target. At equilibrium, the angle of each joint is determined by the length-tension curves of the opposing muscles, together with the loads, internal and external, acting on the limb. Target limb positions could then be specified simply by choosing pairs of length-tension curves for agonists and antagonists at each joint (see Berkinblit *et al.*, 1986, and accompanying commentaries). Clearly, if stiffness is constant for each muscle the computational task is greatly simplified, since only the position of each length-tension curve need be specified to achieve a given displacement (Figure 15.1). Again, if stiffness were variable, a change in joint angle could still be specified by choosing appropriate length-tension curves, but their precise shapes would need to be known to predict how the equilibrium point was displaced.

In the remainder of this section the phenomenon of stiffness invariance will be examined more closely to elaborate a model of the mechanisms by which it may be achieved. Attention will be restricted to the steady-state stiffness of the cat's soleus muscle, since this can be modelled without invoking dynamic properties of muscle, receptors or neurones.

15.2.1 *Control systems modelling*

The model of stiffness regulation outlined by Houk (1979) illustrates the limitations of linear control system modelling (Figure 15.2). According to this model, the length-tension curve of a contracting muscle results from the mechanical properties of the muscle itself, together with spinal feedback loops mediated by mechanoreceptors and their afferents. These are divided into spindle afferents - signalling length changes - and Golgi tendon organs - signalling tension changes. Briefly, if at a given level of contraction, the intrinsic stiffness of the muscle is too low, the load acting on it will cause it to stretch, raising the muscle spindle discharge rate. By virtue of the excitatory action of primary spindle afferents on homonymous alpha motoneurones, motor output will be supplemented and the force in the muscle increased, preventing further stretch. Conversely, if the stiffness is too high, Golgi tendon organs will signal an increase in force. This will then bring about a reduction in motor output, mediated by an inhibitory action on motoneurones. In the steady state, the two influences balance each other at a reference stiffness level. In other words, length feedback mediated by spindle afferents, and force feedback mediated by tendon organs, together make up a stiffness (force/length) servo which compensates for non-linearities in muscle properties.

This model makes many simplifying assumptions about the central actions and sensitivity of muscle receptors. For instance, primary muscle spindle afferents have been shown to converge together with tendon organ afferents on interneurones mediating inhibition of extensor motoneurones (Harrison & Jankowska, 1985). The interaction of the two feedback arcs illustrated in Figure 15.2 is unlikely, therefore, to be linear. The model is also unsatisfactory because neither spindles nor tendon organs, singly or in combination, sense departures of stiffness *per se* from a desired value, so the error signal required for an efficient servo mechanism is lacking. The system could reduce variations in muscle stiffness, but only if length and force feedback both have a high gain, or themselves show non-linearities complementary to those of the muscle. Primary spindle afferents show a weak steady-state length sensitivity (see Matthews, 1972, for a review), so they would appear not to be well suited to signal departures of the length-tension curve from a reference slope. Secondary spindle afferents, on the other hand, appear not to contribute incrementally to the stretch reflex in the soleus muscle of the decerebrate cat (Jack & Roberts, 1978), even though stiffness regulation has been demonstrated in this preparation. Finally, when tendon organ feedback was measured in the same

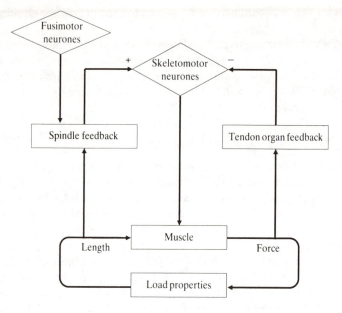

Figure 15.2 Control system model of stiffness regulation. Muscle forces interact with load properties to produce length changes. The relationship between force change and length change (stiffness) is determined by the central actions of muscle receptors: muscle spindle (length) and tendon organ (force) feedback, together with muscle properties, constitute the stiffness servo. Redrawn from Houk (1979).

preparation, its gain was found to be negligible (Houk *et al.*, 1970; Jack & Roberts, 1978).

It has even been suggested that afferent feedback does not significantly affect the stiffness of the contracting muscle at all, since similar length-tension curves have been observed in deafferented muscles of decerebrate cats as in those where the reflex loop was intact (Pompeiano, 1960; Grillner & Udo, 1971; Ellaway & Trott, 1975). To date, parallel shifts of the length-tension curve have not been demonstrated in deafferented muscles of decerebrate animals, but this may reflect the difficulty of obtaining an extensor tone in the absence of motoneurone excitation from spindle afferents in this preparation. Awake monkeys can make accurate reaching and head-positioning movements after deafferentation, indicating that feedback loops are not necessary to achieve desired changes in joint position (Bizzi *et al.*, 1976, 1978). If, as suggested by Feldman and co-workers (Berkinblit *et al.*, 1986), such movements are achieved by shifting length-tension curves without changing their shape, then stiffness regulation does not depend on an intact reflex arc.

It thus appears that afferent feedback may not be necessary for stiffness regulation. But how can this be reconciled with the finding that stiffness varies widely when the contraction is obtained by electrical stimulation of the efferent nerves? The answer appears to be that electrical stimulation does not reproduce the motor output obtained in a physiological contraction.

15.2.2 *An alternative model of stiffness regulation*

When an animal contracts a muscle, tension is increased both by increasing the firing rate of the active motor units and by recruiting more motor units according to the size principle. Initially, alpha motoneurones with small diameter axons, supplying small numbers of muscle fibres, are active. As the contraction develops, their firing rates increase and motoneurones with larger axons, supplying larger numbers of muscle fibres, are brought into action. This is quite different from the pattern achieved by electrical stimulation of the efferent nerves. The natural recruitment cannot easily be reproduced by altering stimulus voltage, so changing the stimulation frequency on its own cannot be compared to physiological modulation of the contraction.

With cathodal stimulation of the cut ventral roots, stiffness varies widely with stimulation frequency (Rack & Westbury, 1969; D.M. Kullmann, unpublished observations). More precisely, as the frequency increases, the length-tension curve is shifted up and becomes shallower, until a tetanic contraction is achieved. This is illustrated in Figure 15.3A. Clearly, as stimulation frequency increases, stiffness, measured as the slope of the length-tension curve, *decreases* over most muscle lengths.

In soleus muscle of the decerebrate animal, motor units which are simultaneously active fire at roughly the same rate (Grillner & Udo, 1971; Clark *et al.*, 1981). In other words, at any level of contraction, motor unit firing rates are tightly grouped, and as new units are recruited they begin to fire at the prevailing discharge frequency. All the active units should therefore be at roughly the same point on a curve relating stiffness to firing rate. Since the contractile tensions of individual motor units add roughly linearly, it follows that recruitment is accompanied by a simple scaling up of the length-tension curve. Stiffness is thus *increased* by recruitment over most firing rates and muscle lengths.

Now, since increases in firing rate and recruitment have opposite effects on stiffness, a change in motor output could be achieved without altering stiffness if the two effects balanced one another. In other words, if an increase in firing rate were accompanied by an appropriate increase in recruitment, the length-tension curve could be shifted up without any change in its slope. This is illustrated in Figure 15.3B, where the length-tension curves in Figure 15.3A have been scaled in such a way that the overall slope remains roughly constant. Stiffness regulation could thus be achieved simply by virtue of the complementary effects of firing rate and recruitment modulation, without invoking feedback arcs.

The model proposed here only applies to the steady-state relationship between muscle length and tension, and does not claim to account for the dynamic changes in force in response to length perturbations. Spindle feedback, carried by primary afferents, is probably essential in linearizing the tension transients seen with such

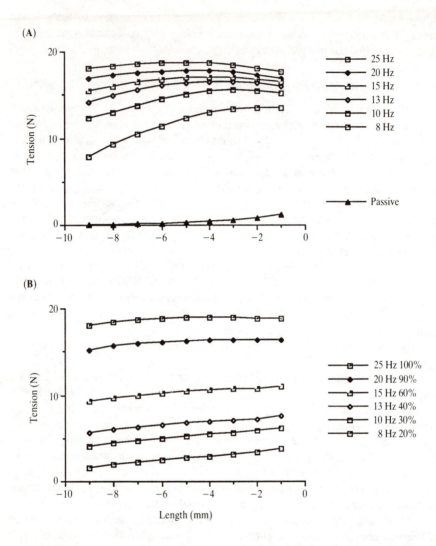

Figure 15.3 A. Length-tension curves obtained in soleus muscle of an anaesthetized cat by electrically stimulating the severed ventral roots at various frequencies (shown at right). Steady-state tension was measured at different muscle lengths, measured from maximal physiological length (MPL). The passive tension obtained without any stimulus (also shown) was subtracted from each curve. **B.** Parallel length-tension curves which could be obtained if different fractions of the total muscle output were active at each stimulation frequency. Each curve was obtained by scaling the length-tension curves in **A** by different amounts (shown at right), and adding the passive tension. This generated a family of curves with constant stiffness at different levels of contraction, apart from some deviations at the longer lengths, near MPL.

perturbations (Nichols & Houk, 1976), but does not form part of the present model. Its principal role in the *steady-state* stretch reflex is to provide a background excitatory drive to the motoneurone pool. This, together with other descending and afferent inputs to the motoneurones, determines the level of motor output, which is reflected in the position of the length-tension curve.

15.3 Implications of the model

According to the model outlined above, firing rate and recruitment must be coupled in a precise relationship for stiffness to remain constant in the face of changes in motor output. In Figure 15.3B, the stiffness at intermediate levels of motor output was chosen arbitrarily to be the same as that at a firing rate of 25 Hz and 100% recruitment, expressed as a percentage of the maximal contractile force available. (Some deviation from stiffness constancy is seen near maximal physiological length, but this may represent the operational limits of the regulatory mechanisms.) A different relationship between firing rate and recruitment could have been chosen to maintain a different value of stiffness. The essence of the model, however, is that whatever relationship actually applies is adhered to in a stereotypic manner.

The regulation of stiffness is achieved by ensuring that the appropriate relationship is respected between firing rate and recruitment, rather than by correcting deviations of the effector from the target performance. This raises the question of whether the phenomenon is one of regulation at all, since the effector is driven by an open loop signal. Some evidence that error correction does take place is discussed later in this chapter (Section 15.4). First, the mechanisms which determine the firing rate-recruitment relationship will be examined to assess whether the model is compatible with available data. Is the motoneurone pool, together with its inputs, organized in such a way that a tight relationship can hold between firing rate and recruitment? And if so, can it account for the observation that, at any level of motor output, soleus motor unit firing rates are closely grouped (Grillner & Udo, 1971; Clark *et al.*, 1981)? If this can be explained on the basis of the organization of the motoneurone pool, then one need not invoke extraneous error signals to account for the firing rate-recruitment relationship.

The motoneurones which supply a postural muscle such as soleus receive a rich synaptic input from primary spindle afferents, as well as from interneurones mediating influences from other peripheral afferents and descending pathways. There appear not to be any major qualitative differences in the projection patterns to individual cells. Several factors which determine neurone firing are, however, continuously graded. These factors, which have recently been reviewed by Burke (1987), can be divided into the strength of the synaptic inputs, and properties intrinsic to the cells.

15.3.1 Synaptic input to the motoneurone pool

The analysis could be greatly simplified if synaptic current were distributed evenly across the motoneurone pool; that is, if cells received the same overall synaptic current irrespective of their recruitment order. Such a pattern may be surprising, since motoneurones recruited late have a relatively larger surface area than ones recruited early, and could be expected to bear more synaptic boutons on their surface (Gelfan & Rapisarda, 1964). There is, nevertheless, some evidence that this pattern does apply, at least for some of the major excitatory and inhibitory influences on motoneurones; what is this evidence?

Excitatory post-synaptic potentials (EPSPs) elicited by stimulating group Ia afferents from homonymous or synergistic nerves are roughly proportional in amplitude to the input resistance of the motoneurone (Burke, 1968; Dum & Kennedy, 1980; Lev-Tov et al., 1983; Luscher et al., 1983). Applying Ohm's law, this implies that the same amount of synaptic current is injected into motoneurones with large or small input resistance. Now, since cells with a high input resistance are recruited earlier than those with a low input resistance (Kernell, 1983), it follows that the synaptic current from group Ia afferents is roughly the same for motoneurones recruited early and late. This has also been shown to hold during continuous synaptic bombardment. Using high frequency stimulation of Ia afferents, the steady-state depolarization in different motoneurones is again distributed in proportion to input resistance (Munson et al., 1982a; Heckman & Binder, 1985).

Data for inhibitory synaptic inputs to motoneurones are less complete, but point to the same conclusion. Inhibitory post-synaptic potentials (IPSPs) elicited by stimulating antagonist group Ia afferents have been shown to co-vary with motoneurone input resistance (Dum & Kennedy, 1980; see also Burke et al., 1973). Similar findings have been obtained by recording group Ib afferent inhibition (Powers & Binder, 1985) and recurrent inhibition from Renshaw cells (Friedman et al., 1981; Lindsay & Binder, 1987) in motoneurones with different input resistances. Again applying Ohm's law, these results are consistent with the principle that synaptic current is independent of recruitment order.

Two exceptions to this rule have been tentatively identified. Monosynaptic EPSPs from vestibulospinal tracts appear not to co-vary with either the after-hyperpolarization (AHP) duration of the motoneurone (Grillner et al., 1971) or the amplitude of monosynaptic Ia EPSPs (Burke et al., 1976). Since both AHP duration and Ia EPSP amplitude are related to motoneurone recruitment order (Kernell, 1983; see above), this would imply that cells recruited late received a larger synaptic current, which was balanced by their lower input resistance. Monosynaptic EPSPs from group II afferents also appear to be independent of input resistance (Munson et al., 1982b).

In summary, it appears that several important sources of excitation and inhibition of the motoneurone pool are organized in such a way that synaptic current is independent of recruitment order. The two exceptions may not invalidate the overall conclusion, since the monosynaptic projections from both vestibulospinal

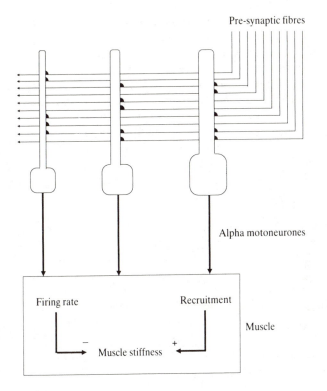

Figure 15.4 The firing rate-recruitment model of stiffness regulation. Three motoneurones of different sizes are shown schematically, together with some pre-synaptic fibres projecting to them, and the synaptic contacts, representing current injecting sites. Excitatory and inhibitory synaptic currents from most sources investigated to date are distributed to motoneurones irrespective of their recruitment order. Thus, the total number of synaptic contacts is shown as being the same on each cell. Motor output varies as a function of both firing rate and recruitment of the motoneurone pool supplying the muscle. Stiffness is varied in opposite directions by modulating firing rate and recruitment.

tracts and group II afferents to motoneurones appear to be of minor importance compared to polysynaptic pathways. The latter pathways are shared with other afferents (reviewed by Baldissera *et al.*, 1981; see also Lundberg *et al.*, 1987), and may well follow the pattern observed for other inputs. The organization of the inputs described above is summarized in Figure 15.4. Three motoneurones of different sizes are shown to indicate the tendency for overall synaptic current to be independent of the recruitment order. Before the above description can be used to derive the relationship between firing rate and recruitment, the distribution of properties intrinsic to the motoneurones must be examined.

15.3.2   Intrinsic motoneurone properties

Spinal motoneurones appear to behave somewhat akin to the units incorporated by McClelland and Rumelhart (1981) into their model of parallel distributed processing: inhibitory synaptic currents subtract linearly from excitatory ones, and the firing rate above a threshold is roughly linearly related to the total injected current (see Kernell, 1983, for a review). Especially relevant to the present model are motoneurones supplying 'type S' motor units. These units, which contract slowly and are fatigue resistant, make up soleus muscle and account for most of the contractile force seen in the hindlimb during postural movements and slow locomotion (Walmsley *et al.*, 1978). In response to a step change in injected current, such motoneurones accommodate rapidly and then fire at a constant rate (Kernell, 1983). The distribution of intrinsic properties across the motoneurone pool can be summarized as follows:

1) Motoneurones are recruited into regular discharge when the injected current exceeds their rheobase, which is inversely related to the input resistance (Kernell, 1983). The product of rheobase and input resistance is the voltage threshold for repetitive firing, roughly 15 mV, and appears not to vary appreciably between motoneurones (Stein & Bertoldi, 1981; Pinter *et al.*, 1983).

2) The initial firing rate of the cell is roughly equal to the inverse of the AHP duration (Kernell, 1983). This is linearly related to the input resistance (Gustafsson, 1979; Luscher *et al.*, 1983), ensuring that motoneurones recruited early fire at a lower initial rate than those recruited later.

3) Once recruited, cells increase their firing rate linearly with injected current, with a slope of approximately 1.5 pps/nA (Kernell, 1979; Gustafsson, personal communication). This quantity shows no consistent relationship to recruitment order, as estimated from the input resistance.

15.3.3   Firing rate-recruitment relationship

The above description has important implications for the behaviour of the motoneurone pool. It confirms that a tight relationship should hold between firing rate and recruitment. This follows since the same excitatory or inhibitory synaptic current appears to be injected into motoneurones irrespective of their recruitment order. Since inhibitory currents subtract from excitatory ones, only one variable is needed to describe the overall input to the motoneurone pool in the steady state. This variable can be equated to the total synaptic current per cell, which, together with motoneurone properties, determines the firing rate and recruitment of the entire pool. Various permutations of excitatory and inhibitory inputs will only increase or decrease the total effective synaptic current.

A deviation from the stereotyped firing rate-recruitment relationship could only be achieved if another synaptic input were distributed according to a different pattern. For instance, if a major source of excitation were distributed in the same way as the monosynaptic vestibulospinal input (Section 15.3.1), then the motoneurone pool could be controlled in two dimensions. Cells normally recruited late could then be brought into activity earlier, because they would receive a relatively larger synaptic current than cells recruited early. According to available evidence, however, this pattern only holds for a small fraction of the total excitatory influences acting on hindlimb motoneurones, at least in the decerebrate cat. It thus appears that a tight firing rate-recruitment relationship results simply from the organization of the motoneurone pool. Is this, however, the same relationship which would maintain constant stiffness?

In order for the contraction strength to be modulated without any change in stiffness, the appropriate trade-off must be maintained between firing rate and recruitment changes. A qualitative indication of what this trade-off might be comes from the observation that in soleus muscle of the decerebrate cat, active motor units all appear to fire at the same rate (Grillner & Udo, 1971; Clark *et al.*, 1981). Does this result from the organization of the motoneurone pool? The close grouping of firing rates implies that newly recruited motoneurones begin to fire at the frequency attained by cells recruited earlier. If this results from motoneurone properties alone, initial firing rates, plotted against rheobase, must be distributed with the same slope as the average firing rate-current relationship.

The initial firing rate-rheobase slope can be estimated by replotting the distribution of AHP duration with input resistance given by Gustaffson (1979 & personal communication), and Luscher *et al.* (1983). Initial firing rate is estimated from the inverse of the AHP duration, while the rheobase is estimated by taking the ratio of threshold depolarization, 15 mV, to input resistance. The result of this manipulation is shown in Figure 15.5. Motoneurones supplying fast-contracting and fatiguing motor units were included in this analysis, but the behaviour of cells typical of soleus muscle can be observed by restricting attention to those with input resistance greater than 1.2 MΩ and AHP longer than 70 ms (roughly corresponding to a rheobase less than 12 nA and an initial firing rate less than 15 pps). This distribution has a slope of approximately 1.5 pps/nA, which agrees with the average firing rate-current slope reported by Kernell (1979) and Gustafsson (personal communication). As synaptic current increases, new motoneurones should indeed begin to fire at approximately the same rate as other cells recruited previously.

If motoneurones with lower input resistance are considered (below 1.2 MΩ, corresponding to a rheobase greater than 12 nA), the gradient of initial firing rate to rheobase becomes shallower, and therefore diverges from the mean firing rate-current slope (Figure 15.5). This predicts that new motor units start to fire at a lower firing rate than that attained by previously recruited ones, and is consistent with the behaviour observed at higher contraction strengths in muscles of 'mixed' motor unit type (Harris & Henneman, 1976). This may reflect different functional strategies, not necessarily concerned with stiffness regulation, and does not invalidate the present conclusions.

To summarize the above discussion, hindlimb motoneurone properties, together with the synaptic organization of the major sources of excitation and inhibition, allow motor unit recruitment and firing rate modulation to be coupled in

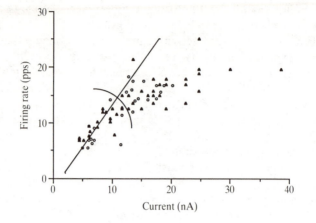

Figure 15.5 Dependence of initial firing rate on rheobase in triceps surae motoneurones, estimated by replotting data from Gustafsson (1979, open symbols) and Luscher *et al.* (1983, filled symbols). Also shown is the average slope (1.5 pps/nA) of the firing rate-current relationship, given by Kernell (1979) and Gustafsson (personal communication). The curved line indicates the approximate limits of motoneurones supplying 'type S' motor units. See text for details.

the stereotypical manner observed in soleus muscle of the decerebrate animal. This firing rate-recruitment relationship, which appears to ensure that stiffness remains constant in the face of changing motor output, is obtained without the intervention of feedback signals. Stiffness regulation, according to this model, results from appropriately setting the strength of synaptic inputs to motoneurones, in relation to their biophysical properties.

15.4   Regulation of synaptic strength

The model described above raises the issue of how synaptic inputs and biophysical properties of motoneurones may be adjusted to ensure the appropriate firing rate-recruitment relationship. It would appear unlikely that they could be specified genetically, because the mechanical properties of muscles may alter with age and training. On the other hand, if stiffness is genuinely *regulated*, an error signal must be generated to correct deviations from a reference value, and transmitted to the spinal apparatus to adjust the variables which control motoneurone discharge patterns. The mechanisms by which this error signal might be generated are unknown, but they may involve supraspinal centres monitoring performance during postural movements. Long term changes in the synaptic organization of the spinal cord could then be produced by descending signals. Some information is, however, emerging which may explain how the strength of synapses onto motoneurones is altered.

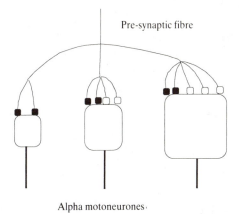

Pre-synaptic fibre

Alpha motoneurones

Figure 15.6 A model of the mechanism by which synaptic current may be distributed equally between motoneurones, irrespective of their recruitment order. Three motoneurones of different sizes are shown, together with the terminal arborization of one pre-synaptic fibre from a primary spindle afferent. Cells recruited late, which tend to be larger and have a lower input resistance than those recruited early, have a larger proportion of silent release sites on their surface. This is indicated by the proportion of open symbols. The number of filled symbols, representing active release sites, is equal in the resting state. Only one release site is shown per contact, for the sake of clarity, although histological evidence shows that several can occur in the same synaptic bouton.

Intriguing results have been reported from studies on post-tetanic potentiation of both EPSPs and IPSPs in motoneurones. The increase in monosynaptic Ia afferent EPSPs is inversely related to motoneurone input resistance (Luscher *et al.*, 1983). This implies that more synaptic current is turned on by a pre-synaptic tetanus in cells recruited late than in cells recruited early. A similar trend has been observed by recording the post-tetanic potentiation of recurrent inhibitory potentials from Renshaw cells (Binder & Lindsay, 1987). A simple explanation for this phenomenon is that cells with low input resistance, which tend to be larger, normally have a number of silent synaptic release sites on their surface. Smaller cells, with high input resistance, have a smaller total number of release sites, as might be expected, but a larger proportion of these are active. This could account for the even distribution of synaptic current between motoneurones prior to tetanization, irrespective of recruitment order. When pre-synaptic fibres are tetanized, however, more release sites are available to be activated on large cells than on small ones. This proposal is illustrated in Figure 15.6. In essence, the roughly even distribution of synaptic current normally observed in motoneurones results from plastic changes, which are temporarily reversed by tetanic stimulation.

The experimental evidence for this scheme is indirect, but it does provide a mechanism by which synaptic strength can be modulated differentially between motoneurones, depending on their biophysical properties.

Conclusion

The above discussion stresses the importance of distributing activity across the entire motoneurone pool to obtain an appropriate motor output. Only if firing rate and recruitment vary according to a strict relationship can motor output alter without any change in stiffness. For this to be achieved, synaptic inputs must be precisely adjusted, in relation to the biophysical parameters controlling cell firing, across the entire motoneurone pool. By extrapolation, other networks in the central nervous system may employ a similar strategy to optimize performance. If so, a full understanding of their computational capacity will only be achieved if synaptic strengths are related to cell properties across the breadth of each neurone pool.

Acknowledgement

I am indebted to Dr. J.J.B. Jack for helpful comments.

References

Baldissera F., Hultborn H. & Illert M. (1981) Integration in spinal neuronal systems. In: **Handbook of Physiology Sec. 1. Vol. II. Part 1.** pp. 509-595, V.B. Brooks (ed.) Am. Physiol. Soc., Bethesda.

Berkinblit M.B., Feldman A.G. & Fukson O.I. (1986) Adaptability of innate motor patterns and motor control mechanisms. **Behav. Brain Sci. 9,** pp. 585-638

Binder M.D. & Lindsay A.D. (1987) Post-tetanic potentiation of recurrent IPSPs in cat motoneurons. **Soc. Neurosci. Abstr. 13,** p. 1695

Bizzi E., Dev P., Morasso P. & Polit A. (1978) Effect of load disturbances during centrally initiated movements. **J. Neurophysiol. 41,** pp. 542-556

Bizzi E., Polit A. & Morasso P. (1976) Mechanisms underlying achievement of final head position. **J. Neurophysiol. 39,** pp. 435-444

Burke R.E. (1968) Group Ia synaptic input to fast and slow twitch motor units of cat triceps surae. **J. Physiol. 196,** pp. 605-630

Burke R.E. (1987) Synaptic efficacy and the control of neuronal input-output relations. **TINS 10,** pp. 42-45

Burke R.E., Rymer W.Z. & Walsh J.V. (1973) Functional specialization in the motoneuron population of cat medial gastrocnemius muscle. In: **Control of Posture and Locomotion.** pp. 29-44, R.B. Stein, K.B. Pearson & J.B. Redford (eds.) Plenum, NY.

Burke R.E., Rymer W.Z. & Walsh J.V. (1976) Relative strength of synaptic inputs from short latency pathways to motor units of defined types in medial gastrocnemius. **J. Neurophysiol. 39,** pp. 447-458

Clark F.J., Matthews P.B.C. & Muir R.B. (1981) Motor unit firing and its relation to tremor in the tonic vibration reflex of the decerebrate cat. **J. Physiol. 313,** pp. 317-334

Dum R.P. & Kennedy T.T. (1980) Synaptic organization of defined motor-unit types in cat tibialis anterior. **J. Neurophysiol. 43,** pp. 1631-1644

Ellaway P.H. & Trott J.R. (1975) The mode of action of 5-hydroxytryptophan in facilitating a stretch reflex in the spinal cat. **Exp. Brain Res. 22,** pp. 145-162

Feldman A.G. & Orlovsky G.N. (1972) The influence of different descending systems on the tonic stretch reflex in the cat. **Exp. Neurol. 37,** pp. 481-494

Friedman W.A., Sypert G.W., Munson J.B. & Fleshman J.W. (1981) Recurrent inhibition in type-identified motoneurons. **J. Neurophysiol. 46,** pp. 1349-1359

Gelfan S. & Rapisarda A.F. (1964) Synaptic density on spinal neurones of normal dogs and dogs with experimental hindlimb rigidity. **J. comp. Neurol. 123,** pp. 73-95

Grillner S., Hongo T. & Lund S. (1971) Convergent effects on alpha motoneurones from the vestibulospinal tract and a pathway descending in the medial longitudinal fasciculus. **Exp. Brain Res. 12,** pp. 457-479

Grillner S. & Udo M. (1971) Motor unit activity and stiffness of the contracting muscle fibres in the tonic stretch reflex. **Acta Physiol. Scand. 81,** pp. 422-424

Gustafsson B. (1979) Changes in motoneurone electrical properties following axotomy. **J. Physiol. 293,** pp. 197-215

Harris D.A. & Henneman E. (1976) Identification of 2 species of alpha motoneurons in the cat's plantaris pool. **J. Neurophysiol. 40,** pp. 16-25

Harrison P.J. & Jankowska E. (1985) Organization of input to interneurones mediating group I non-reciprocal inhibition of motoneurones in the cat. **J. Physiol. 361,** pp. 403-418

Hasan Z. & Stuart D.G. (1988) Animal solutions to the problem of movement control: the role of proprioceptors. **Ann. Rev. Neurosci. 11,** pp. 199-223

Heckman C.J. & Binder M.D. (1985) Analysis of steady-state Ia synaptic potentials and synaptic currents in cat motoneurons. **Soc. Neurosci. Abstr. 11,** p. 402

Hoffer J.A. & Andreassen S. (1981) Limitations in the servoregulation of soleus muscle stiffness in premamillary cats. In: **Muscle Receptors and Movement.** pp. 311-324, A. Taylor and A. Prochazka (eds.) Macmillan, London.

Houk J.C. (1979) Regulation of stiffness by skeletomotor reflexes. **Ann. Rev. Physiol. 41,** pp. 99-114

Houk J.C., Singer J.J. & Goldman M.R. (1970) An evaluation of length and force feedback to soleus muscles of decerebrate cats. **J. Neurophysiol. 34,** pp. 1051-1065

Jack J.J.B. & Roberts R.C. (1978) The role of muscle spindle afferents in stretch and vibration reflexes of the soleus muscle of the decerebrate cat. **Brain Res. 146,** pp. 366-372

Kernell D. (1979) Rhythmic properties of motoneurones innervating muscle fibres of different speed in m. gastrocnemius medialis of the cat. **Brain Res. 160,** pp. 159-162

Kernell D. (1983) Functional properties of spinal motoneurones and the gradation of muscle force. In: **Motor Control Mechanisms in Health and Disease. Adv. Neurol. Vol. 39.** pp. 213-226, J.E. Desmedt (ed.) Raven Press, NY.

Lev-Tov A., Pinter M.J. & Burke R.E. (1983) Post-tetanic potentiation of group Ia EPSPs: Possible mechanisms for differential distribution among medial gastrocnemius motoneurons. **J. Neurophysiol. 50,** pp. 379-398

Lindsay A.D. & Binder M.D. (1987) Analysis of steady-state recurrent IPSPs and their underlying effective synaptic currents in cat motoneurons. **Soc. Neurosci. Abstr. 13,** p. 1695

Lundberg A., Malmgren K. & Schomburg E.D. (1987) Reflex pathways from group II muscle afferents. 1. Distribution and linkage of reflex actions to alpha-motoneurones. **Exp. Brain Res. 65,** pp. 271-281

Luscher H.-P., Ruenzel P. & Henneman E. (1983) Composite EPSPs in motoneurons of different sizes before and during post-tetanic potentiation: implications for transmission failure and its relief in Ia projections. **J. Neurophysiol. 49,** pp. 269-289

McClelland J.L. & Rumelhart D.E. (1981) An interactive activation model of context effects in letter perception: Part 1. An account of basic findings. **Psychol. Rev. 88,** pp. 375-407

Matthews P.B.C. (1959) A study of certain factors influencing the stretch reflex of the decerebrate cat. **J. Physiol. 147,** pp. 547-564

Matthews P.B.C. (1972) **Mammalian Muscle Receptors and their Central Actions.** Arnold, London.

Munson J.B., Morales F.R., Sypert G.W. & Zengel J.E. (1982a) Steady state depolarization in spinal motoneurons: relation to input resistance and motor unit type. **Soc. Neurosci. Abstr. 8,** p. 792

Munson J.B., Sypert G.W., Zengel J.E., Lofton S.A. & Fleshman J.W. (1982b) Mono-synaptic projections of individual spindle group II afferents to type-identified medial gastrocnemius motoneurons in the cat. **J. Neurophysiol. 48,** pp. 1164-1174

Nichols T.R. & Houk J.C. (1976) Improvement in linearity and the regulation of stiffness that results from the actions of the stretch reflex. **J. Neurophysiol. 39,** pp. 199-242

Nichols T.R. & Steeves J.D. (1986) Resetting of resultant stiffness in ankle flexor and extensor muscles in the decerebrate cat. **Exp. Brain Res. 62,** pp. 401-410

Pinter M.J., Curtis R.L. & Hosko M.J. (1983) Voltage threshold and excitability among variously sized cat hindlimb motoneurons. **J. Neurophysiol. 50,** pp. 644-657

Pompeiano O. (1960) Alpha types of 'release' studied in tension-extension diagrams from cat's forelimb triceps. **Arch. Ital. Biol. 98,** pp. 92-117

Powers R.K. & Binder M.D. (1985) Distribution of oligosynaptic group I input to the cat medial gastrocnemius motoneuron pool. **J. Neurophysiol. 53,** pp. 497-517

Rack P.M.H. & Westbury D.R. (1969) The effect of length and stimulation rate on tension in the isometric cat soleus. **J. Physiol. 204,** pp. 443-460

Stein R.B. (1982) What muscle variable(s) does the nervous system control in limb movements? **Behav. Brain Sci. 5,** pp. 535-577

Stein R.B. & Bertholdi R. (1981) The size principle: a synthesis of neurophysiological data. In: **Motor Unit Types, Recruitment and Plasticity in Health and Disease. Prog. Clin. Neurophysiol. Vol. 9.** pp. 85-96, J.E. Desmedt (ed.) Karger, Basel.

Walmsley B., Hodgson J.A. & Burke R.E. (1978) Forces produced by medial gastrocnemius and soleus muscles during locomotion in freely moving cats. **J. Neurophysiol. 41,** 1203-1216

Windhorst U. (1988) **How Brain-like is the Spinal Cord?** Studies in Brain Function. Vol. 17. Springer, Berlin.

16
The Modelling of Pyramidal Neurones in the Visual Cortex

Ken Stratford, Adrian Mason, Alan Larkman, Guy Major &
Julian Jack

Summary

Pyramidal cells from layers 2/3 and 5 of the visual cortex of the rat have been studied using intracellular recording and horseradish peroxidase (HRP) injection in slices maintained *in vitro*. These data have been used to develop compartmental models of their dendritic electrical geometry. Computationally efficient, simplified representations of these cells have been developed. Values for the biophysical parameters of the model were estimated by comparing the model's predicted voltage response to a brief pulse of injected current with that recorded experimentally. It was found that many combinations of parameter values could fit the experimental data equally well. The effects of these various combinations on the time courses and relative efficacies of synaptic inputs are explored, and some implications for the possible computational capabilities of these neurones are discussed.

16.1 Introduction

Recent developments in connectionist modelling techniques (e.g. Rumelhart & McClelland, 1986) have led to the development of network models capable of providing elegant solutions to a number of difficult problems (e.g. Hopfield & Tank, 1985; Lehky & Sejnowski, 1988; Zipser & Andersen, 1988). Typically, these networks are constructed from assemblies of individual units, each of which has the following properties:

1) An integrating function, which sums the contributions from other connected units.

2) An output function, which transforms the output from the integrator into a pattern of activity which is then transmitted to other units. This transform may take the form of a step function, or some continuously graded response.

3) Some pattern of modifiable connections.

Although the individual units of artificial networks are not necessarily intended to correspond to 'real' neurones, many neurobiologists have noted that the above specification is a somewhat impoverished description of a neurone (e.g. Crick & Asanuma, 1986). Inputs to a neurone (perhaps $10^3 - 10^5$) are distributed over the soma and dendrites, which form an extended, geometrically complex structure. The neuronal membrane contains a dozen or so different voltage and time dependent ionic conductances (Adams & Galvan, 1986), some of which are also modulated by neurotransmitters and molecular messengers. The interplay of these ionic channels leads to complex non-linearities in electrical behaviour, not only above but also below the threshold for action potential firing. Furthermore, any given neural circuit is likely to involve many different types of neurone, each with its own distinctive morphological and electrophysiological 'personality'.

It could be argued that, despite their complexity, neurones have no greater computational ability than the simple units presently used in artificial networks. This complexity might only be a solution to the constraints imposed by the nature of biological structures, evolution, embryonic development, etc. However, it seems more likely to us that 'real' neurones might possess greater computational resources than the units of present artificial networks, and thus that an assembly of biologically more realistic units might have information processing capabilities in excess of those demonstrated by present artificial networks.

What information about 'real' neurones would be required to construct such a network? In principle, the electrical behaviour of a neurone could be completely specified if its morphology and membrane properties (which would include a precise description of the behaviour of the ion channels) were known. The supreme example of this approach is, of course, the account of the electrical excitability of the squid giant axon by Hodgkin and Huxley. (The further step of joining the units together would require equally detailed knowledge about the distribution, polarity, strength and modifiability of synaptic connections.) Unfortunately, because of their greater complexity and the technical difficulties of recording from them *in vivo*, one has had to be content with less fundamental descriptions of mammalian CNS neurones, with the properties of the underlying ionic conductances being inferred from intracellular recordings of current/voltage relations, action potential shape and after-potentials, etc.

However, the development of *in vitro* brain slice techniques (Dingledine, 1984; Kerkut & Wheal, 1981) has not only greatly facilitated high-quality intracellular recordings but, when combined with the single electrode voltage clamp (SEVC) technique suitable for small neurones (Wilson & Goldner, 1975), has led to more direct measurements of ionic conductances (albeit with certain limitations). More recently, the combination of patch clamp (Hamill *et al.*, 1981) and cell disaggregation techniques (Kay & Wong, 1986) has enabled preliminary studies of single ion channels from freshly isolated mammalian CNS neurones.

Partly because of its relatively simple structure, with most neuronal somata in a single, densely packed layer, and partly because of its relevance to important topics such as epilepsy (Schwartzkroin & Wheal, 1984) and long term potentiation (Landfield & Deadwyler, 1988), the hippocampus is the brain area which has been most intensively studied using *in vitro* slice techniques over the last decade. As a result, a huge amount of information has been amassed on the properties of hippocampal neurones (Schwartzkroin & Mueller, 1987). For example, of particular relevance to the subject of this chapter, details of active properties (e.g. Wong *et al.*, 1979; Johnston *et al.*, 1980; Wong & Prince, 1981) have been combined with passive models of electrical geometry (Turner & Schwartzkroin, 1984) to produce computer models which simulate many aspects of the electrical behaviour of hippocampal neurones (Traub & Llinas, 1979; Traub, 1982). Estimates of the pattern and strength of connections between neurones, including the rarer, inhibitory cell classes, are available from dual-impalement studies (e.g. Miles & Wong, 1984, 1986; Lacaille *et al.*, 1987). Much of this information has recently been incorporated into network models composed of 520 or 1020 biologically realistic units (Traub *et al.*, 1987a,b). The models successfully mimic the characteristics of some spontaneous and evoked events seen in experimental recordings from hippocampal slices.

In comparison to the hippocampus, studies on the neocortex have lagged somewhat behind. Although the same techniques are applicable, analysis of neocortical neurones and their connections is hindered by additional biological and technical complexities. In the rat the neocortex is a six layered structure containing a wide variety of neuronal types (Peters & Jones, 1984) and the cell bodies are not aligned in dense bands. However, on the positive side, it is possible to define fairly precisely the function of at least some neocortical areas, and this should prove of considerable benefit for attempts to construct and validate network models. Additionally, the importance of understanding neocortical function hardly needs stating and so an increasing number of laboratories are exploiting the technical advantages of *in vitro* preparations in order to study neocortical neurones. As a result, information is beginning to emerge about the basic electrophysiological properties of some cell types, (e.g. Stafstrom *et al.*, 1984a; McCormick *et al.*, 1985), their electrical geometry (Stafstrom *et al.*, 1984b) and ionic conductances (e.g. Stafstrom *et al.*, 1985; Spain *et al.*, 1987; Huguenard *et al.*, 1988; Schwindt *et al.*, 1988). Thus, by analogy with the hippocampus, it should be feasible to acquire sufficient information about individual neocortical neurones and their connections, to permit the construction of network models using biologically realistic units.

As a first step in this endeavour we have begun to characterize the morphology and electrophysiology of pyramidal neurones in brain slices of the rat visual cortex. Using a combination of these two kinds of data obtained from the same neurones we have derived models of neuronal electrical geometry. Although based on passive assumptions, our models are capable of incorporating active conductances as data become available. One important, interim goal of this type of modelling is to answer questions about synaptic integration by individual cortical neurones. For example, what are the likely relative efficacies of synaptic inputs on different parts of the dendritic tree? To date we have studied over fifty neurones in layers 2/3 and 5, and have been able to group them into three major classes on the basis of their morphology and electrophysiology. These results will be presented in detail elsewhere. In this chapter we will illustrate our approach using results obtained from a single neurone in layer 5.

16.2   Experimental data

16.2.1   *Methods*

Details of slice preparation, recording and HRP injection are given elsewhere (Larkman *et al.*, 1988; Mason *et al.*, 1988). Briefly, 0.4 mm thick slices of rat visual cortex were cut and maintained in an interface-type recording chamber at 34.5 °C for 6 - 8 hours. Individual neurones were impaled with HRP-containing glass micropipettes, and their voltage responses to current injection investigated using standard bridge-balance techniques. After HRP injection, slices were fixed, reacted and embedded in resin. In this way, morphology and electrophysiological data were obtained from the same neurone, allowing detailed correlations to be made. Using a light microscope, stained neurones were drawn, reconstructed and the lengths and diameters of their dendrites measured. The number of spines per unit length was measured for those dendrites, of different types and of a range of diameters, which lay in the plane of focus and so could be counted reliably. These values were then used to estimate the spine numbers on dendrites which were not favourably oriented. The mean membrane area per spine was estimated from our own and previously published material. Thus the total membrane area, including dendritic spines, of each cell could be estimated. Preliminary data collection and analysis was performed using IBM/PCs. Computer modelling of neuronal electrical geometry was performed using a SUN 3/280 with Floating Point Accelerator or a CONVEX vector processor. Most programs were written by the authors, but the basis of the compartmental modelling system was kindly supplied by Drs Clements and Redman of the Australian National University.

16.2.2   *Morphology*

Our sample of cells from layer 2/3 showed some variation in their dendritic branching depending on their depth within the layer, but appeared to conform to a single basic pattern. The layer 5 cells, on the other hand, were more variable. Based on features such as the thickness and length of the apical dendrite, we subdivided the layer 5 cells into two main classes. The cell we shall use as an example in this paper was from the class of cells with slender apical dendrites which did not form a visible terminal arbour in layer 1, as opposed to the other class which had thicker apical dendrites giving rise to an obvious terminal arbour in layer 1. A *camera lucida* reconstruction of the example cell is shown in Figure 16.1A. Its soma was squat, and the apical dendrite arose abruptly from its upper surface. It had five primary basal dendrites, each of which branched repeatedly near the soma. The mean length of the basal dendrites was 140 μm (±16 μm SD). The apical dendrite ascended towards the pia and terminated, without apparently arbourizing, in layer 2/3 at a

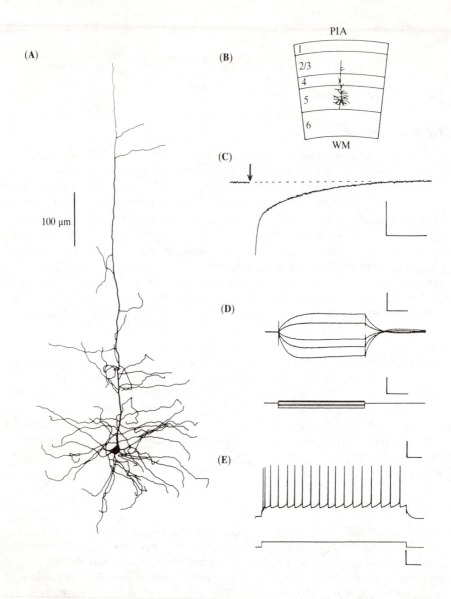

Figure 16.1 Morphological and electrophysiological data from a pyramidal neurone in layer 5 of the rat visual cortex. All data in this and subsequent figures are from this neurone. **A.** *Camera lucida* reconstruction of somadendritic morphology. Dendritic spines not shown. **B.** Survey diagram indicating laminar position of cell within cortex. WM - White matter. (Distance from pia to white matter = 1.5 mm). **C.** Voltage response to a 0.44 ms, 1.36 nA hyperpolarizing current pulse at time indicated by arrow. Average of 66 sweeps. For clarity, stimulus artefacts at onset and offset of pulse have been deleted. (Scale bars = 2 mV, 10 ms). **D.** Current / Voltage relationship. Upper trace - voltage; lower trace - current. Each trace is the average of 24 (**Cont. opposite**)

distance of 730 μm from the soma. As the apical dendrite ascended, it gave off a total of 22 oblique branches, mainly in the proximal third of its length. The more proximal obliques usually branched at least once, but the more distal obliques were unbranched. All but the most proximal parts of the basal and apical arbours were covered in dendritic spines. The cell was estimated to have a total of 8300 spines, of which 3200 were on the basal dendrites, 1400 were on the apical trunk and 3700 were on the apical oblique dendrites. Since the vast majority of excitatory synaptic inputs to neocortical pyramidal cells are made via dendritic spines and most spines bear only one such synapse, spines can be used as indicators to quantify the pattern of distribution of excitatory inputs to these cells.

16.2.3   Electrophysiology

Brief (0.5 ms) current pulses were applied through the micropipette, and the membrane voltage decay after the end of the pulse was recorded and averaged (Figure 16.1C). This voltage transient contains information about the electrical geometry of the neurone and was used, along with morphological data, to develop electrical models of the neurones (see below, and Figure 16.4).

In addition, we characterized neurones by their current-voltage relationships and repetitive firing properties. Current-voltage relationships were investigated using 150 ms current pulses (Figure 16.1D) and the apparent input resistance (38 MΩ for the cell illustrated) was measured over a voltage range just negative to rest. All neurones had distinctly non-linear current-voltage relationships, showing inward rectification both positive and negative to rest (not illustrated). In layer 5 neurones the presence of active conductances operating at potentials sub-threshold to firing level was also indicated by the 'sag' of the voltage back towards the resting value during hyperpolarizing or depolarizing current pulses, and the temporary 'overshoot' or 'undershoot', respectively, after the end of the current pulse (Figure 16.1D). Repetitive firing was examined using supra-threshold current pulses of 0.5 s duration (Figure 16.1E). Action potentials were produced throughout the duration of the pulse but their frequency diminished with time; i.e. the neurone showed spike frequency adaptation. Electrophysiological studies on pyramidal neurones from other neocortical areas have reported properties similar to those described here (e.g. McCormick *et al.*, 1985; Stafstrom *et al.*, 1984a) but detailed, correlated morphological information has usually been lacking. Amongst the entire sample of neurones studied we found differences in several aspects of sub- and supra-threshold properties, and these electrophysiological differences correlated closely with the cell types defined morphologically.

(**Fig. 16.1 Cont.**) sweeps. Note sag during and overshoot following current pulse. (Scale bars = 5 mV, 1 nA, 25 ms). **E.** Action potentials elicited by a 0.5 s supra-threshold depolarizing current pulse. Upper trace voltage, lower trace current. Note decrease in spike frequency during pulse. (Scale bars = 25 mV, 2 nA, 50 ms).

16.3 Models of neurones

Deriving a model which describes the passive electrical properties of the soma and dendritic tree of a neurone is a necessary first step in modelling its overall electrical behaviour. The objective of such a model is a representation which encompasses variations in morphology and physiology, but is streamlined enough for ultimate incorporation into a network simulation (e.g. Traub *et al.*, 1987a). A number of passive modelling strategies have been employed for different types of neurone, some of which are more suitable than others for cortical pyramidal cells. Some also facilitate the subsequent incorporation of active properties such as voltage and transmitter sensitive conductances. A brief review of some of the major approaches, as well as our experience in applying them to cortical pyramidal cells, is now given.

16.3.1 Equivalent cylinder models

Rall has demonstrated that certain classes of dendritic tree could be collapsed into single, unbranched 'equivalent cylinders' (for review see Rall, 1977). Such simple structures are tractable mathematically, and equations describing voltage responses to both current injection and synaptic inputs at different locations have been derived. It has been shown that the somatic voltage transient following a current impulse to the soma can be expressed as the sum of a series of exponentials, whose amplitudes and time constants provide information about the electrotonic structure of the cell (Rall, 1969). Techniques similar to these have been applied to the modelling of motoneurones (see Jack & Redman, 1971; Rall, 1977), hippocampal cells (Brown *et al.*, 1981; Johnston, 1981; Turner & Schwartzkroin, 1983) and certain classes of neocortical pyramidal cells (Lux & Pollen, 1966; Stafstrom *et al.*, 1984b).

At least two basic criteria must be met before a dendritic structure can be collapsed into an equivalent cylinder :

1) All the dendritic branches must terminate at the same electrotonic distance from the soma.

2) The '3/2 Power Law' must be obeyed at all dendritic branch points - in other words, the diameter of the parent segment raised to the power of 3/2 must equal the sum of the diameters of the daughter segments each raised to the same power.

Our morphological findings clearly indicate that: (i) although the basal dendrites of a given cell are of similar electrotonic length, the apical trunk and terminal arbour dendrites are usually considerably longer; (ii) some dendritic branch points follow the 3/2 Power Law, but many do not. In particular, the points where oblique dendrites branch off the apical trunk often deviate from this relationship, with the trunk showing little or no reduction in diameter after such a branch. We therefore concluded that the neocortical pyramidal cells in our sample did not meet the above criteria for collapse into a single equivalent cylinder.

16.3.2   Segmental cable models

A number of methods have been devised for the implementation of cable model solutions which can cope with dendritic structures of arbitrary geometry (Barrett & Crill, 1974; Butz & Cowan, 1974; Horwitz, 1981; Koch & Poggio, 1985; Turner, 1984; Wilson, 1984). These techniques can thus be used for cells which do not satisfy the criteria for equivalent cylinder collapse. They involve solving the cable equations in the Laplace domain, with the voltage responses of the cell being computed from transfer functions using numerical methods such as the fast Fourier transform (FFT) (Koch *et al.*, 1982; Koch & Poggio 1983a,b; Turner, 1984). These methods, however, become cumbersome when multiple synaptic conductance changes must be computed (Holmes, 1986), and cannot cope with active electrical properties over the full physiological voltage range.

16.3.3   Compartmental modelling

An alternative method of coping with arbitrary geometries is to divide the dendritic tree into a large number of 'compartments', each of which is sufficiently small to be regarded as isopotential. Each compartment is modelled using a parallel capacitance and resistor with adjacent compartments being joined by axial link resistances. In this way a set of coupled differential equations encapsulating the geometry form the model and may be solved using numerical integration (Traub, 1977) including, for example, matrix methods (Perkel *et al.*, 1981) or simple iteration (Clements, 1984). Further equations describing voltage-sensitive ionic conductances and synaptic inputs can be added to compartments if required (Dodge & Cooley, 1973; Pellionisz & Llinas, 1977; Traub & Llinas, 1979). Compartmental models are thus highly flexible and well suited to our approach. The compartmental model we have employed is specified, in its simplest form, by the geometry of the cell's soma and dendrites, together with three biophysical membrane parameters - specific membrane resistivity (R_m), specific membrane capacitance (C_m) and cytoplasmic resistivity (R_i). We also considered two further complications, the dendritic spines and a somatic shunt; and we then explored various simplifications of the dendritic geometry to reduce the computational cost of the model.

Dendritic spines

Cortical pyramidal cells bear large numbers of dendritic spines which may account for as much as half of the total membrane area of the cell. These must therefore be incorporated into any accurate model of the cell. Each spine and neck could be modelled by separate compartments, but this will generate massive systems of differential equations (>20 000).

Our calculations suggest that for many purposes the membrane area of the spines can be incorporated into the parent dendritic shaft membrane. The membrane area of each dendritic segment is increased using the following transformation:

$$l' = l\,F^{2/3} \quad \text{and} \quad d' = d\,F^{1/3}$$

where l and d are the dimensions of the original dendritic shaft, l' and d' their transformations, and F, the folding factor, is given by:

$$F = \frac{(area_{sh} + N_{sp}(area_{sp} - area_{sn}))}{area_{sh}} \tag{16.1}$$

where $area_{sh}$ refers to the area of the dendritic shaft without spines, N_{sp} is the number of spines on the segment, $area_{sp}$ is the membrane area of a spine, and $area_{sn}$ is the cross sectional area of the spine neck - this is generally small enough to be disregarded. This transformation preserves the area, input resistance, axial resistance and effective electrotonic length of the spiny segment. The resultant transformed segment behaves like the spiny original under most circumstances. However, in certain situations it may not be appropriate to incorporate all spine membrane into shafts in this way. Particular spines which are receiving synaptic inputs, and perhaps their near neighbours, may be left 'unincorporated' and modelled in full, so that the effects of spine neck resistances, synaptic conductance changes (Jack et al., 1975; Koch et al., 1982; Koch & Poggio, 1983a; Brown et al., 1988) and possible active conductances in spine heads (Miller et al., 1985; Perkel & Perkel, 1985; Shepherd & Brayton, 1987) can be investigated.

Somatic shunt

A common modelling assumption is that the neuronal membrane properties are constant over both the soma and the entire dendritic arbour. This may be an oversimplification. In particular, attention has been drawn to the possibility that the membrane resistivity at or close to the soma may be lower than in the dendrites, giving rise to what is sometimes known as a somatic shunt (Iansek & Redman, 1973). A somatic shunt might be caused by a number of factors, one of the most obvious being the lack of a perfect electrical seal between the somal membrane and the micropipette. Additionally, impalement damage may result in the activation of ion channels close to the soma, possibly as a result of the ingress of calcium. Such channels may tend to restore the cell's resting potential, but will contribute to a reduced membrane resistivity at the soma. The possible effects of a somatic shunt on the passive properties of a neurone have been explored (Durand, 1984; Kawato, 1984; Gnam, 1987), and it is straightforward to include such a shunt into a compartmental model. We have done so by introducing a fourth biophysical parameter to the model, the somatic shunt conductance, G_{sh}.

Simplified representations

Compartmental models which encompass all biophysical and morphological details can represent the passive features of the cortical pyramidal cell accurately. However, even when the spines have been incorporated into the shaft membranes, this type of model suffers from the disadvantage that it is extremely costly in terms of computing resources, since the set of differential equations must be solved for each compartment at every time step during a simulation. We have therefore explored further simplified representations of the dendritic geometry which reduce the numbers of compartments but still retain the essential descriptive features.

Profiles Dendritic trees which do not satisfy equivalent cylinder criteria may nonetheless be collapsed by similar means into an 'equivalent profile' - sometimes called the 'equivalent dendrite' (Clements, 1984). Unlike a cylinder, this profile may vary in diameter along its length. The lengths of all the dendritic segments are normalized by:

$$l_i' = l_i \sqrt{(D/d_i)} \tag{16.2}$$

where l_i is the length of the dendritic section, d_i its diameter, D an arbitrary normalizing constant and l_i' its normalized length. The segments are then divided into short subsections of length l_s (typically 1 micron) and subsections at the same normalized distance from the soma are combined using the transformation:

$$d_c = \left(\sum d_i^{3/2} \right)^{2/3} \tag{16.3}$$

where d_c refers to the diameter of the combined subsection. To return from arbitrarily normalized to real lengths, and thereby conserve membrane surface area, we perform a further transformation:

$$l_c = l_s \sqrt{(d_c/D)} \tag{16.4}$$

where l_c refers to the length of the combined subsection.

Such profiles need much less computer time than full compartmental models, but for cortical pyramidal cells, which have apical and basal dendrites of very different lengths, they show significant departures from the full model behaviour, particularly when dendritic synaptic inputs are simulated. A more accurate representation can be achieved by collapsing all the basal dendrites together separately from the apicals to yield a 'double profile' (see Figure 16.2A). However, the apical oblique dendrites, which originate at various distances along the apical trunk, still provide a complication which cannot be incorporated accurately into profile representations.

Cartoons 'Cartoon' representations are our attempt to make use of the potential speed of profile representations while preserving more features of the dendritic

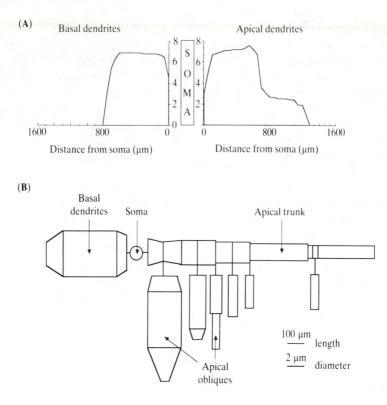

Figure 16.2 Simplified representations of dendritic geometry. **A.** 'Double profile' representation. Basal and apical dendrites have been collapsed separately into equivalent profiles, each linked to the soma (see text). Vertical axis is the diameter of the equivalent profile in μm. **B.** 'Cartoon' representation. Basal dendrites have been collapsed into an equivalent profile. Apical obliques originating at similar electrotonic distances are collapsed together and the resulting equivalent profiles are located at the appropriate electrotonic distances along the apical trunk.

geometry. The cartoon representation of a typical pyramidal cell is shown in Figure 16.2B and consists of: a) a soma; b) a profile representation of the basal dendrites; c) an apical trunk from which emerge the apical obliques, and d) a profile of the terminal arbour. In most cases, apical obliques emerging close to each other on the trunk can be profiled together for greater speed, although a degree of subjectivity may be involved in such a procedure. Cartoon representations occupy significantly less computer resources. A typical full compartmental model, with spines incorporated as described above, takes of the order of 6000 cpu seconds (SUN 3/280 with FPA) to simulate a single 30 ms voltage transient. The cartoon representation takes 15 cpu seconds, which is about the same as the double profile. The voltage response, recorded at the soma, to current injections and synaptic conductance changes is virtually identical to that shown by the full model and clearly superior to the double profile (see Figure 16.3). However, the voltage

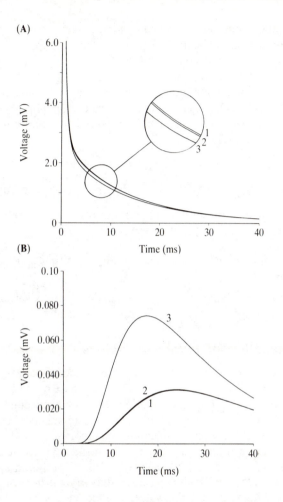

Figure 16.3 Performance of simplified representations compared with the full model of dendritic geometry. 1 - full model, 2 - cartoon, 3 - double profile. Model parameter values : R_m = 15 000 Ωcm^2, R_i = 250 Ωcm, C_m = 1.0 μFcm^{-2}, G_{sh} (somatic shunt conductance) = 0.0 nS. Note that the responses of the cartoon representation closely match those of the full model, whereas those of the double profile do not. **A.** Voltage response to a brief (0.44 ms, 1.36 nA) current pulse at soma. **B.** Voltage response at soma to a current injection (α-function) at the distal apical trunk. α = 1 ms^{-1}, Q_0 = 0.1 pC.

response in an equivalent, profiled dendritic branch receiving input is smaller than would be the case in the original dendritic segment in the full model. In situations where these differences are important, the branch receiving input can be 'unwrapped' from the profile and modelled in full. Otherwise the voltage distribution throughout the cartoon representation is the same as that in corresponding parts of the full model. Since only the parts of the tree experiencing virtually the same voltage are modelled by a given compartment, active properties can be incorporated conveniently. This requires the assumption that the density of channels at the same electrotonic distance from the soma is the same for each dendrite in the group to be collapsed.

The cartoon would therefore appear to be the most suitable representation for neocortical pyramidal cells. It can combine speed and simplicity with the ability to represent complex morphologies, active properties and non-uniform membrane properties (e.g. somatic shunt).

16.4   Modelling pyramidal cells in the rat visual cortex

Having made the choice of compartmental models with cartoon simplifications, the model may now be used:

1) to estimate values of the biophysical parameters (R_m, C_m, R_i, G_{sh}) for a given cortical pyramidal cell
2) to investigate the relative efficacy of synaptic inputs at various points on the dendritic arbour for a given set of parameter estimates.

16.4.1   Estimation of parameter values

The values for the biophysical parameters of the model may be explored by comparing the model's prediction of the voltage response of the cell to a brief pulse of injected current to that recorded experimentally. Our procedure was to derive a cartoon representation of a given cell from the measurements of its soma-dendritic morphology as revealed by HRP injection, incorporating the dendritic spines as described above. We initially set C_m and R_i to their widely accepted values of 1 μFcm^{-2} and 70 Ωcm respectively, and G_{sh} to zero. For this case with no somatic shunt, R_m can be calculated from the measured membrane time constant (τ_m) using $R_m = \tau_m/C_m$, and R_m was set to this value. The model was then given a brief pulse of current of the same amplitude and duration as had been given to the real neurone during the experiment. For most cells, including the cell used as an example in this paper, the prediction of the model with these parameter values failed to fit the recorded data closely (Figure 16.4A). From this semi-log plot, it can be seen that the model prediction is in error both at later times, when the potential is decaying as a single exponential (the straight-line portion of the semi-log plot) and at early times when the potential is falling more rapidly.

Given this initial failure, we then allowed R_m, G_{sh} and R_i to vary as free parameters under the direction of a simplex optimization routine (Nelder & Mead, 1965) until an optimal least-squares fit to the experimental waveform was obtained. This 'direct fitting' approach (Clements, 1984) differs from that of several previous workers (e.g. Brown *et al.*, 1981; Stafstrom *et al.*, 1984b) who have used the method of 'peeling' (Rall, 1969). By peeling, the predicted and experimental voltage transients are each decomposed into a series of exponential time constants

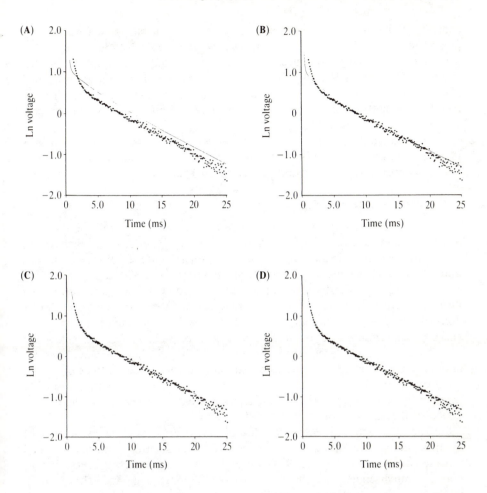

Figure 16.4 Comparisons of simulated voltage responses, using different sets of model parameter values, with the experimentally recorded voltage response. Each panel shows a semi-log plot of the voltage response to a brief current pulse (0.44 ms, 1.36 nA) delivered to the soma. Experimental data represented by points, model output by solid line. **A.** Model parameters calculated using conventional values (R_i = 70 Ωcm, C_m = 1.0 μFcm^{-2}). No somatic shunt conductance and no neuronal membrane area adjustment. R_m (derived from τ_m) = 12 100 Ωcm^2. Note the lack of fit over the full time course. **B.** Simplex optimization used to determine values for R_m and G_{sh}. R_i fixed at 70 Ωcm, C_m fixed at 1.0 μFcm^{-2}, with no area adjustment. Computed parameter values are R_m = 16 400 Ωcm^2, G_{sh} = 5.6 nS. Note that the model waveform does not match the experimental data at early times. **C.** Simplex optimization used to determine values for R_m, R_i and G_{sh}. C_m fixed at 1.0 μFcm^{-2}, with no area adjustment. Computed parameter values are R_m = 21 000 Ωcm^2, R_i = 306 Ωcm, G_{sh} = 5.6 nS. Model waveform matches experimental data closely over the full time course. **D.** Simplex optimization used to determine values for R_m, R_i and G_{sh}. C_m fixed at 0.9 μFcm^{-2}, area adjusted by a factor of 0.9. Computed parameter values are R_m = 52 940 Ωcm^2, R_i = 336 Ωcm, G_{sh} = 13.4 nS. Note that the model waveform is indistinguishable from that shown in Figure 16.4C.

and amplitudes, which may then be compared. For our sample of neocortical pyramidal cells we found peeling unsatisfactory. The presence of dendrites of very unequal electrical lengths produces transients containing low amplitude exponential components (Holmes & Rall, 1987). Given inevitable noise in the experimental data, we were unable to resolve these components reliably. The 'direct fitting' method compares the actual waveforms and avoids the difficulties we encountered with exponential peeling.

By allowing R_m, G_{sh} and R_i to vary, we were able to obtain satisfactory fits to the data for most of the cells in our sample, including the example cell (see Figure 16.4C). However, two serious difficulties became apparent.

Cytoplasmic resistivity (R_i)

We were unable to fit the early parts of the experimental voltage transients using conventional values for R_i of 70-100 Ωcm (see Figure 16.4B). When R_i was made a free parameter in the simplex routine, optimal fits of the full waveform were obtained with R_i values of 200-400 Ωcm (median about 300 Ωcm; see Figure 16.4C). It is possible that our experimentally recorded transients have been distorted at early times, either by the micropipette and the recording system, or by non-passive behaviour of the cell membrane. Using cell analogues, we have checked the performance of our micropipettes and recording system and have found no behaviour likely to account for the problem. There is, however, evidence for non-passive membrane behaviour, since all our cells displayed a degree of inward rectification, even at potentials close to rest. Unfortunately, there are insufficient data presently available about the conductances responsible to assess their likely impact on the transient waveform.

The conventional values of 70-100 Ωcm are based on estimates of cytoplasmic composition and a single experimental determination in the spinal motoneurone (Barrett & Crill, 1974). Recently there have been suggestions that R_i could be much higher than this (Rall, personal communication; Shelton, 1985), which would be consistent with our findings. R_i represents a major difficulty in our modelling effort, and the possibility that its value might be higher than is presently accepted should be investigated.

Non-uniqueness

The direct fitting procedure outlined above involved specifying the measured soma-dendritic morphology of the neurone and a value for C_m, then allowing R_m, G_{sh} and R_i to vary as free parameters. However, both the morphological measurements and the value for C_m are subject to uncertainty. In our opinion, it is impossible to measure dendritic lengths, diameters, spine numbers and areas to an accuracy of better than 5%. Thus errors of ±10% in estimates of neuronal membrane area are entirely plausible. The value for C_m for cortical pyramidal cells has not been established. Based on detailed studies of the squid giant axon (Takashima, 1976; Haydon *et al.*, 1980), the likely range of C_m for biological membranes is 0.6 - 1.1 μFcm^{-2}.

We therefore explored the effect of systematically varying both the dimensions of the dendrites and the value of C_m within the above ranges, while allowing R_m, R_i and G_{sh} to be determined by the simplex procedure. Lengths and diameters were all reduced or incremented by 5%. Other combinations, such as increasing lengths while decreasing diameters, had less dramatic effects and are not illustrated here. It was found that for many combinations of values for C_m and morphological adjustment, widely different values for R_m and G_{sh} could be obtained which generated waveforms which all matched the experimental data equally well (Figures 16.4C-D). A table of results for our example cell is given in Table 16.1, and these are typical for the sample as a whole.

Table 16.1 Table showing effect of altering C_m and neuronal membrane area on the values of R_m, R_i and G_{sh} obtained by direct fitting (see text). All sets of model parameter values result in predictions which are consistent with the experimental data (see Figure 16.4)

| C_m | Neuronal membrane area adjustment factor | | | | | | | | |
| | 1.1 | | | 1.0 | | | 0.9 | | |
	R_m	G_{sh}	R_i	R_m	G_{sh}	R_i	R_m	G_{sh}	R_i
1.1	12 400	1.2	286	15 020	4.7	287	19 440	8.1	289
1.0	16 520	4.7	304 *a	21 000	7.9	306	29 290	10.8	310
0.9	23 910	8.1	326	32 870	10.9	330	52 940	13.4	336 *b
0.8	40 040	11.3	355	65 900	13.7	362	162 390	15.5	378

For most cells, including the example in Table 16.1, fits to the data could not be obtained for the entire range of C_m values and morphological adjustments described above. Lower and upper limits are set by the value of G_{sh}, which could vary between zero and the recorded input conductance of the cell. Nevertheless, given the likely errors in measurement and the uncertainty about C_m, our data for this pyramidal neurone are consistent with values for R_m ranging between about 12 000 and 160 000 Ωcm^2. Lower values for C_m and downward adjustments to the dendritic measurements give high values for G_{sh} and R_m and vice versa. The values obtained for R_i, however, are less sensitive to these changes than those for R_m, and range between 286 and 378 Ωcm. This modelling procedure demonstrates that there are many sets of parameter values which will allow the model to predict the experimentally recorded transient response of the cell. At present we have no objective criteria for selecting between the different possibilities. An additional source of uncertainty is the extent to which the somatic shunt is caused by impalement damage. If all or most is caused by the experimental procedure, then the intact cell is more accurately modelled with the shunt conductance removed.

However, if a sizeable proportion of the shunt is physiological, the cell should be modelled with at least part of the shunt in place. Finally, the possibility that our high values for R_i are the result of some distortion of the recorded waveform cannot be excluded. This means that sets of parameter values including conventional, lower R_i values should also be considered, even though these are not consistent with the early portion of the recorded waveforms.

16.4.2   Simulation of synaptic inputs

Given that there are many sets of parameter values that could be consistent with the recorded data for each cell, we have explored the implications of each set for the integrative properties of the neurone. For each set, we simulated synaptic inputs at many different points on the dendritic arbour and computed the synaptic potentials produced at the soma. We were interested in both the time course of these potentials and the degree of attenuation experienced during propagation through the dendritic tree. For simplicity, we will show results for just two sets of parameter values for our example cell, indicated by asterisks in Table 16.1. In both cases, it was assumed that the somatic shunt was caused by impalement damage, and the cell was modelled with the shunt conductance removed.

Time course of synaptic potentials

Small, brief conductance changes can be approximated by current injections whose time course, $I(t)$, can be described by an alpha function (Jack *et al.*, 1975). We used:

$$I(t) = Q_0\, \alpha^2\, t\, e^{-\alpha t} \quad \text{with } Q_0 = \text{total charge (usually 0.1pC)} \tag{16.5}$$
$$\text{and } \alpha = 1 \text{ ms}^{-1}$$

Examples of the synaptic waveforms obtained are shown in Figure 16.5. The same synaptic current has been injected at four different points on the dendritic arbour of the cell, for each of the two sets of parameter values indicated by asterisks in Table 16.1. In Figure 16.5A the R_m value was about 16 500 Ωcm^2, and in Figure 16.5B it was 53 000 Ωcm^2. In both cases, the synaptic inputs on the basal and proximal oblique dendrites all produced potentials at the soma with similar, relatively rapid, time courses. Inputs on the distal apical dendrites, on the other hand, produced dramatically slower waveforms. As Dr J. Hopfield points out, the range of synaptic time courses produced by the dendritic arbour might enhance the cell's computational power and lead to new emergent properties in a neural network composed of such units. The high-R_m case is of additional interest due to the very slow decay of the synaptic waveforms, which do not reach baseline until well after 200 ms. In this case, the membrane would retain a decrementing electrical 'trace' of past synaptic activity for what may be, in physiological terms, a considerable period of time. Such a trace might also increase the range of computational possibilities for the neurone.

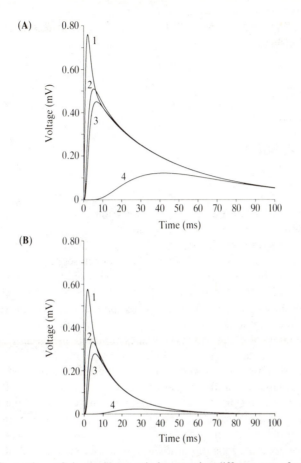

Figure 16.5 Comparison of simulated synaptic inputs using different sets of model parameter values (both consistent with the experimental data, see Table 16.1). Current injections (α-function, $Q_0 = 0.1$ pC, $\alpha = 1$ ms^{-1}) on soma (1), basal dendrite (2), proximal apical oblique dendrite (3) and distal apical trunk (4). **A.** Voltage response at soma with parameters : $R_m = 52\,940$ Ωcm^2, $R_i = 336$ Ωcm, $C_m = 0.9$ μFcm^{-2}, $G_{sh} = 0.0$ nS, area adjusted by factor of 0.9 ('b' in Table 16.1). Note the prolonged decay of the waveforms. **B.** Voltage response at soma with parameters : $R_m = 16\,520$ Ωcm^2, $R_i = 304$ Ωcm, $C_m = 1.1$ μFcm^{-2}, $G_{sh} = 0.0$ nS, area adjusted by factor of 1.1 ('a' in Table 16.1). Note the more rapid decay of the waveforms and extreme attenuation of the distal apical input.

Efficacy of synaptic potentials

The efficacy (or weight) of a synaptic input depends on some combination of peak voltage, rate of rise and the time integral (area) of the voltage response at the soma. Area efficacy is less dependent on the precise time course of the injected current, and may be more important than peak voltage in influencing the firing rate of the cell in cases where small inputs occur against a noisy background (Fetz &

Gustafsson, 1983; Kirkwood, 1979). We have therefore used 'relative area efficacy', defined as:

$$E = \frac{\displaystyle\int_0^\infty V_{ds}(t)\,dt}{\displaystyle\int_0^\infty V_{ss}(t)\,dt} \qquad\qquad (16.6)$$

where V_{ds} is the voltage response measured at the soma to a synaptic current at a given location on a dendrite, and V_{ss} is the voltage response at the soma to an identical synaptic current injected at the soma.

As in the previous section, identical synaptic currents were injected at many different points on the model dendritic arbour for each set of parameter values. The relative area efficacy was calculated for each, and used to construct 'iso-efficacy contour plots'. Plots for the same two example sets of parameter values used previously are shown in Figure 16.6. Some features of the plots are sensitive to the values of model parameters selected, but others, surprisingly, are highly robust. For the whole range of combinations of values explored, the basal dendrites and the proximal apical oblique dendrites were electrically highly compact. Even synapses located at the extreme tips showed relative area efficacies of >70%. The precise position of a synapse along these dendrites has little effect on its efficacy or time course, and thus all the synapses on these dendrites may be functionally equivalent. Interestingly, of the 8300 spines on the example cell, some 6500 were estimated to lie within this proximal category.

For most combinations of parameter values, including both those in Figure 16.6 and all others with a high R_i, the efficacies of the distal synapses were lower, and their time courses much slower, than those of the proximal synapses. A relatively abrupt decline in efficacy often occurred along the proximal part of the apical dendrite. This might lead to a stratification of classes of inputs, such that inputs to different parts of the cell, possibly from different sources, would have very different efficacies.

Some combinations using a low value for R_i, combined with a very high R_m and the somatic shunt removed, could produce a cell with the entire dendritic system being highly compact electrically. All the synaptic inputs, regardless of location, would have very similar efficacies and time courses. Such a cell could functionally resemble a simple connectionist model unit.

The inclusion or removal of the somatic shunt conductance, while keeping the other parameters constant, alters the time course of all synaptic inputs, but was found to make no difference to the iso-efficacy contour plot for the cell. This may be of functional importance in keeping the relative efficacies of synapses on a given cell constant in the face of conductance changes at the soma, such as might occur during spike firing activity.

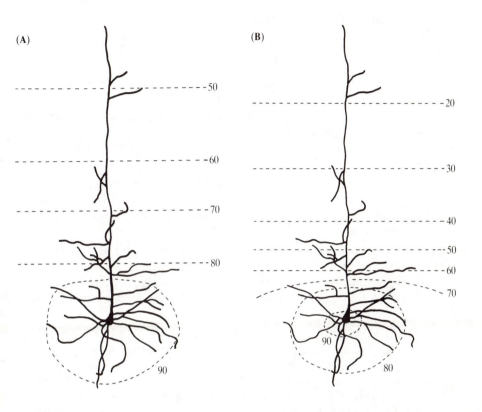

Figure 16.6 Iso-efficacy plots for synaptic inputs distributed over the dendritic arbour for different sets of model parameter values (see Table 16.1). Synaptic inputs simulated as in Figure 16.5. Contour lines show percentage relative area efficacy. **A.** Model parameters : R_m = 52 940 Ωcm2, R_i = 336 Ωcm, C_m = 0.9 µFcm−2, G_{sh} = 0.0 nS, area adjusted by factor of 0.9 ('b' in Table 16.1). Note that inputs on all basal and proximal apical oblique dendrites have relative efficacies of at least 90%, whereas distal apical inputs have efficacies of about 50%. **B.** Model parameters : R_m = 16 520 Ωcm2, R_i = 304 Ωcm, C_m = 1.1 µFcm−2, G_{sh} = 0.0 nS, area adjusted by factor of 1.1 ('a' in Table 16.1). Note that inputs on basal and proximal apical oblique dendrites still have efficacies greater than 70%, whereas distal inputs now have efficacies of about 20%.

Although it appears to be impossible to predict fully the passive properties of the dendritic arbours of neocortical pyramidal cells at present, it seems very likely that these cells are capable of more complex computation than the units used commonly in connectionist network models. As more data concerning the active properties of these cells becomes available, further levels of sophistication may become apparent.

Summary and conclusions

1) In the rat visual cortex several types of pyramidal cell could be distinguished on the basis of their soma-dendritic morphology. Each of the types studied in detail displayed distinctive electrophysiological properties which will influence their input/output relationships.

2) Most cells in our sample could not be modelled as single equivalent cylinders. Using compartmental modelling techniques we devised simplified 'cartoon' representations of the dendritic geometry which are both accurate and computationally efficient.

3) We used a method of direct fitting of model predictions to experimentally-recorded voltage transients in order to estimate values for biophysical parameters. This avoided the difficulties associated with exponential peeling for these cells.

4) Our data were not consistent with the conventionally used values for R_i of 70-100 Ωcm, and could only be fitted by models with values for R_i nearer to 300 Ωcm. Although this may be a result of non-passive behaviour of the cell membrane, we suggest that the possibility of R_i being greater than previously thought should be investigated.

5) The results of the fitting procedure suffered from 'non-uniqueness'. Given the possibility of a somatic shunt, uncertainty about the value for specific membrane capacitance and the inaccuracy of morphological measurements, a wide range of values for R_m was found which fitted the data equally well. Coupled with the uncertainty over the value for R_i, we were forced to consider a number of different model scenarios, all consistent with the data.

6) If the somatic shunt is caused by micropipette damage, then our data indicate that cortical pyramidal cells, prior to impalement, might have much longer membrane time constants than previously estimated - possibly greater than 100 ms. Thus the membrane could retain an electrical 'trace' of past synaptic activity, decrementing over periods of 200 ms or more.

7) For all the possibilities we have investigated, the basal and proximal apical oblique dendritic trees are electrically very compact. The precise position of a synaptic input along a basal or proximal apical oblique dendrite makes little difference to its relative area efficacy or time course.

8) For most models, and all those using high R_i values, synaptic inputs on the distal part of the apical trunk, the terminal arbour and the distal obliques will experience substantially more attenuation and will have a slower time course than similar inputs on the basal and proximal oblique dendrites. The existence of multiple classes of synaptic inputs with different time courses could enhance the computational power of these neurones.

Acknowledgements

This research was supported by grants from the Wellcome Trust, the Medical Research Council and the University of Oxford. A.U.L. is a Beit Memorial Research Fellow. SUN workstations were obtained through a grant from the Wellcome Trust. We would like to thank Drs Clements and Redman of the Australian National University for allowing us to use their compartmental model simulation program.

References

Adams P.R. & Galvan M. (1986) Voltage-dependent currents of vertebrate neurons and their role in membrane excitability. **Adv. Neurol. 44**, pp. 137-171

Barrett J.N. & Crill W.E. (1974) Specific membrane properties of cat motoneurones. **J. Physiol. 239**, pp. 301-324

Brown T.H., Fricke R.A. & Perkel D.H. (1981) Passive electrical constants in three classes of hippocampal neurons. **J. Neurophysiol. 46,** pp. 812-827

Brown T.H., Chang V.C., Ganong A.H., Keenan C.L. & Kelso S.R. (1988) Biophysical properties of dendrites and spines that may control the induction and expression of long-term synaptic potentiation. In: **Long-Term Potentiation: from biophysics to behaviour.** pp. 201-264, P.W. Landfield & S.A. Deadwyler (eds.) Alan R. Liss, NY.

Butz E.G. & Cowan J.D. (1974) Transient potentials in dendritic systems of arbitrary geometry. **Biophys. J. 14**, pp. 661-689

Clements J.D. (1984) Ph.D. dissertation. Experimental Neurology Unit, John Curtin School of Medical Research, Australian National University.

Crick F. & Asanuma C. (1986) Certain aspects of the anatomy and physiology of the cerebral cortex. In: **Parallel Distributed Processing: Explorations in the Microstructure of Cognition, Vol. 2**. pp. 333-371, D.E. Rumelhart & J.L. McClelland (eds.) MIT Press, Cambridge, MA.

Dingledine R. (ed.) (1984) **Brain Slices**. Plenum, NY.

Dodge F.A. & Cooley J.W. (1973) Action potential of the motoneurone. **IBM Research and Development 17**, pp. 219-229

Durand D. (1984) The somatic shunt cable model for neurons. **Biophys. J. 46**, pp. 645-653

Fetz E.E. & Gustafsson G. (1983) Relation between shapes of post-synaptic potentials and changes in firing probability of cat motoneurones. **J. Physiol. 341**, pp. 387-410

Gnam W. (1987) **The Two Time Constant Model of the Neurone**. M.Sc. dissertation, Department of Physiology, University of Oxford

Hamill O.P., Marty A., Neher E., Sakmann B. & Sigworth F.J. (1981) Improved patch-clamp techniques for high-resolution current recording from cells and cell-free membrane patches. **Pflugers Arch. 391**, pp. 85-100

Haydon D.A., Requena J. & Urban B.W. (1980) Soma effects of aliphatic hydrocarbons on the electrical capacity and ionic currents of the squid giant axon membrane. **J. Physiol. 309**, pp. 229-245

Holmes R.W. (1986) **Cable theory modelling of the effectiveness of synaptic inputs in cortical pyramidal cells.** Ph.D. dissertation. University of California, Los Angeles.

Holmes W.R. & Rall W. (1987) Estimating the electrotonic structure of neurons which cannot be approximated as equivalent cylinders. **Soc. Neurosci. Abstr.**, 422.7

Hopfield J.J. & Tank D.W. (1985) 'Neural' computation of decisions in optimisation problems. **Biol. Cybern. 52**, pp. 141-152

Horwitz B. (1981) An analytical method for investigating transient potentials in neurons with branching dendritic trees. **Biophys. J. 36**, pp. 155-192

Huguenard J.R., Hamill O.P. & Prince D.A. (1988) Developmental changes in Na^+ conductances in rat neocortical neurons: Appearance of a slowly inactivating component. **J. Neurophysiol. 59**, pp. 778-795

Iansek R. & Redman S.J. (1973) The amplitude, time course and charge of unitary excitatory post-synaptic potentials evoked in spinal motoneurone dendrites. **J. Physiol. 234**, pp. 665-688

Jack J.J.B., Noble D. & Tsien R.W. (1975) **Electric Current Flow in Excitable Cells.** Oxford University Press, Oxford.

Jack J.J.B. & Redman S.J. (1971) An electrical description of the motoneurone and its application to the analysis of synaptic potentials. **J. Physiol. 215**, pp. 321-352

Johnston D. (1981) Passive cable properties of hippocampal CA3 pyramidal neurons. **Cell. Molecular Neurobiol. 1**, pp. 41-55

Johnston D., Hablitz J.J. & Wilson W.A. (1980) Voltage clamp discloses slow inward current in hippocampal burst-firing neurones. **Nature 286**, pp. 391-393

Kawato M. (1984) Cable properties of a neuron model with non-uniform membrane resistivity. **J. Theor. Biol. 111**, pp. 149-169

Kay A.R. & Wong R.K.S. (1986) Isolation of neurons suitable for patch-clamping from adult mammalian central nervous systems. **J. Neurosci. Meth. 16**, pp. 227-238

Kerkut G.A. & Wheal H.V. (eds.) (1981) **Electrophysiology of Isolated Mammalian CNS Preparations.** Academic Press, NY.

Kirkwood P.A. (1979) On the use and interpretation of cross-correlation measurements in the mammalian central nervous system. **J. Neurosci. Meth. 1**, pp. 107-132

Koch C. & Poggio T. (1983a) Electrical properties of dendritic spines. **TINS 6**, pp. 80-83

Koch C. & Poggio T. (1983b) A theoretical analysis of electrical properties of spines. **Proc. Roy. Soc. London B 218**, pp. 455-477

Koch C. & Poggio T. (1985) A simple algorithm for solving the cable equation in dendritic trees of arbitrary geometry. **J. Neurosci. Meth. 12**, pp. 303-315

Koch C., Poggio T. & Torre V. (1982) Retinal ganglion cells: a functional interpretation of dendritic morphology. **Phil. Trans. Roy. Soc. B 298**, pp. 227-264

Lacaille J.-C., Mueller A.L., Kunkel D.D. & Schwartzkroin P.A. (1987) Local circuit interactions between oriens/alveus interneurons and CA1 pyramidal cells in hippocampal slices: Electrophysiology and morphology. **J. Neurosci. 7**, pp. 1979-1993

Landfield P.W. & Deadwyler S.A. (eds.) (1988) **Long-term potentiation: From Biophysics to Behavior**. Alan R. Liss, NY.

Larkman A.U., Mason A.J.R. & Blakemore C. (1988) The in vitro slice preparation for combined morphological and electrophysiological studies of the rat visual cortex. **Neurosci. Res. 6**, pp. 1-19

Lehky S.R. & Sejnowski T.J. (1988) Network model of shape-from-shading: neural function arises from both receptive and projective fields. **Nature 333**, pp. 452-454

Lux H.D. & Pollen D.A. (1966) Electrical constants of neurons in the motor cortex of the cat. **J. Neurophysiol. 29**, pp. 207-220

Mason A.J.R., Larkman A.U. & Eldridge J.L. (1988) A method for intracellular injection of horseradish peroxidase by pressure. **J. Neurosci. Meth. 22**, pp. 181-187

McCormick D.A., Connors B.W., Lighthall J.W. & Prince, D.A. (1985) Comparative electrophysiology of pyramidal and sparsely spiny stellate neurons of the neocortex. **J. Neurophysiol. 54**, pp. 782-806

Miles R. & Wong R.K.S. (1984) Unitary inhibitory synaptic potentials in the guinea-pig hippocampus in vitro. **J. Physiol. 356**, pp. 97-113

Miles R. & Wong R.K.S. (1986) Excitatory synaptic interactions between CA3 neurones in the guinea pig hippocampus. **J. Physiol. 373**, pp. 397-418

Miller J.P., Rall W. & Rinzel J. (1985) Synaptic amplification by active membrane in dendritic spines. **Brain Res. 325**, pp. 325-330

Nelder J.A. & Mead R. (1965) A geometric technique for optimisation. **Computer J. 7**, pp. 308-327

Pellionisz A. & Llinas R. (1977) A computer model of cerebellar Purkinje cells. **Neurosci. 2**, pp. 37-48

Perkel D.H., Mulloney B. & Budelli R.W. (1981) Quantitative methods for predicting neuronal behaviour. **Neurosci. 6**, pp. 823-837

Perkel D.H. & Perkel D.J. (1985) Dendritic spines: role of active membrane in modulating synaptic efficacy. **Brain Res. 325**, pp. 331-335

Peters A. & Jones E.G. (eds.) (1984) **Cerebral Cortex. Vol. 1**. Plenum, New York.

Rall W. (1969) Time constants and electrotonic length of membrane cylinders and neurons. **Biophys. J. 9**, pp. 1483-1508

Rall W. (1977) Core conductor theory and cable properties of neurons. In: **Handbook of Physiology. The Nervous System, Section 1, Vol 1**. pp. 39-97, E.R. Kandel (ed.) American Physiological Society, Bethesda, MD.

Rumelhart D.E. & McClelland J.L. (1986) **Parallel Distributed Processing: Explorations in the microstructure of cognition, Vol. 1 & 2**. MIT Press, Cambridge, MA.

Schwartzkroin P.A. & Mueller A.L. (1987) Electrophysiology of hippocampal neurons. In: **Cerebral Cortex, Vol. 6**. pp. 295-342, A. Peters & E.G. Jones (eds.) Plenum, NY.

Schwartzkroin P.A. & Wheal H.V. (eds.) (1984) **Electrophysiology of Epilepsy**. Academic Press, London.

Schwindt P.C., Spain W.J., Foehring R.C., Stafstrom C.E., Chubb M.C. & Crill W.E. (1988) Multiple potassium conductances and their functions in neurons from cat sensorimotor cortex in vitro. **J. Neurophysiol. 59**, pp. 424-449

Shelton D.P. (1985) Membrane resistivity estimated for the Purkinje neuron by means of a passive computer model. **Neurosci. 14**, pp. 111-131

Shepherd G.M. & Brayton R.K. (1987) Logic operations are properties of computer-simulated interactions between excitable dendritic spines. **Neurosci. 21**, pp. 151-165

Spain W.J., Schwindt P.C. & Crill W.E. (1987) Anomalous rectification in neurons from cat sensorimotor cortex in vitro. **J. Neurophysiol. 57**, pp. 1555-1576

Stafstrom C.E., Schwindt P.C., Chubb M.C. & Crill W.E. (1985) Properties of persistent sodium conductance and calcium conductance of layer V neurons from cat sensorimotor cortex in vitro. **J. Neurophysiol. 53**, pp. 153-170

Stafstrom C.E., Schwindt P.C., Flatman J.A. & Crill W.E. (1984a) Properties of subthreshold response and action potential recorded in layer V neurons from cat sensorimotor cortex in vitro. **J. Neurophysiol. 52**, pp. 244-263

Stafstrom C.E., Schwindt P.C. & Crill W.E. (1984b) Cable properties of layer V neurons from cat sensorimotor cortex in vitro. **J. Neurophysiol. 52**, pp. 278-289

Takashima S. (1976) Membrane capacity of squid giant axon during hyper- and depolarizations. **J. Membrane Biol. 27**, pp. 21-39

Traub R.D. (1977) Motoneurones of different geometry and the size principle. **Biol. Cybern. 25**, pp. 163-176

Traub R.D. (1982) Simulation of intrinsic bursting in CA3 hippocampal neurons. **Neurosci. 7**, pp. 1233-1242

Traub R.D. & Llinas R. (1979) Hippocampal pyramidal cells: significance of dendritic ionic conductances for neuronal function and epileptogenesis. **J. Neurophysiol. 42**, pp. 476-496

Traub R.D., Miles R. & Wong R.K.S. (1987a) Models of synchronized hippocampal bursts in the presence of inhibition. I. Single population events. **J. Neurophysiol. 58**, pp. 739-751

Traub R.D., Miles R., Wong R.K.S., Schulman L.S. & Schneiderman J.H. (1987b) Models of synchronized hippocampal bursts in the presence of inhibition. II. Ongoing spontaneous population events. **J. Neurophysiol. 58**, pp. 752-775

Turner D.A. (1984) Segmental cable evaluation of somatic transients in hippocampal neurones (CA1, CA3 and dentate). **Biophys. J. 46**, 73-84

Turner D.A. & Schwartzkroin P.A. (1983) Electrical characteristics of dendrites and dendritic spines in intracellularly stained CA3 and dentate hippocampal neurones. **J. Neurosci. 3**, pp. 2381-2394

Turner D.A. & Schwartzkroin P.A. (1984) Passive electrotonic structure and dendritic properties of hippocampal neurons. In: **Brain Slices**, pp. 25-50, R. Dingledine (ed.) Plenum, NY

Wilson C.J. (1984) Passive cable properties of dendritic spines and spiny neurons. **J. Neurosci. 4**, pp. 281-297

Wilson W. & Goldner M.A. (1975) Voltage-clamping with a single microelectrode. **J. Neurobiol. 4**, pp. 411-422

Wong R.K.S. & Prince D.A. (1981) Afterpotential generation in hippocampal pyramidal cells. **J. Neurophysiol. 45**, pp. 86-97

Wong R.K.S. Prince D.A. & Basbaum A.I. (1979) Intradendritic recordings from hippocampal neurons. **Proc. Nat. Acad. Sci. USA 76**, pp. 986-990

Zipser D. & Andersen R.A. (1988) A back-propagation programmed network that simulates response properties of a subset of posterior parietal neurones. **Nature 331**, pp. 679-684

17
The Reliability of Single Neurons and Circuit Design: A Case Study
Simon Laughlin

17.1 Introduction

It has long been recognized that the speed of response and the reliability of neurons are important factors in the design of nervous systems, and this is one reason why the architectures and operations of brains differ from the computers that we use to model them (von Neumann, 1958). When compared with integrated circuits, neurons are slow and unreliable. These disadvantages are directly attributable to the materials from which neurons are constructed. Response speed is limited by the relatively lengthy opening times of channels, in the order of 0.1 to 1 ms, and by the time constants of neural membranes. Unreliability stems from the fact that neural signals are generated by controlling the mean rates of molecular or sub-cellular processes that are essentially stochastic. For example, both the opening and closing of the molecular channels in the cell membrane, and the release of chemical neurotransmitter vesicles at synapses, are probabilistic processes (review: Stevens, 1987). The unreliability associated with generating electrical responses in single cells will ultimately limit accuracy, irrespective of whether coding is by means of graded potentials (analogue signals) or action potentials (pulse coded signals). However, in some situations these single cell limits are secondary to properties of the network, such as the non-coherent barrage of impulses converging on a neuron (Stevens, 1987).

The limitations imposed on accuracy when information is transmitted by a stochastic process are well known in vision and image processing. Optical information is carried by photons which are absorbed at the eye or camera according to Poisson statistics. The variance in absorption rate equals the mean rate, consequently the signal-to-noise ratio improves as the square root of intensity - the square root law (review: Rose, 1972). When translated to neurons, the implication is that the fewer the channels or synaptic vesicles generating a signal, the less reliable that signal will be. Although precise data are scarce, single nerve cells generate signals using relatively small numbers of vesicles and channels. For example, about 300 synaptic vesicles are released when an action potential stimulates the motor endplate: a large synapse connecting a motoneuron to a muscle (Kuffler *et al.*, 1984, pp. 280). In the fish central nervous system, a single action potential in one afferent fibre releases between 5 and 25 vesicles to generate a post-synaptic response in the Mauthner neuron (Korn & Faber, 1987). These numbers should be compared with the 10 000 or so Poisson events required to give an r.m.s. noise that is 1% of the mean output.

Given the stochastic nature of molecular and sub-cellular processes and the relatively small numbers of events involved, how reliable can neurons be? I will address this question by examining data from our recent work on the reliability of phototransduction and neural coding in the fly compound eye (Howard *et al.*, 1987; Laughlin *et al.*, 1987). Because our findings indicate that this system has been designed to minimize noise contamination, these photoreceptors and neurons probably operate close to the upper limits of the performance of single cells. Consequently they provide a convenient yardstick for assessing the performance of neurons in general.

17.2 The experimental approach

The fly visual system has proved favourable material for studying the fundamentals of visual processing, and we have been able to draw upon a wealth of behavioural, anatomical and physiological data accumulated over the last 20 years (reviews: Reichardt, 1970; Ali, 1984; Stavenga & Hardie, 1989). In our experiments we have examined the accuracy of two fundamental retinal processes, the transduction of light energy to electrical potential in photoreceptors and the synaptic transfer of these signals from photoreceptors to interneurons. Both the photoreceptors and the post-synaptic (second order) neurons of the blowfly are well characterized (Shaw, 1984; Hardie, 1985). The particular interneurons that we work with are the large monopolar cells (LMCs). They are the largest interneurons in the lamina and are a major pathway for conveying information from the photoreceptors to the brain. Our experiments provide accurate measurements of signal and noise in this well characterized neural system. These measurements allow us to estimate the information transmitted by single neurons and to identify the factors that limit this bit rate. This quantitative analysis was made possible by three favourable circumstances.

1) We can define the signal to be transmitted because we are working at the front end of a visual system. Signals are evaluated in terms of behaviourally significant optical parameters. In the fly, as in our own eye, the photo-receptors code stimulus intensity as the amplitude of receptor potential. As shown in Figure 17.1, the LMCs extract from this photoreceptor input a graded voltage signal that depends on stimulus contrast, defined as $\Delta I/I$, where ΔI is the change in intensity about the mean level I. In our experiments, stimuli of known contrast were generated by suddenly changing the intensity of a large spatially uniform stimulus. The change was a pulse, lasting 100 ms, and for the rest of the time the stimulus was maintained at one of a number of background light levels. We then define the signal generated by a

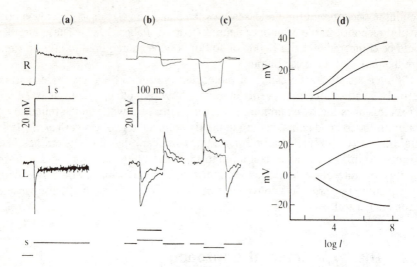

Figure 17.1 The responses of a photoreceptor and an LMC to identical stimuli showing (**a**) the response to the onset of a steady intense background light, (**b**) the responses to intensity increments and (**c**) the response to intensity decrements about the background level. (**d**) shows the envelopes of graded responses generated in a photoreceptor and an LMC by a stimulus of contrast 0.4 (the mean environmental contrast) presented over a wide range of background intensities. Whereas receptors code both the background level and intensity fluctuations, the LMCs code the fluctuations alone and, at high light levels, response amplitude depends on stimulus contrast, independent of background intensity. Adapted from Laughlin *et al.*, 1987, and Laughlin, 1987.

photoreceptor or an LMC as the amplitude of the response to the sudden intensity change.

2) We can measure the noise and express it as a fraction of the signal. Photoreceptors and LMCs are accessible to intracellular recording in an intact preparation. Stable recordings can be made from single identified cells, sometimes for an hour or more. The cells produce an analogue signal, known as a graded response, which increases in amplitude with contrast. The noise is the standard deviation of the fluctuations in membrane potential recorded in the absence of any contrast signal. The system is sufficiently linear with respect to small signals to allow one to measure signal-to-noise ratios by the following direct means. First the noise is recorded. Next a stimulus is chosen which produces a response of about the same amplitude as the peak-to-peak noise. This stimulus is repeated 200 times, the responses averaged, and the peak response amplitude measured. This measured amplitude is then converted to response per unit contrast by dividing by the contrast of the stimulus. We call this normalized parameter the contrast response. It is the slope of the curve relating stimulus contrast to intracellular response amplitude. We then divide the contrast response by the r.m.s. noise amplitude

to give a signal-to-noise ratio (SNR). Using this definition, the signal-to-noise ratio is the reciprocal of the contrast required to generate a response that is equal in amplitude to the r.m.s. noise.

3) We can identify the noise generated during neural processing because we know the neural circuitry responsible for signal processing. The noise measured in the LMC can be separated into two components: (i) noise generated in the photoreceptors during transduction and fed into the LMCs, and (ii) intrinsic noise generated by the visual system as the signal passes from the site of transduction to the LMC. Precise anatomical, physiological and optical studies show that six identical photoreceptors, looking at the same point in space, converge upon 2 almost identical LMCs (review: Shaw, 1984). Each photoreceptor makes over 200 chemical synapses with each LMC (Nicol & Meinertzhagen, 1982). From this pattern of convergence the signal-to-noise ratio, with respect to transduction noise, should improve by a factor of $\sqrt{6}$ as one passes from photoreceptor to LMC. Any shortfall in this expected improvement indicates the addition of intrinsic noise during transmission.

17.3 The circuit connecting receptor and LMC is designed to reduce noise

Before we examine our results, it is worth emphasizing that the LMCs are designed to code the contrast component of photoreceptor signals efficiently. A comparison between the responses of photoreceptors and LMCs (Figure 17.1) shows that two basic processes are involved in coding (Laughlin & Hardie, 1978). The first is the subtraction of the steady background component (the DC-bias) from the photoreceptor input. The second is the amplification of the remaining contrast component. Through the collaborative action of subtraction and amplification, the contrast signal is extracted from the background and expanded to fill the limited dynamic range of the LMC response (Figure 17.1). To ensure that full use is made of the LMC response range, the processes of subtraction and amplification are optimized to deal with the natural signals. The design principles underlying this optimization have recently been reviewed (Laughlin, 1987). Briefly, the value of the background signal subtracted away is a statistical prediction of the signal expected at the particular set of 6 photoreceptors. This prediction is derived from correlated components in surrounding regions of the retina and in the same region of the retina at immediately preceding times (Srinivasan *et al.*, 1982). This procedure corresponds to predictive coding, as used in digital image processing (Gonzalez & Wintz, 1977). In addition, the gain for amplification follows the cumulative probability distribution in natural scenes so that all LMC response levels are used equally often (Laughlin, 1981). This procedure corresponds to another digital image enhancement technique, histogram equalization (Gonzalez & Wintz, 1977). The matching of subtraction and amplification to signal statistics serves to maximize the permissible level of amplification and so makes full use of the LMC graded response range.

Why is it so important to maximize amplification? As we shall see below, synaptic amplification protects the signal from intrinsic noise contamination, and in particular protects it from the synaptic noise generated as the signal is transferred from photoreceptors to LMC. Synaptic noise reduction also explains the large number of parallel synapses used to convey the signal from photoreceptors to LMCs. The large area of synaptic contact helps maximize the number of vesicles carrying the signal and so reduces shot noise (Laughlin, 1973). Note that it is logical for noise protection to be the first step in vision. Moreover, we can expect the processes reducing noise to be optimized because the lower the noise, the lower are behavioural thresholds and the more flies can see. Male flies hunt female flies and engage in aerobatic dog-fights during courtship (Land & Collett, 1974), during which the females try to escape, perhaps to ensure that the successful males are fit. The fly visual system has a spatial resolving power of 2 to 3 degrees: consequently the image of another fly will be a small blurred grey spot, often moving rapidly across the retina (Land & Collett, 1974). The resulting photoreceptor signal must be rather small. Thus there is ample evolutionary pressure to reduce intrinsic noise levels in the retina, because this noise can mask the small retinal signals generated by prospective mates.

Given the biological importance of noise reduction and the way in which coding has been engineered to increase efficiency, we expect that the performance of the neurons involved, the LMCs, will approach the upper limit with which information can be coded. How well do these retinal cells work, and what limits their performance? We will first consider the quality of photoreceptor signals and then examine the reliability of LMC responses.

17.4 Photoreceptors and the limitations imposed by molecular events

Photoreceptor responses are band-limited in the temporal frequency domain and contaminated by noise. Both limitations are primarily determined by the molecular process of phototransduction. Photons are absorbed by visual pigment molecules according to Poisson statistics and, in invertebrate photoreceptors, are transduced to generate a depolarizing receptor potential (e.g. Wong, 1978). At low light levels, single quantum events are seen which last tens of milliseconds. As intensity rises these events fuse to produce a continuous noisy response. Shot noise analysis shows that the event rate increases with intensity up to the highest natural light levels and this increase in rate is accompanied by a decrease in event duration and a consequent decline in overall gain (Dodge *et al.*, 1968; Howard *et al.*, 1987). Essentially the photoreceptor is trading response amplitude (sensitivity) against temporal resolving power. Voltage clamp studies show that this trade-off depends more upon the light level (i.e. the mean event rate), than the photoreceptor membrane potential (Wong, 1978). It follows that the chemical reactions involved in phototransduction determine the temporal resolving power of the photoreceptors, and set the upper limit to the resolution of moving objects or flicker.

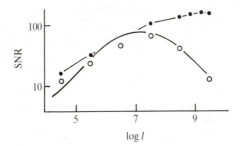

Figure 17.2 The signal-to-noise ratios measured in the photoreceptors of the white eyed mutant of the fly *Lucilia cuprina* (o) and from photoreceptors of the dorsal retina of dragonfly *Hemicordulia tau* (•) at a number of different light intensities. The curve shows the signal-to-noise ratio expected in a fly photoreceptor containing 30 000 transduction units, each unit producing a response with an effective duration derived from the measured power spectrum of the noise (Howard *et al.*, 1987).

How seriously are the responses of fly photoreceptors contaminated by noise and what factors determine noise levels? The fundamental determinant of signal quality is the shot event triggered by a photon absorption. If, at any one mean light intensity, all shot events were of the same amplitude, the signal-to-noise ratio (SNR) would be set solely by the number of photons, rising with the square root of light intensity according to Poisson statistics. However, at any one mean intensity, the individual shot events vary in amplitude, in duration, and in latency, so reducing the signal-to-noise ratio. Nonetheless, at low intensities the SNR still rises in proportion to the square root of intensity at a rate that is about half that predicted from the photon catch (Lillywhite & Laughlin, 1979). At high intensities the SNR of photoreceptors levels out (Figure 17.2), even though the number of shot events carries on increasing (Howard & Snyder, 1983; Howard *et al.*, 1987). This ceiling could be imposed because the shot noise generated during transduction falls below the level of noise generated by other channels in the photoreceptor membrane. Alternatively the large number of photon absorptions could be saturating intermediate processes in phototransduction (Howard & Snyder, 1983).

To test the saturation hypothesis, advantage was taken of a mutant fly. Normal fly photoreceptors contain a screening pigment that is brought close to the photopigment at high light intensities to attenuate light and prevent saturation (Kirschfeld & Franceschini, 1969). The pigment acts like a pair of dark glasses which the fly puts on to avoid being dazzled. The white eyed mutant fly lacks this pigment, consequently we can saturate the photoreceptor's response. In the white eyed fly the signal-to-noise ratio rises progressively with intensity to reach a maximum and then declines again as the response saturates (Figure 17.2). This intensity dependence of the SNR is of the form expected when each photoreceptor contains 30 000 sites for phototransduction, or transduction units (Figure 17.2); a figure that is tantalizingly close to the number of ultrastructural membrane units (microvilli) in the photoreceptor membrane, but is orders of magnitude less than the number of photopigment molecules. Thus the number of phototransduction units packed into a fly photoreceptor appears to limit the signal-to-noise ratio. With 30 000 such units (and this is an estimate of the minimum number required) the fly can resolve a contrast of just over 1%, and the SNR is about 90:1 (Howard *et al.*, 1987).

Is this 1% accuracy close to the upper limit that one can expect for single cells of this size? Photoreceptors are long and thin, and it has usually been assumed that their length allows them to catch most of the available light while their narrowness reduces the blurring effect of their sampling aperture. A comparison between the photoreceptors of different species suggests that photoreceptor size is not wholly determined by optical performance. The longer photoreceptors tend to be in fast flying insects that are active during the day, such as flies, butterflies and bees. Nocturnal animals, such as moths, often have shorter cells. It is possible that the diurnal insects have longer photoreceptors in order that they might accommodate more transduction units, and hence make full use of the available light. The strictly day-active dragonflies have some of the longest photoreceptors known - in the dorsal eye region the cells are almost 1 mm long (Laughlin & McGinness, 1978). Dragonflies are voracious aerial predators and during their evolution they have pushed their compound eyes to the limit, having some of the largest and most acute insect eyes. If one measures the maximum signal-to-noise ratio in their dorsal photoreceptors under daylight conditions it is almost exactly twice that of the fly (Figure 17.2). This is the improvement one expects if the number of transduction units increases with length, because their photoreceptors are four times longer than those of the fly and SNR is proportional to the square root of the number of transduction units. Apparently, these dragonfly photoreceptors have grown longer to accommodate more transduction units, so supporting the suggestion (Howard & Snyder, 1983) that photoreceptor performance is ultimately limited by the amount of molecular machinery that can be packed into a cell. In conclusion, insect photoreceptors provide a good example of the limitations imposed upon neural coding by the essentially particulate (i.e. molecular) nature of signal generation in the nervous system. We can now examine other cellular factors that determine the neural performance and, in particular, ask how the process of synaptic transfer from photoreceptors to LMCs influences signal quality.

17.5 Interneuronal performance: the effects of bandwidth and noise

In the time domain, LMC performance is indicated by their frequency response (Figure 17.4) which peaks at around 80 Hz. The decrease in response below 80 Hz reflects the high pass filter properties of signal transmission from receptor to LMC (Järvilehto & Zettler, 1971; Laughlin *et al.*, 1987). This high pass characteristic is related to the observation that the correlated signal components received at earlier times are subtracted away (Srinivasan *et al.*, 1982). The decline in response at high frequencies is determined by the photoreceptors. As found in vertebrate retina (e.g. Copenhagen *et al.*, 1983), synaptic transfer is much faster than phototransduction. In the fly, the minimum duration of the phototransduction event is about 2 ms (Howard *et al.*, 1987) but the time constant of synaptic transmission is less than 0.5 ms (Laughlin *et al.*, 1987). Thus the photoreceptors band-limit the input to such an extent that synaptic processes, and the properties of the post-synaptic membrane, have no effect on the cut-off frequency of the signal.

When we look at signal-to-noise ratios, the limitations imposed by synaptic processes become more apparent. As with photoreceptors, the LMC SNR rises steadily with intensity to reach a maximum (Figure 17.3a). However, the maximum is only slightly better than the corresponding best photoreceptor SNR and falls far below the levels expected from the convergence of six photoreceptors. This shortfall in SNR indicates that intrinsic noise has been added and allows us to estimate its amplitude (Figure 17.3b).

Let us look at the effects of this added noise in more detail. The absolute level of noise is relatively large in comparison with the LMC's dynamic response range. At the highest intensities, where performance is best, the r.m.s. intrinsic noise is about 0.75 mV. This is 1/80 of the total response range of 60 mV. Components of the noise lie at frequencies higher than the signal (Figure 17.4b) and these can be attributed, by virtue of their power spectrum, to synaptic events at the LMC membrane. Consequently some of the noise could be stripped from the signal by filtering it. If we removed all the noise above the effective cut off of the photoreceptors, the intrinsic r.m.s. noise would be approximately halved.

Despite these relatively high absolute noise levels, the LMC still codes small input signals extremely effectively. With respect to an optical signal of unit contrast, the interneuron SNR is 50:1 (Figure 17.3) and this corresponds to the resolution of a 2% modulation in light intensity. The signal generated in each of the 6 photoreceptor inputs by this 2% modulation is less than 200 µV. The seeming paradox of good signal resolution in a noisy cell comes about because synaptic amplification improves the signal-to-noise ratio by recruiting more vesicles to carry the signal and this also increases the absolute level of noise.

We have analysed the effect of amplification on the synaptic SNR using a simple model of synaptic transmission (Falk & Fatt, 1972) that fits our data. According to the simple model, neurotransmitter release rises exponentially with pre-synaptic depolarization. Thus:

$$T = ae^{bR} \tag{17.1}$$

where T is the number of neurotransmitter molecules activating post-synaptic conductance channels at any one time, R is the pre-synaptic membrane potential and a and b are constants. If the transmitter activated conductance channels are solely responsible for changes in LMC potential, then the effective transmitter dose T determines the post-synaptic membrane potential, L, according to the familiar hyperbolic function:

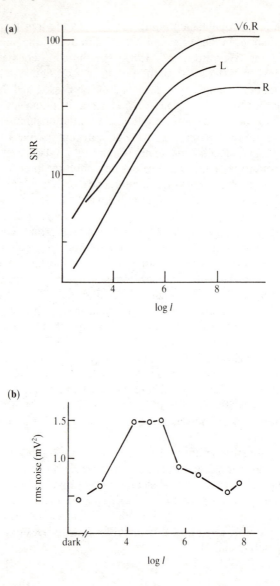

Figure 17.3 (a) A logarithmic plot of the signal-to-noise ratios recorded in fly photoreceptors (R) and LMCs (L) at a number of background light levels. The upper curve is the $\sqrt{6}$ improvement in SNR expected in the LMCs if no extra (intrinsic) noise were added during signal transfer. **(b)** The r.m.s. voltage amplitude of the added intrinsic noise as a function of background light levels. Data in **(a)** and **(b)** replotted from Laughlin *et al.*, 1987.

$$\frac{L}{L_m} = \frac{T}{T + c} \qquad (17.2)$$

where c is a constant determined by the relative sizes of the synaptic conductance channels relative to the passive load conductance of the cell, and L_m is the maximum response, corresponding to the reversal potential. Substituting for T from Equation 17.1, and differentiating, gives the gain for synaptic transmission:

$$\frac{dL}{dR} = bL\left[1 - \frac{L}{L_m}\right] \qquad (17.3)$$

and this is a maximum of $bL_m/4$ when $L = L_m/2$ (Falk & Fatt, 1972). Note that the gain is proportional to b, the exponential transmitter release constant defined in Equation 17.1.

We now use this model to derive the signal-to-noise ratio (Laughlin *et al.*, 1987). Analysis is simplified by assuming that all noise is generated during transmitter release (i.e. it results from the random discharge of transmitter vesicles). Thus for relatively small signals and low noise amplitudes, we can compute the signal-to-noise ratio by considering the effective transmitter concentration, T. If the signal to be transmitted is a small change in receptor potential, ΔR, the resulting transmitter signal ΔT is given by

$$\Delta T = \frac{dT}{dR}\Delta R = Tb\Delta R \qquad (17.4)$$

where T is the mean effective transmitter dose upon which ΔT is superimposed. Assuming Poisson statistics for the noise, the r.m.s. noise is $\sqrt{T}$. Thus the signal-to-noise ratio for the synapse, SNR_s, is given by

$$SNR_s = b\Delta R\sqrt{T} \qquad (17.5)$$

Note that both the synaptic signal-to-noise ratio and the synaptic gain (Equation 17.4) are proportional to b. Thus the higher the gain, the better the signal-to-noise ratio. SNR_s is also proportional to the square root of the number of synaptic vesicles involved.

This simple relationship between synaptic gain and signal-to-noise ratio follows from the particular model we used. However, our conclusion that one should generate synaptic signals with the highest possible gain, so using the greatest number of vesicles and channels, is not tied to this particular model. The following argument suggests that a high gain system usually enhances the signal-to-noise ratio. Consider the intrinsic noise generated in a neuron which produces graded membrane potential responses, either for direct transmission (as in LMCs) or for conversion into a train of action potentials. Taking the simplest of cases, a cell contains two types of conductance, one hyperpolarizing the cell and the other depolarizing it. Within the total range of response amplitudes set by the reversal

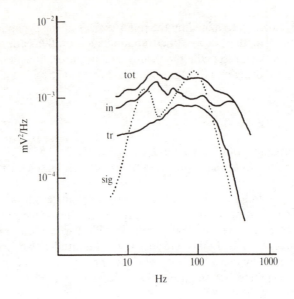

Figure 17.4 The power spectra of signal and noise in fly LMCs. The dotted curve (sig) is the power spectrum of the LMC signal, computed by taking the Fourier transform of an impulse response of low amplitude and is scaled to arbitrary units. The top curve (tot) is the power spectrum of the total noise measured in the LMCs. An estimate of the transduction noise (tr) injected into an LMC by the photoreceptors is subtracted from the total to give the power spectrum of the intrinsic noise (in). Replotted from the data of Laughlin *et al.*, 1987.

potentials of these two conductances, the membrane potential is determined by the ratio between the two conductances (e.g. Kuffler *et al.*, 1984, p.563). When generating a particular amplitude of response, the cell should use as many conductance channels as possible, to minimize shot noise. In this case, any particular value of membrane potential is associated with a unique pair of values for the numbers of hyperpolarizing and depolarizing conductance channels activated. These channel numbers also determine the noise because channel activation is stochastic. It follows that every value of membrane potential is associated with a particular value of voltage noise power. With the voltage noise determined by the cell's voltage response, the only way to improve the signal-to-noise ratio is to ensure that incoming signals produce the largest possible changes in membrane potential. It follows from this simple observation that the amplification of the signal should be maximized within the constraints of the neuron's limited dynamic range if intrinsic noise effects are to be minimized.

17.6 The efficiency of single neurons and simple circuits

In conclusion, our data demonstrate some of the factors that limit the fidelity of neural coding. Biochemical rate constants band-limit transduction, and the essentially particulate processes of signal generation, in both phototransduction and synaptic transfer, generate shot noise. Using our data we can say that a neuron in an efficiently designed circuit can achieve signal-to-noise ratios in the region of 50 to 100:1. These values are achieved in a system that seems to have gone to some trouble to reduce the effects of noise. Redundancy is stripped away, amplification is maximized by matching it to signal statistics, and the signal is produced by a formidable array of over 1200 synapses, responding in parallel to 6 highly correlated signals from identical photoreceptors. It follows that any model that requires a numerical accuracy in single nerve cells of better than a few percent in its individual neurons is really pushing its luck in terms of practicality, particularly if it does not follow the fly's example and design the circuit to minimize noise.

We can also use our data to estimate the bit rate for our fly LMC, using Shannon's classic expression for a noisy band-limited channel (Shannon & Weaver, 1949)

$$H = \int_0^\infty \log_2 \left[1 + \frac{S(f)^2}{N(f)^2} \right] df \tag{17.6}$$

With respect to this expression, we have measured the noise power spectrum, $N(f)$, (Figure 17.4). If we assume that the system is linear and that all response levels are used equally often, we can use the power spectrum for small signals (Figure 17.4) to derive the total available signal power as a function of frequency, $S(f)$, and this gives us the channel capacity, H, of approximately 3000 bits/second. This estimate has been confirmed using random stimuli (de Ruyter & Laughlin, in prep.). Given that an LMC is not linear and noise levels probably change with response amplitude, the simple linear treatment (Equation 17.6) is likely to overestimate the information capacity. This overestimate is offset by the fact that the LMC's natural signal has been band-limited by the photoreceptors' 2 ms time constant. The LMC's membrane time constant is less than 1.0 ms (Laughlin & Osorio, 1989.) so this cell could accommodate a bandwidth twice that of the receptor. Thus our two errors will tend to cancel, and 3000 bits per second cannot be far from the maximum information transmission rate attainable in a neuron of this size. Seeing that the LMC is only 2 - 3 μm in diameter this is good going and it is difficult to see how action potential codes, limited to about 1000 spikes per second in maximum rate, can exceed this bit rate. In this context, note that the process of graded signal transmission is a more basic constraint than action potential coding, because graded synaptic responses generally constitute the cellular inputs and outputs to spike codes.

Our findings also show that, in the fly retina, accuracy is promoted by designing the circuit to handle visual signals efficiently. Tailoring circuit performance to function complements the more commonly considered means of enhancing accuracy in the nervous system: replicating parallel channels and averaging their outputs. Replication essentially recruits extra particles to carry the signal. By comparison, a well designed circuit matches coding to the signal in order to use the available particles most effectively. In the fly eye, the use of particles is optimized by matching signal amplification to signal statistics. It is interesting to note that this amplification is non-linear. For best performance the relationship between input amplitude and output amplitude should be approximately sigmoidal (Laughlin, 1981). This non-linearity is provided by chemical synaptic transmission, illustrating that neuronal non-linearities not only provide computational power, but can be used to improve accuracy.

Does our data on neural accuracy have any implications for neural network modelling? It is dangerous to presume the goals of a field that is expanding rapidly, and in many different directions. Nonetheless, I will make three simple observations. If one goal of neural modelling is to create neural analogues that solve problems, then the accuracy of real wet neurons is not relevant. However, if one uses analogues to explain the function of wet circuits, then accuracy should be considered. For example, if a particular neural model is prone to noise contamination (e.g. it performs a multiplication by using one noisy synapse to shunt another noisy synapse) its validity must be questioned. Indeed susceptibility to noise could well be used as a benchmark of performance to choose between rival models. Moreover, if noise is generated during neural processing, noise suppression could well be a valid goal for neural modelling (e.g. Stevens, 1987), capable of providing insight into the structure and function of wet networks.

References

Ali M.A. (ed.) (1984). **Photoreception and Vision in Invertebrates.** NATO ASI Series A, Vol. 74. Plenum, NY.

Copenhagen D.R., Ashmore J.F. & Schnapf J.K. (1983) Kinetics of synaptic transmission from photoreceptors to horizontal cells in turtle retina. **Vision Res. 23**, pp. 363-369

Dodge F.A., Knight B.W. & Toyoda J. (1968) Voltage noise in *Limulus* cells. **Science 160**, pp. 88-90

Falk G. & Fatt P. (1972) Physical changes induced by light in the rod outer segment of vertebrates. In: **Handbook of Sensory Physiology**, vol. VII/1 pp. 200-244, H.J.A. Dartnall (ed.) Springer, Berlin.

Gonzalez R.C. & Wintz P. (1977) **Digital Image Processing**. Addison-Wesley, Reading, Mass.

Hardie R.C. (1985) Functional organization of the fly retina. In: **Progress in Sensory Physiology Vol. 5**, pp. 1-79, D. Ottoson (ed.) Springer, Berlin.

Howard J. & Snyder A.W. (1983) Transduction as a limitation on compound eye function and design. **Proc. R. Soc. Lond. B217**, pp. 287-307

Howard J., Blakeslee B. & Laughlin S.B. (1987) The intracellular pupil mechanism and the maintenance of photoreceptor signal-to-noise ratios in the blowfly *Lucilia cuprina*. **Proc. R. Soc. Lond. B231**, pp. 415-435

Järvilehto M. & Zettler F. (1971) Localized intracellular potentials from pre- and post-synaptic components in the external plexiform layer of an insect retina. **Z. vergl. Physiol. 75**, pp. 422-440

Kirschfeld K. & Franceschini N. (1969) Ein Mechanismus zur Steuerung des Lichtflusses in den Rhandomeren des Komplexauges von *Musca*. **Kybernetik 6**, pp. 13-22

Korn H. & Faber D.S. (1987) Regulation and significance of probabilistic release mechanisms at central synapses. In: **Synaptic Function**. pp. 57-108, G.M. Edelman, W.E. Gall & W.M. Cowan (eds.) Wiley, NY.

Kuffler S.H., Nicholls J.G. & Martin A.W. (1984) **From Neuron to Brain**. Sinauer, Sunderland, Mass.

Land M.F. & Collett T.S. (1974) Chasing behaviour of houseflies (*Fannia canicularis*). A description and analysis. **J. comp. Physiol. 89**, pp. 331-357

Laughlin S.B. (1973) Neural integration in the first optic neuropile of dragonflies. I. Signal amplification in dark-adapted second order neurons. **J. comp. Physiol. 84**, pp.335-355

Laughlin S.B. (1981) A simple coding procedure enhances a neuron's information capacity. **Z. Naturforsch. 36c**, pp. 910-912

Laughlin S.B. (1987) Form and function in retinal processing. **TINS 10**, pp. 478-483

Laughlin S.B. & Hardie R.C. (1978) Common strategies for light adaptation in the peripheral visual systems of fly and dragonfly. **J. comp. Physiol. 128**, pp. 319-340

Laughlin S.B., Howard J. & Blakeslee B. (1987) Synaptic limitations to contrast coding in the retina of the blowfly *Calliphora*. **Proc. R. Soc. Lond. B231**, pp. 437-467

Laughlin S.B. & McGinness S. (1978) The structures of dorsal and ventral regions of a dragonfly retina. **Cell Tissue Res. 188**, pp. 427-447

Laughlin S.B. & Osorio D. (1989) Mechanisms for neural signal enhancement in the blowfly compound eye. **J. exp. Biol.**, in press.

Lillywhite P.G. & Laughlin S.B. (1979) Transducer noise in a photoreceptor. **Nature (Lond.) 277**, pp. 569-572 von Neumann J. (1958) **The Computer and the Brain**. Yale University Press, New Haven.

Nicol D. & Meinertzhagen I.A. (1982) An analysis of the number and composition of the synaptic populations formed by photoreceptors of the fly. **J. comp. Neurol. 207**, pp. 29-44

Reichardt W. (1970) The insect eye as a model for the uptake, transduction and processing of optical data in the nervous system. In: **The Neurosciences**. 2nd study programme, F.O. Schmitt (ed.) Rockefeller University Press, NY.

Rose A. (1972). **Vision: Human and Electronic**. Plenum Press, NY.

Shannon C.E. & Weaver W. (1949) **The Mathematical Theory of Communication**. University of Illinois Press, Urbana.

Shaw S.R. (1984) Early visual processing in insects. **J. exp. Biol. 112**, pp. 225-251

Srinivasan M.V., Laughlin S.B. & Dubs A. (1982) Predictive coding: a fresh view of inhibition in the retina. **Proc. R. Soc. Lond. B216**, pp. 427-459

Stavenga D.G. & Hardie R.C. (eds.) (1989) **Facets of Vision**. Springer, Berlin.

Stevens C.F. (1987) Specific consequences of general brain properties. In: **Synaptic Function**. pp. 699-709, G.M. Edelman, W.E. Gall & W.M. Cowan (eds) Wiley, NY.

Wong F. (1978) Nature of the light induced conductance changes in ventral photoreceptors of *Limulus*. **Nature (Lond.) 276**, pp. 76-79

18
Designing Synaptic Connections in the Outer Retina
David Attwell & Marc Tessier-Lavigne

Summary

In the salamander retina there are electrical synapses between adjacent rods, and between adjacent rods and cones. We review work providing a rationale for the existence of these synapses. The chemical output synapse from rods has extremely non-linear properties, and clips large signals during synaptic transmission. The electrical synapses reduce this signal clipping, and improve the signal-to-noise ratio in post-synaptic bipolar cells. Quantitatively, the strength of the rod-rod and rod-cone synapses can be predicted from the non-linearity of the chemical output synapse.

18.1 Introduction

A common theme in the theoretical modelling of neural networks is the adjustment of synapse strengths to allow the network to carry out particular functions, such as pattern retrieval or classification. In this chapter we describe how synapse strengths in the outer retina may have been adjusted, by evolutionary selection, to improve the information coding capacity of the retina.

As essential background to this work, we will review briefly how visual information is coded in the outer retina, and suggest what one might naively expect for the properties of outer retinal synapses, before describing the rather unexpected properties of the real synapses.

18.1.1 Information coding in the outer retina

When light is absorbed by a vertebrate photoreceptor, the receptor responds by hyperpolarizing: the cell's membrane potential (potential inside the cell minus potential outside the cell) becomes more negative to an extent determined by the amount of light absorbed. Large spots of bright light can produce a hyperpolarization of up to 25 mV from the potential in the dark (–40 mV). Thus, the pattern of light intensities incident on the retina is converted into a pattern of graded

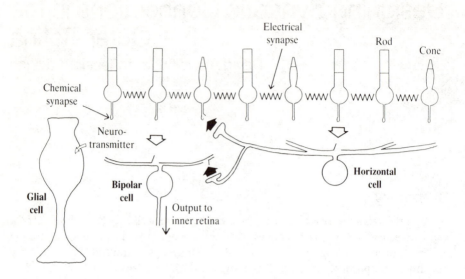

Figure 18.1 Schematic diagram of the outer retina of the salamander (*Ambystoma*). Light hyper-polarizes the photoreceptors (rods and cones) and thus suppresses release of neurotransmitter (probably glutamate, open arrows) from their chemical output synapses. This neurotransmitter acts on ion channels (shown as small 'gates' in the cell membrane) in post-synaptic bipolar and horizontal cells, altering these cells' membrane potentials. Bipolar cells send their output to the inner retina. Horizontal cells mediate lateral inhibition in the outer retina by releasing an inhibitory neurotransmitter (probably GABA, filled arrows) which acts on bipolar and/or cone cells. The post-synaptic action of neurotransmitter glutamate released from photoreceptors is terminated by the glutamate being taken up (curved open arrow) into glial cells. Gap junctions (shown as resistors) form electrical synapses between adjacent photoreceptors.

potentials in the photoreceptors. These signals are then transmitted through the receptors' chemical output synapses (by release of a neurotransmitter), to two types of post-synaptic cell: bipolar cells, which transmit the visual signal to the inner retina, and horizontal cells, which mediate lateral inhibition in the outer retina (Figure 18.1). In both these cell types different light intensities are coded as graded changes in membrane potential. In addition to the chemical output synapses from photoreceptors (open arrows in Figure 18.1), there can also be electrical synapses between adjacent receptors (shown as resistors in Figure 18.1), the function of which will be described below.

18.1.2 Expected properties of retinal synapses

If the outer retina is to code visual information efficiently, one might have the following naive expectations for the properties of the photoreceptor synapses.

1) *The operating range of the photoreceptor chemical output synapse should be matched to that of the cell's phototransduction machinery.* If the synapse cannot generate changes in neurotransmitter release over all of the range of voltages induced in the receptor by light, then information will be lost as the visual signal leaves the photoreceptor layer.

2) *There should be no 'crosstalk' between different photoreceptors.* To maximize the ability of the retina to encode spatial information, one would expect the photoreceptors to behave as independent signal transducers, each measuring the light intensity at one point on the retina.

3) *There should be no synaptic convergence from receptors to bipolar cells.* If each bipolar cell received an input synapse from just one photoreceptor, the visual signal being passed to the inner retina by the bipolar cells could contain as much high spatial frequency information as was present in the array of photoreceptor membrane potentials. Convergence of synaptic inputs from receptors to bipolar cells would lead to a loss of high spatial frequency information.

As will be described in detail below, none of these expectations is borne out in practice. We will review work showing:

1) that the chemical output synapse from photoreceptors can operate only over a small fraction of the voltage response range of the receptors, so that large signals are clipped;

2) that electrical synapses between photoreceptors are advantageous in that they reduce signal clipping by the chemical output synapse (although they introduce 'crosstalk' between receptors and result in the loss of high spatial frequency information);

3) that consideration of how signals and noise are transmitted through the chemical output synapse can lead to predictions for the strengths of the electrical synapses between adjacent rods and between rods and cones, and to an understanding of how synaptic convergence from receptors to bipolar cells can be advantageous.

We will argue below that the limited operating range of the chemical synapse is determined by the properties of the calcium channels which control neurotransmitter release from the synapse, and that evolutionary selection has had to 'design' the outer retina to avoid the constraints imposed on information coding by the properties of these channels.

18.2 The rod chemical output synapse is extremely non-linear

By recording simultaneously from a pre-synaptic photoreceptor and a post-synaptic bipolar or horizontal cell, the input-output relationship for the photoreceptor chemical output synapse can be investigated (Attwell *et al.*, 1987; Belgum & Copenhagen, 1988). Figure 18.2 shows recordings made from a rod and a horizontal cell in the retina of the tiger salamander (chosen for the large size of its photoreceptors, which facilitates impalement with recording microelectrodes). To obtain an approximation to the steady-state input-output relationship for the rod / horizontal cell synapse, a very bright light flash was applied to the retina. This stimulus covered a large area of the retina, illuminating uniformly all the rods with synapses to the horizontal cell. All these rods will undergo the same voltage change in response to light, so the pre-synaptic signal occurring in all the rod synapses to the horizontal cell will be the same (facilitating interpretation of the post-synaptic signal recorded). This pre-synaptic voltage change is shown in Figure 18.2A. When the light is switched on, the rod hyperpolarizes from –40 to –60 mV, but then partly repolarizes to reach a maintained plateau potential of about –50 mV. (On the time scale of the figure the larger initial transient hyperpolarization, which lasts only 150 ms, appears as a vertical line.) When the light is switched off (after about 1 second) the rod does not repolarize immediately (this corresponds, psychophysically, to an after-image being generated by the retina after looking at a bright light), but after about 10 seconds the potential slowly recovers to its dark level. This slow depolarization provides a naturally occurring pre-synaptic voltage ramp which can be used to obtain an approximation to the steady-state input-output relation for the synapse.

The trace in Figure 18.2B shows the voltage change in the horizontal cell which results from light-induced changes of neurotransmitter release from pre-synaptic photoreceptors. While the light is applied the horizontal cell is hyperpolarized from its dark potential (–32 mV) to –103 mV, but after the light is turned off the potential returns to a plateau level of –70 mV. The extra hyperpolarization, below the plateau level, during illumination can be shown (by varying the wavelength of the light) to be due to input to the horizontal cell from cones (Marshall & Werblin, 1978). However, after the light is turned off the cones repolarize to their dark level rapidly, and the changes in horizontal cell voltage after $t = 10$ seconds in Figure 18.2B reflect changes in the voltage of pre-synaptic rods. (As will be discussed later, some of the rod signal leaving the photoreceptor layer actually reaches post-synaptic bipolar and horizontal cells via the *cone* output synapse: nevertheless, this signal is driven by the voltage change generated in rods.)

As the rods slowly depolarize to their dark potential (after $t = 10$ s in Figure 18.2), their chemical synapses start to release more neurotransmitter, resulting in a corresponding slow depolarization of the horizontal cell. By plotting the horizontal cell potential as a function of the rod potential during this slow voltage ramp (eliminating the time variable), the input-output relation for the synapse is obtained.

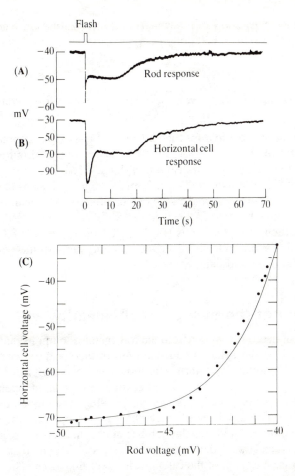

Figure 18.2 Input-output relation for transmission of signals from rods to horizontal cells. **A.** Voltage response of a rod to a 2 mm spot of 500 nm light (3×10^4 photons/μm^2/s, timing shown by top trace). **B.** Voltage response (recorded simultaneously with that in **A**) of a post-synaptic horizontal cell. **C.** Horizontal cell voltage as a function of rod voltage from the data in **A** & **B** for $t > 10$ seconds. Since some of the signal reaching horizontal cells from rods passes via the *cone* output synapse (see Section 18.4), the input-output relation for the rod / horizontal cell chemical synapse must be even more non-linear than the curve shown here: at very negative rod potentials (where the rod's own synapse is no longer releasing transmitter) rod hyperpolarization still generates a horizontal cell hyperpolarization by reducing transmitter release from cones.

This is shown in Figure 18.2C. Near the dark potentials (–40 mV for the rod, -32 mV for the horizontal cell) the synapse has a high gain: changing the rod potential by 1 mV generates a 13 mV change in post-synaptic potential. However, at more negative rod potentials the gain of the synapse is much lower: light-induced hyperpolarization of the rod from –40 to –45 mV hyperpolarizes the horizontal cell from –32 to –68 mV, while further rod hyperpolarization from –45 to –50 mV generates only a further 2 mV of horizontal cell hyperpolarization. The entire input-output relation in Figure 18.2C can be approximated by an exponential curve (continuous line) with the form:

$$\Delta V_{post\text{-}synaptic} = G\left[\exp\left(\frac{\Delta V_{pre\text{-}synaptic}}{2.1 \text{ mV}}\right) - 1\right] \quad \text{where } G \text{ is a constant} \quad (18.1)$$

which increases its slope e-fold for each 2.1 mV of pre-synaptic depolarization.

The effect of the non-linear input-output relation in Figure 18.2C is to strongly clip, during synaptic transmission, large signals occurring in the rods. Although the rods can be hyperpolarized 25 mV by light, it appears that only signals in the first 5 mV of this response range can be effectively transmitted across the rods' chemical output synapse (Attwell *et al.*, 1987). A similar result is obtained for signal transmission to bipolar cells (Belgum & Copenhagen, 1988). Thus, there seems to be a severe mismatch between the operating range of the synapse and that of the phototransduction machinery.

18.3   Origin of the synaptic non-linearity

Release of neurotransmitter from the rod chemical output synapse is thought to be controlled by the calcium concentration in the synaptic terminal (but see Schwartz, 1986), which is in turn determined by the calcium channels in the membrane of the synaptic terminal. The voltage-dependent opening of these channels has been investigated by Bader *et al.* (1982). They found that at the dark potential of –40 mV only 2.5% of these channels are open (in the steady state). Hyperpolarizing the rod reduces the number of channels open, reducing calcium entry into the cell and thus reducing transmitter release. At potentials more negative than –45 mV essentially all of the calcium channels are closed. Thus, the voltage-dependence of calcium entry into the rod seems appropriate to explain the non-linear behaviour of the chemical output synapse. Hyperpolarization of the rod from –40 to –45 mV will close the calcium channels which are open at the dark potential, and reduce transmitter release, but further hyperpolarization from –45 mV cannot further reduce release because all the calcium channels are already closed. The voltage-dependence of the calcium channels in cones is similar to that in rods (Kaneko & Tachibana, 1986), suggesting that the cones' chemical output synapse is likely to behave in a similar non-linear manner.

In addition to the pre-synaptic source of non-linearity described above, there are two other mechanisms which may contribute to the non-linear behaviour of the synapse. First, two or more molecules of the rod neurotransmitter (glutamate) may be needed to open ion channels in the post-synaptic cell membrane (Shiells *et al.*, 1986). Secondly, a mechanism which removes neurotransmitter from the extracellular space, glutamate uptake into glial cells (Figure 18.1), is known to saturate at high extracellular glutamate concentrations (Brew & Attwell, 1987). Both of these effects will tend to result in a given change of rod voltage having a greater

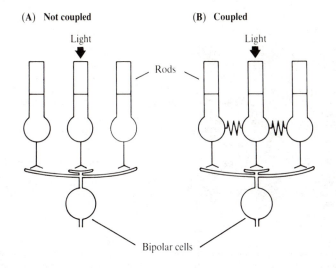

Figure 18.3 For localized stimuli, signal clipping at the rod chemical output synapse is reduced by rod-rod electrical synapses. **A.** Schematic diagram showing synaptic input to a bipolar cell from pre-synaptic rods that are not electrically coupled. Bright localized light will polarize a single illuminated rod by an amount greater than the operating range of the rod output synapse, leading to signal clipping. **B.** Schematic diagram for the case where the pre-synaptic rods are electrically coupled. During bright illumination of one rod, current will flow from the illuminated rod to the unilluminated rods. Consequently, all the coupled rods will undergo a small voltage change, rather than one rod undergoing a large voltage change, and signal clipping during synaptic transmission will be reduced.

post-synaptic effect (i.e. a higher synaptic gain) when the rate of transmitter release is higher (i.e. when the rod is more depolarized).

18.4   Electrical coupling of photoreceptors reduces signal clipping by the chemical output synapse

We suggested above that photoreceptors ought to behave as independent units if high spatial frequency information is not to be lost in the retina. In fact, histological work has shown that there are gap junctions forming electrical synapses between adjacent photoreceptors (Uga *et al.*, 1970; Custer 1973). Physiological recording has demonstrated that these anatomically observed structures do indeed allow current to flow between adjacent photoreceptors (Baylor *et al.*, 1971), resulting in 'crosstalk' which decreases the spatial resolution of the system.

In the tiger salamander retina there are two types of electrical synapse between photoreceptors (reviewed by Attwell, 1986). First, each rod is quite strongly electrically coupled to the four rods around it. Second, each cone is weakly electrically coupled to the four rods around it (see Figure 18.4). We will now

(A)   **(B)**

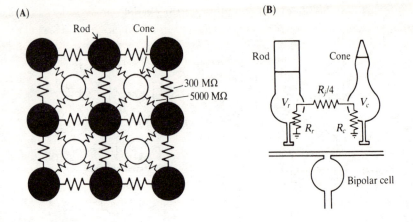

Figure 18.4 For large area stimuli, signal clipping at the rod chemical output synapse is reduced by rod-cone electrical synapses. **A.** Wiring diagram of the photoreceptor layer in the salamander retina (reviewed by Attwell, 1986). Each rod is coupled to 4 surrounding rods by an electrical synapse of resistance 300 MΩ. Each cone is coupled to 4 surrounding rods by an electrical synapse of resistance 5000 MΩ. There are no cone-cone electrical synapses. Rod-cone coupling is sufficiently weak that, to a first approximation, it can be ignored when considering the effects of rod-rod coupling. **B.** Simplification of the diagram in **A** for large area stimuli, when all the rods have the same potential (so there is no current flow through rod-rod electrical synapses), and all cones have the same potential. The receptor network can then be represented as one rod (of resistance R_r) coupled to one cone (resistance R_c) through a resistance which is one quarter of that of one rod-cone electrical synapse (because there are 4 such synapses coupling each cone to the surrounding rods), i.e. $R_j/4 = 1250$ MΩ. When light polarizes the rods by an amount V_r, a reduced version of this signal will be transmitted to the cones, modulating release of neurotransmitter from the cone chemical output synapse even if V_r is larger than the operating range of the rod chemical output synapse. The change in cone potential, V_c, is related to that in the rods by $V_c/V_r = R_c/\{R_c+R_j/4\} \approx 1/5$ for $R_j/4 = 1250$ MΩ and $R_c = 300$ MΩ. In the salamander retina, bipolar and horizontal cells receive chemical synaptic input from both rods and cones, so rod-driven changes in neurotransmitter release from cones will produce voltage changes in the same post-synaptic cells that receive direct input from rods.

explain how these two types of electrical synapse can, in different circumstances, partly mitigate the signal clipping which would otherwise occur at the rod chemical output synapse.

Consider first the case of localized illumination (e.g. when only one rod is illuminated) and, for simplicity, let us initially ignore the weak electrical coupling that exists between rods and cones. If there were no rod-rod coupling (Figure 18.3A), localized illumination of greater than a certain intensity (sufficient to polarize the rod beyond the 5 mV operating range of the chemical output synapse) would produce an almost maximum response in the post-synaptic cell: over much of the intensity range where the rod generates responses of different sizes, the post-synaptic voltage change would be of almost constant size. In the presence of rod-rod coupling (Figure 18.3B), current will spread from the illuminated rod to the surrounding rods. Thus, instead of a large voltage change occurring in just one rod, a smaller change will occur in several rods, each of which will have its chemical output synapse operating at a higher gain. In this way, less information will be lost during transmission of the visual signal out of the receptor layer, because there will be less signal clipping at the output synapse.

In the case of broad-field (large area) illumination, rod-rod coupling does not serve to avoid signal clipping at the chemical output synapse: all the rods undergo the same voltage change, there is no current flow between them, and pre-synaptic signals larger than about 5 mV in amplitude will be clipped. In this situation, however, the electrical coupling of adjacent rods and cones can partly avoid the effects of signal clipping (Figure 18.4). In the retina of the tiger salamander, post-synaptic bipolar and horizontal cells receive input from both rods and cones. When large area stimuli hyperpolarize the rods, a reduced version of the rod potential change is transmitted through the rod-cone electrical synapses to cones, modulating transmitter release from their chemical output synapses. (The cones, which are less light sensitive than the rods, will still be near their dark potential if the light intensity is not too high.) In this way, light-induced changes in rod voltage which are in the voltage range negative to the operating range of the rod chemical output synapse can still generate a voltage change in the post-synaptic cell.

18.5 How strong should the rod-rod and rod-cone electrical synapses be?

If one reason for the evolution of electrical synapses between photoreceptors is to avoid signal clipping at the photoreceptors' chemical output synapse, it is natural to ask how strong such synapses should be. The photoreceptors can (in principle) vary the strengths of such synapses by altering the number of gap junctional particles (connexons) they insert into each electrical synapse. For example, the rod-rod synapses have approximately 25 times the number of junctional particles as there are in rod-cone junctions (in toad: Gold & Dowling, 1979), in reasonable agreement with the relative strengths of these synapses (17:1 in salamander, Attwell *et al.*, 1984). In principle, then, evolutionary selection might have resulted in adjustment of the electrical synapse strengths to optimize the coding of information by the outer retina.

Consider first how the strength of rod-rod synapses might be set, to avoid signal clipping during localized illumination. For an isolated rod (or for broad-field illumination when no current flows through the rod-rod synapses), the maximum light-induced voltage change is about 25 mV, i.e. 5 times greater than the synapse operating range of about 5 mV. The effect of rod-rod coupling is to reduce the maximum voltage change induced by bright localized illumination. Clearly, if the strength of the rod-rod synapses were such that the input resistance of a rod in the retina were 5 times smaller than that of an isolated rod, then the maximum response evoked by localized illumination of just one rod would be 25 mV / 5 = 5 mV. With this strength of synapse, the range of responses to different intensities of illumination of just one rod would map exactly onto the synapse operating range, and no information would be lost as a result of signal clipping. Stronger rod-rod synapses would result in a maximum response that was less than the chemical synapse operating range, and the coding range would not be optimally used (because of noise, as discussed below). Thus, if detection of localized stimuli is important, we expect the strength of rod-rod synapses to be such that the resistance of an isolated rod is about 5 times that of a rod in the retina (Attwell *et al.*, 1987). Experimentally, this ratio is found to be about 7 (Attwell & Wilson, 1980).

A similar calculation can be done to predict the strength of the rod-cone electrical synapses. If, for broad-field illumination, signal clipping at the rod chemical output synapse is to be avoided by transmitting information via the cone output synapse, how strong should the rod-cone synapses be? Let us assume that the cone chemical output synapse has a similar operating range to that of the rod (because calcium channels with similar properties may control neurotransmitter release). It would seem appropriate, then, to set the strength of the rod-cone synapses so that the maximum light response occurring in the rods (25 mV) is reduced by a factor of 5 during transmission to cones, so that the largest rod-evoked signal occurring in the cones is matched in amplitude to the operating range of the cone chemical output synapse. Experimentally, rod signals are reduced in amplitude by a factor of about 5 during transmission to cones (Figure 18.4; Attwell *et al.*, 1984; Attwell 1986).

These predictions are presented in Table 18.1. Given that there is a 5-fold mismatch between the voltage operating range of the rod phototransduction machinery and that of the rod chemical output synapse, we predict that the rod-rod electrical synapses will have a strength sufficient to reduce the rod input resistance by a factor of 5, and that the rod-cone electrical synapses will have a strength sufficient to attenuate rod signals by a factor of 5 during transmission to cones. Experimentally, these predictions are found to be approximately correct.

Table 18.1 Predictions of electrical synapse strengths

	Theory	Experiment
Maximum rod light response / chemical synapse operating range	?	5
Isolated rod input resistance / rod network input resistance	5	7
Maximum rod light response / rod response transmitted to cones	5	5

18.6 Setting the peak rod light response

An obvious problem arising from this analysis is highlighted by the question mark in Table 18.1: there is no theoretical prediction for the mismatch between the operating range of the phototransduction machinery and of the chemical output synapse. If the properties of calcium channels limit the synapse operating range to 5 mV, why has evolutionary selection not set the maximum rod response (to broad-field illumination) at 5 mV? In this case there would be no signal clipping, and apparently no need for electrical synapses between photoreceptors or the consequent loss of spatial information entailed by such synapses. The theory presented so far gives no answer to this because, in predicting the strengths of the electrical synapses, we have taken as given the range of amplitudes of the light-induced signals and considered only how this range might be mapped onto the chemical synapse operating range. Insight into why there is a mismatch between these two ranges can be obtained by considering one factor that we have not, so far, included in our analysis, and which severely limits the efficiency of information coding by the outer retina, that is, the levels of voltage noise in the cells.

In what follows, we will review theory showing that the existence of voltage noise in rods actually provides a rationale for electrical synapses between the rods. The existence of electrical synapses provides, in turn, a reason for having a mismatch between the rod light response range and the chemical synapse operating range, as follows. In the presence of electrical synapses, if the peak rod response (to broad-field illumination) were matched to the synapse operating range (5 mV) then the peak response to localized illumination would use only a small fraction of this operating range, resulting in a loss of information coding capacity (see below). Making the peak rod response much greater than the synapse operating range allows the peak response to localized illumination (reduced by the electrical coupling) to be better matched to the synapse operating range. On this basis, if it is more important for the animal to detect localized than large area stimuli (see Section 18.10), one would predict the rod light response range (for broad-field stimuli) to be greater than the synapse operating range by a factor equal to the ratio of input resistances of an isolated rod and a rod in the intact retina. (Conversely, the response range mismatch will be smaller than this maximum value if large area stimuli are also important to the animal.)

18.7 Noise

Voltage noise is generated in the photoreceptors (and other retinal neurones) by fluctuations in the number of ion channels open in the cell membrane. In photoreceptors a significant fraction of this noise results from the occurrence of photon-like events in the receptor outer segment: visual pigment molecules can occasionally break down and trigger the phototransduction machinery even though they have not absorbed a photon (Ashmore & Falk, 1977; Lamb, 1980). In the presence of background illumination, random absorption of photons (photon noise) also generates noise in the membrane potential. Unless a change in light intensity is large enough to alter the membrane potential by more than the noise level, reliable detection of that change in intensity will not be possible. Thus, noise effectively divides up the response range of the cell into a set of discrete levels. If the range of

(A)   (B)

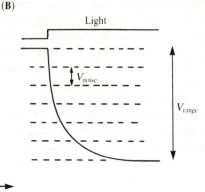

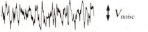

Time

Figure 18.5 Noise divides the rod response range into a finite number of distinguishable signal categories. **A.** Schematic diagram of noise in the membrane potential as a function of time. Fluctuations in membrane current due to thermal breakdown of visual pigment molecules, fluctuations in the number of photons absorbed, and opening and closing of ion channels, cause fluctuations in the membrane potential around its mean value. The size of this voltage noise (twice the standard deviation) is labelled V_{noise}. **B.** Schematic diagram showing the rod light response with voltage noise omitted (solid line) as a function of time, with superimposed dashed lines showing how the response range, V_{range}, is divided up into different signal categories separated by V_{noise} (assuming that V_{noise} is the same over all of the response range). Two potentials that are closer together than V_{noise} cannot be reliably distinguished because of the noise in the membrane potential. Thus, the total number of distinguishable signal categories is V_{range}/V_{noise}. (Although the different categories are shown in this figure as having well-defined boundaries, it should be understood that this is only a schematic way of counting the number of voltage ranges which are separated by more than V_{noise}.)

possible signals is V_{range}, and the magnitude of the noise (roughly twice its standard deviation) is V_{noise}, the signal range is effectively divided up into a number of independent voltage ranges

$$N_{signal\ categories} = \frac{V_{range}}{V_{noise}} \tag{18.2}$$

(i.e. separated by more than the noise level) which code different signals (Figure 18.5: see also Snyder *et al.*, 1977). Clearly, the amount of information that can be encoded is determined by the number of different signal categories possible. Thus, from Equation 18.2, the larger the noise is, the less information can be encoded.

18.8 Electrical synapses and noise in the photoreceptor layer

The existence of electrical synapses between photoreceptors reduces voltage noise in the photoreceptors (Lamb & Simon, 1976) and thus increases the number of signal categories that they can encode (Equation 18.2). In addition the electrical synapses can improve the signal-to-noise ratio in the photoreceptors for certain stimuli, thus improving the detectability of those stimuli (Lamb & Simon, 1976).

These points can be seen as follows. Suppose that a number, N, of rods are *perfectly* electrically coupled to each other (i.e. the electrical synapses between them are sufficiently strong that the cells become isopotential). If current noise is generated independently in each rod, the total current variance in the network of coupled rods will be N times larger than that in an isolated rod. Thus, the standard deviation of the total current noise will be increased $\sqrt{N}$-fold by the electrical synapses. However, the input resistance of the coupled rods will be N times lower than for an isolated rod, and so the standard deviation of the *voltage* noise in the rods will be lower than that in an isolated rod by a factor of $\sqrt{N}$ (i.e. by $N/\sqrt{N}$). For the tiger salamander, the standard deviation of the voltage noise in an isolated rod in the dark is about 0.2 mV (Attwell & Tessier-Lavigne, 1987), so V_{noise} is 0.4 mV (twice the standard deviation). Thus, for a maximum response range of 25 mV, the number of signal categories available is roughly 25 mV/0.4 mV = 62 (or 12 if the response range is taken as the 5 mV operating range of the chemical output synapse), assuming the noise level is the same over all of the response range. The input resistance of a rod in the intact salamander retina is about 1/7 of that of isolated rods, due to the electrical synapses between the rods (see above). Taking 7 as an estimate of the number of rods which are effectively coupled together, we therefore predict that the effect of the electrical synapses is to produce a 2.6-fold (i.e. $\sqrt{7}$-fold) reduction of V_{noise}, and a corresponding increase in the number of signal categories to 164 (or 32 for a 5 mV response range).

This calculation, assuming perfect rod coupling, gives only a rough estimate of the decrease in noise produced by electrical coupling in the salamander retina for two reasons. Firstly, the rods are not segregated into groups of perfectly coupled cells. Instead, the rods must be treated as a distributed network of cells coupled by electrical synapses of finite (rather than zero) resistance. In fact, for a given reduction of input resistance produced by electrical coupling, distributed rod coupling produces a greater reduction of noise than does perfect coupling (over two-fold greater for the salamander retina: Tessier-Lavigne & Attwell, 1988). Secondly, the existence of electrical synapses between rods and cones in the salamander retina also alters the noise levels in rods, in two ways: by reducing the input resistance of the rod network, this coupling reduces the noise level in rods, but noise generated in cones can be transmitted through these synapses and can increase the noise level in rods. The combination of these effects decreases slightly the standard deviation of the voltage noise in salamander rods (by about 9%: Attwell & Tessier-Lavigne, in preparation). Seven per cent of the standard deviation of the rod voltage noise is attributable to noise generated in cones and transmitted to rods through the electrical synapses coupling these cells (Attwell & Tessier-Lavigne, 1987).

18.9   Trading-off spatial information capacity and the number of signal categories

The stronger are the electrical synapses between rods, the more they will reduce noise in the receptor layer, but the more they will result in the loss of spatial information. Is some compromise possible between these two effects? Snyder *et al.* (1977) have analysed this situation in the case where all the noise in the photoreceptors is photon noise. They found that, for optimal information coding, the effective area of a photoreceptor (i.e. the effective number of rods coupled in our case) should be inversely proportional to the average light intensity (so long as diffraction by the pupil was not important). This implies an inverse variation in the strength of rod-rod electrical synapses with mean light intensity. Such a variation has not been detected: rod-rod coupling has a similar strength in relatively light adapted preparations (Attwell & Wilson, 1980) and in dark adapted retinae studied under infra-red illumination (Attwell *et al.*, 1985). It remains an attractive hypothesis, however, that the actual strength of rod-rod coupling has been set, by evolutionary selection, to maximize the information coding capacity of the outer retina by generating the optimum trade-off (perhaps averaged over all illumination conditions) between spatial information capacity and number of signal categories codable by the receptors. Once this electrical synapse strength has been set, the apparent mismatch between the rod response range and the chemical synapse operating range, and the strength of rod-cone synapses are also set (see Sections 18.6 and 18.5 above).

18.10   Electrical synapses and signal-to-noise ratio in the receptor layer

Electrical synapses between photoreceptors will not affect the voltage response produced by large area stimuli which illuminate all the coupled receptors: the voltage change occurring will be the same in all receptors and there will be no current flow through the rod-rod synapses. Thus, if N rods are perfectly coupled, reducing the voltage noise standard deviation by a factor of $\sqrt{N}$ relative to that in an isolated rod, the effect of the electrical synapses will be to increase the signal-to-noise ratio for large area stimuli by a factor of $\sqrt{N}$.

For small area stimuli, however, rod-rod coupling decreases the signal-to-noise ratio (Lamb & Simon, 1976). If only one rod is illuminated, the voltage response generated in N perfectly coupled rods will be N times smaller than the response in an isolated rod (because of the reduced input resistance). Thus, the signal-to-noise ratio for this stimulus will be $\sqrt{N}$ times smaller than for an isolated rod.

Considering the signal-to-noise ratio in the photoreceptor layer, therefore, one might conjecture that the strength of rod-rod coupling set by evolutionary selection ought to depend on whether it is more important for the animal to have a good signal-to-noise ratio for large area stimuli or for localized stimuli. This is an approach to determining the strength of rod-rod coupling which is conceptually different to that described in Section 18.9, where we assumed that the key determinant of electrical synapse strength was the information coding capacity of the retina. Here, by considering whether large or small area stimuli should have a better signal-to-noise ratio, we are implicitly assuming that some stimuli are more important than others to the animal, and thus that the total information capacity may not be the sole determinant of retinal wiring (see also Section 18.6). At present it is uncertain which of these approaches is more useful.

18.11 Electrical synapses and bipolar cell signal-to-noise ratio

The situation becomes more complex when the signal-to-noise ratio in post-synaptic bipolar cells is considered. As detailed above, light-induced hyperpolarizations are clipped as they pass through the rod chemical output synapse. However, the smaller amplitude noise will not be so clipped. Thus, the synapse non-linearity shown in Figure 18.2 reduces the signal-to-noise ratio in post-synaptic bipolar cells. In this situation, the electrical synapses which couple rods projecting to one bipolar cell improve the bipolar signal-to-noise ratio for localized stimuli (e.g. illuminating only one receptor), by spreading the pre-synaptic signal over a large number of receptors, each of which undergoes only a small voltage change and thus has its chemical output synapse operating at a high gain (Tessier-Lavigne & Attwell, 1988). This post-synaptic improvement occurs despite the fact that rod-rod synapses decrease the *pre-synaptic* signal-to-noise ratio for stimuli illuminating a single receptor (Section 18.10 above).

Furthermore, for detecting spatially localized stimuli, the existence of synaptic non-linearity can make it advantageous to have synaptic convergence from many electrically coupled rods to each bipolar cell (rather than having just one rod project to each bipolar as was suggested in Section 18.1.2). Figure 18.6 shows the signal-to-noise ratio occurring in a bipolar cell receiving synaptic input from N perfectly coupled rods when one of the rods is illuminated (from Equations 32 & 37 of Tessier-Lavigne & Attwell, 1988). The chemical synapse from each rod to the bipolar cell is assumed to have the (experimentally determined) non-linearity of Equation 18.1, and no noise is assumed to be introduced during synaptic transmission (i.e. all post-synaptic noise originates pre-synaptically). For low intensity stimuli, e.g. when only one photon is absorbed, the highest post-synaptic signal-to-noise ratio is obtained when only one rod projects to the bipolar cell. However, for brighter stimuli (e.g. when 20 photons are absorbed by one rod) a larger post-synaptic signal-to-noise ratio is obtained if the bipolar cell receives input from a number of perfectly coupled rods.

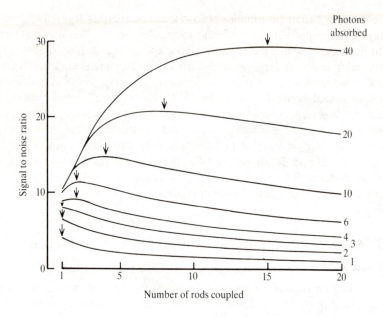

Figure 18.6 Signal-to-noise ratio (ordinate) predicted for a bipolar cell receiving synapses from different numbers (abscissa) of perfectly coupled rods, when just one rod absorbs a certain number of photons (shown by each curve), calculated from equations 32 and 37 of Tessier-Lavigne & Attwell (1988; the parameter A in these equations is set to 5 times the number of photons absorbed). Each synapse is assumed to be non-linear as in Figure 18.2 (i.e. $b = 0.095$ in the equations of Tessier-Lavigne & Attwell, 1988), and to introduce no noise itself. The number of coupled rods projecting to the bipolar cell which gives the best signal-to-noise ratio is shown by an arrow on each curve. For less than 3 photons absorbed by a single rod, the best post-synaptic signal-to-noise ratio is obtained if only one rod projects to each bipolar cell. For larger numbers of photons absorbed by a single rod, the post-synaptic signal-to-noise ratio is larger if the bipolar cell receives input from more than one perfectly coupled rod.

Although the mathematical model used for this analysis (N perfectly coupled rods) is oversimplified, it illustrates another manner in which electrical synapses between photoreceptors (and synaptic convergence from rods to bipolar cells) can be advantageous, that is, to increase the bipolar signal-to-noise ratio for localized stimuli.

Conclusion

The work that we have reviewed suggests that the strengths of rod-rod and rod-cone electrical synapses in the salamander retina are related to the non-linear behaviour of the rod's chemical output synapse. This non-linear behaviour arises from the voltage-dependence of the calcium channels controlling neurotransmitter release from the rod synaptic terminal. This work has provided some insight into how electrical synapses between photoreceptors help avoid signal clipping that would otherwise occur at the rod chemical output synapse, and help improve the signal-to-noise ratio in the outer retina.

Acknowledgements

This work was supported by the MRC, the Wellcome Trust, the Royal Society and the British Council.

References

Ashmore J.F. & Falk G. (1977) Dark noise in retinal bipolar cells and the stability of rhodopsin in rods. **Nature 270**, pp. 69-71

Attwell D. (1986) The Sharpey-Schafer Lecture: Ion channels and signal processing in the outer retina. **Quart. J. Exp. Physiol. 71**, pp. 497-536

Attwell D., Borges S., Wu S. & Wilson M. (1987) Signal clipping by the rod output synapse. **Nature 328**, pp. 522-524

Attwell D. & Tessier-Lavigne M. (1987) Transmission of noise between rods and cones in the isolated retina of the salamander. **J. Physiol. 384**, 22P

Attwell D. & Wilson M. (1980) Behaviour of the rod network in the tiger salamander retina mediated by membrane properties of individual rods. **J. Physiol. 309**, pp. 287-315

Attwell D., Wilson M. & Wu S. (1984) A quantitative analysis of interactions between photoreceptors in the salamander retina. **J. Physiol. 352**, pp. 703-737

Attwell D., Wilson M. & Wu S. (1985) The effect of light on the spread of signals through the rod network of the salamander retina. **Brain Res. 343**, pp. 79-88

Bader C.R., Bertrand D. & Schwartz E.A. (1982) Voltage-activated and calcium-activated currents studied in solitary rod inner segments from the salamander retina. **J. Physiol. 331**, pp. 253-284

Baylor D.A., Fuortes M.G.F. & O'Bryan P.M. (1971) Receptive fields of single cones in the retina of the turtle. **J. Physiol. 214**, pp. 265-294

Belgum J.H. & Copenhagen D.R. (1988) Synaptic transfer of rod signals to horizontal and bipolar cells in the retina of the toad. **J. Physiol. 396**, pp. 225-245

Brew H. & Attwell D. (1987) Electrogenic glutamate uptake is a major current carrier in the membrane of axolotl retinal glial cells. **Nature 327**, pp. 707-709

Custer N.V. (1973) Structurally specialised contacts between the photoreceptors of the retina of the axolotl. **J. comp. Neurol. 151**, pp. 35-56

Gold G.H. & Dowling J.E. (1979) Photoreceptor coupling in the retina of the toad (*Bufo marinus*). I. Anatomy. **J. Neurophysiol. 42**, pp. 311-328

Kaneko A. & Tachibana M. (1986) Blocking effects of cobalt and related ions on the GABA-induced current in turtle retinal cones. **J. Physiol. 373**, pp. 463-479

Lamb T.D. (1980) Spontaneous quantal events induced in toad rods by pigment bleaching. **Nature 287**, pp. 349-351

Lamb T.D. & Simon E.J. (1976) The relation between intercellular coupling and electrical noise in turtle photoreceptors. **J. Physiol. 263**, pp. 257-286

Marshall L.M. & Werblin F.S. (1978) Synaptic transmission to the horizontal cells in the retina of the larval tiger salamander. **J. Physiol. 279**, pp. 321-346

Schwartz E.A. (1986) Synaptic transmission in amphibian retinae during conditions unfavourable for calcium entry into presynaptic terminals. **J. Physiol. 376**, pp. 411-428

Shiells R.A., Falk G. & Naghshineh S. (1986) Iontophoretic study of excitatory amino acids on rod horizontal cells of the dogfish retina. **Proc. Roy. Soc. Lond. B. 227**, pp. 121-135

Snyder A.W., Laughlin S.B. & Stavenga D.G. (1977) Information capacity of eyes. **Vision Res. 17**, pp. 1163-1175

Tessier-Lavigne M. & Attwell D. (1988) The effect of photoreceptor coupling and synapse non-linearity on signal-to-noise ratio in early visual processing. **Proc. Roy. Soc. Lond. B. 234**, pp. 171-197

Uga S., Nakao F., Mimura M. & Ikui H. (1970) Some new findings on the fine structure of human photoreceptor cells. **J. Electron Micr. 19**, pp. 71-84

19
Optical Flow: Computational Properties and Networks, Biological and Analog
Tomaso Poggio, Woodward Yang & Vincent Torre

Summary

The computation of motion is an important task for biological and machine vision. Until now, progress has been steady, but without any drastic changes in perspective. In the past few months, however, three papers have appeared that represent a minor revolution in our view of the initial steps of the computation of motion (Verri & Poggio, 1987; Reichardt *et al.*, 1988; Verri *et al.*, 1988). We review the present understanding of the computational problem of the optical flow and discuss some implementations of parallel analog networks. We also propose some conjectures about how real neurons may compute some form of optical flow.

19.1 Introduction

The computational analysis of motion represents a good example of what a computational analysis of a visual task can tell us about its implementation in terms of either real neurons or artificial networks. The main point that will emerge from this example is that computational constraints are not sufficient to constrain the implementation enough. Properties and limitations of the hardware (or 'wetware') are at least as important as the computational goal itself in determining which of the feasible computational schemes is used.

19.1.1 *Velocity field and optical flow*

One can associate a 3D velocity field with moving objects. This 3D velocity field cannot be measured directly (consider a white rotating sphere) by any mechanism or algorithm that has access only to the time-dependent brightness distribution in the image plane. If features in the image were identifiable that correspond to locations on the surface of the objects, the 2D *velocity* field could be computed from image data. The 2D velocity field is the projection of the true 3D velocity field (one can show that the correct 3D velocity field can be computed from its perspective 2D projection if the latter is available exactly and without noise, see

355

Longuet-Higgins & Prazdny, 1980). It is possible, however, to define an 'optical flow' just from the time-dependent intensities in the image, in such a way that it will be as close as possible to the 'true' 2D velocity field most of the time.

Fennema & Thompson (1979), Horn & Schunck (1981) and others have defined such optical flow in terms of the 'image constraint equation':

$$\frac{dE}{dt} = 0 \tag{19.1a}$$

which defines a component of the optical flow $\mathbf{u}^{FT}$ as (by the chain rule of derivatives):

$$\nabla E \cdot \mathbf{u}^{FT} + \frac{\partial E}{\partial t} = 0 \tag{19.1b}$$

Though Horn makes it clear that this optical flow is generally different from the true velocity field, several authors seem to have assumed that this is not the case. The flow defined by Equation 19.1 has often been referred to in the literature as *the* optical flow, although it is not based on any constraint that is generally valid in the physical world. Equation 19.1 imposes the constraint that the luminance associated with each point of the object remains constant. This is generally incorrect, since the brightness on the image plane of a point on the surface varies with its 3D position relative to the viewer and the image plane. However, Equation 19.1 does satisfy the requirements of (i) simplicity and (ii) providing the true velocity field for an important special case, that is translation of a Lambertian surface (see Verri & Poggio, 1987, for more details).

This discussion suggests therefore that there are several possible definitions of optical flow and not just one. In particular, *optical flows are observable fields* $\mathbf{u}$ *that are usually close to the true velocity field* $\mathbf{v}$ *at least qualitatively*. The choice of the appropriate definition to use will depend on its closeness to the motion field (for the given task) but also on ease and robustness of computation for a given implementation.

19.2 Two steps in the computation of the optical flow

Whatever definition of the optical flow is used there must be another step in order to obtain a satisfactory field: regularization - that is the use of *a priori* constraints to make the result well-behaved and unique - is needed, possibly in such a way as to preserve discontinuities in the field. The reasons for the regularization step are because the initial data provided by the local detectors (we will call the mechanisms implementing the local *definitions* of optical flow *detectors*) may be (i) noisy, (ii) sparse and (iii) non-unique. Condition (i) is always true in practice and is therefore the main motivation for regularization. Depending on the definition the initial motion data may be sparse and even non-unique as in the case of Equation 19.1 (they are unique for other definitions of the optical flow; discussed later).

Thus the computation of the optical flow requires two conceptually separate stages:

1) local evaluation of the chosen definition of optical flow *via* a corresponding motion detector and

2) regularization of these initial motion data.

In this paper we will first analyze stage (1) by listing several possible detectors, that is definitions of the optical flow, characterizing some of their properties and discussing some possible implementations. We will then briefly discuss stage (2). We will first introduce the *aperture problem*.

19.2.1   The aperture problem

Marr & Ullman (1981) recognized a problem in the initial computation of motion: if a straight contour is observed through a small aperture, only the component of velocity normal to the contour can be measured: the tangential component is invisible. They called this the 'aperture problem'. The problem is intrinsic to the situation, and is valid for any mechanism, detector or definition of the optical flow that has access to data through the aperture. Notice, however, that the problem may disappear if the contour is not straight, or if other distinctive features are available within the aperture. We call this the *weak* aperture problem (see Figure 19.1).

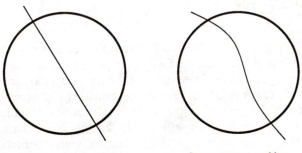

Weak aperture problem   Strong aperture problem

Figure 19.1 Any motion detector - that is, any definition of optical flow - fails to recover the motion component along the straight line edge, as seen through an aperture - since only the motion component perpendicular to the straight line is physically observable. This is the *weak aperture problem* and cannot be overcome by any physical mechanism or definition of optical flow. If a motion detector can only recover one component of motion for a curved edge, it is said to suffer from the *strong aperture problem* since both components of motion are physically observable through an aperture when the image is not simply a straight edge.

The optical flow defined by Equation 19.1 suffers, of course, from the same problem. In fact, the problem for this definition is considerably worse: only the component of **v** which is tangential to the intensity gradient is defined by Equation 19.1 for any intensity distribution, not only for straight edges. This is a very pathological case of the aperture problem, which holds for this particular definition of optical flow. We call this the *strong* aperture problem (see Figure 19.1).

It should be clear that the weak aperture problem cannot be avoided: any definition of the optical flow and therefore any physical detector will suffer from it. The strong form of the aperture problem, however, exists only for special definitions of the optical flow, as we will see later. In practice the weak form is not a serious problem: straight segments without additional features are rare and isolated (see later).

19.3   The first step: definitions of the optical flow

We consider here four main definitions:

19.3.1   The Fennema-Thompson optical flow

This is the same definition as used by Horn & Schunck (1981) and is given by Equation 19.1, that is:

$$\frac{dE}{dt} = 0 \tag{19.1a}$$

which defines an optical flow $\mathbf{u}^{FT}$ as:

$$\nabla E \cdot \mathbf{u}^{FT} + \frac{\partial E}{\partial t} = 0 \tag{19.1b}$$

Verri & Poggio (1987) showed in detail that Equation 19.1 does not in general provide the correct velocity field. They proved that $\mathbf{u}^{FT}$ is the physically correct 2D projection of the 3D velocity field only for translations (in 3D) of a Lambertian surface. For rotations, for instance, Equation 19.1 provides $\mathbf{u}^{FT}$ which is different from the true **v**. If the surface reflectance contains a specular component, $\mathbf{u}^{FT}$ is never the true velocity: Verri & Poggio provide formulae for the discrepancy. They argue that because of this situation, several definitions of optical flow could be considered, as long as they are usually close to the correct velocity. There is no reason for ascribing privileged status to Equation 19.1. Though the authors did not fully realize it, their paper effectively opened the search for a better definition of optical flow.

Equation 19.1 suffers from the strong aperture problem since it is a single scalar equation, while the field it defines is a two-dimensional vector field. Thus the initial data represented by $\mathbf{u}^{FT}$ are non-unique and require regularization, in the form suggested by Horn & Schunck and others (see later).

19.3.2 The Verri-Girosi-Torre flow

The new definition is given by Equation 19.2:

$$\frac{d}{dt}\nabla E = 0 \tag{19.2a}$$

and defines a new optical flow $\mathbf{u}^{VTG}$ as:

$$\nabla\frac{\partial E}{\partial x}\cdot\mathbf{u}^{VTG} + \frac{\partial^2 E}{\partial x \partial t} = 0$$

$$\nabla\frac{\partial E}{\partial y}\cdot\mathbf{u}^{VTG} + \frac{\partial^2 E}{\partial y \partial t} = 0 \tag{19.2b}$$

This definition has, of course, the weak aperture problem (for a straight line the *det[Hessian E]* is zero and only the component tangential to the intensity gradient is recoverable), but usually provides the two components of $\mathbf{u}^{VTG}$, not just one.

This new optical flow is identical to the true velocity field for translation in the image plane, and is otherwise different (an exact calculation similar to that of Verri & Poggio has yet to be carried out). The definition seems to be in practice a good approximation to the velocity field. Other definitions with the same flavor as Equation 19.2 have been proposed (Verri *et al.*, 1988).

19.3.3 The correlation model

Correlation models, mainly associated with the name of Reichardt (Hassenstein & Reichardt, 1956), some of which are shown in Figure 19.2, define a class of optical flows - and, in an equivalent way, they define a class of motion detectors - that may be a first order approximation to what biological organisms use. Reichardt *et al.* (1988) show that a 2D network of correlation detectors will have an output response $\mathbf{u}^R$ given by:

$$u_x^R = h\left(\frac{\partial E}{\partial x}\frac{\partial E}{\partial t} - E\frac{\partial^2 E}{\partial x \partial t}\right)$$

$$u_y^R = h\left(\frac{\partial E}{\partial y}\frac{\partial E}{\partial t} - E\frac{\partial^2 E}{\partial y \partial t}\right) \tag{19.3}$$

in the continuous approximation limit. If $E(x, y, t) = E(x + w_x t, y + w_y t)$ then $\mathbf{u}^R$ is undetermined only when the *det[Hessian(log E)]* is zero. This means that in the most interesting pathological case $(E(x, y) = E(x + ky))$ both Equations 19.3 and 19.2 are undetermined. In particular, both definitions suffer from the weak aperture problem but not from the strong one. For this very special case of rigid translation in the image plane, the 2D continuous approximation to the correlation model is essentially equivalent to the definition given by Equation 19.2 in the following sense: they both fail for 1D patterns but they can both compute the correct velocity

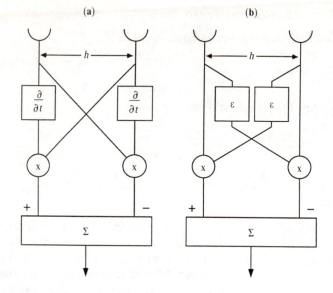

Figure 19.2 Two types of Reichardt's correlation detectors. The detectors compute the product of the time signals measured by neighboring photosensors after they have been filtered in different ways. The time average of the output is direction selective in the sense that inversion of the direction of motion will give a different average output. In the case of the detectors shown here the output for motion in one direction is exactly the opposite of the output for motion in the opposite direction (because of their antisymmetry). The first model (a) contain a high-pass filter in the direct channels, the second model (b) contains a delay in the cross channels. The delay can be replaced by a low pass filter.

otherwise (provided that appropriate derivatives of E are available). Thus for the simple case of translation in the image plane (corresponding to parallel translation of a Lambertian surface in space under orthographic projection), the measurements provided by the correlation network plus Equation 19.3 are equivalent to the new definition of optical flow given by Equation 19.2. Under the same condition, the 'old' definition, Equation 19.1, provides only one correct component of the flow. Under more general conditions, all three definitions are expected to provide values that are not equal to the true 2D velocity field and are different from each other. All three definitions suffer, of course, from the weak form of the aperture problem (see Figure 19.1). In practice, this is not a problem for Equations 19.2 and 19.3, since the $det[Hessian\ E]$ will rarely be zero (i.e., locally straight segments are rare and constant regions of grey-level values are rare).

There are several other variants of the correlation model:

1) F model (low-pass filters instead than delays).

2) F-H (low-pass filters and high-pass filters).

3) The model of Adelson & Bergan (1982).

4) The model of Watson (Watson & Ahumada, 1985) and Fahle & Poggio (1980).

5) The modified Reichardt model by van Santen & Sperling (1985).

Figures 19.2 and 19.3 show some of these models and other ones. All of these models are essentially equivalent to the correlation model in its basic form. Models such as Equations 19.1, 19.2, 19.3, introduced earlier, and 19.4, to be introduced, are approximations of the correlation model. In fact, the following *universality* result holds (Poggio & Reichardt, 1973):

'All motion detectors with negligible nonlinearities of order higher than 2 (order 2 is needed for Direction Selective properties) are equivalent to the correlation model in terms of their time-averaged output.'

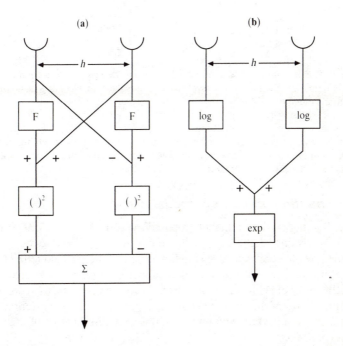

Figure 19.3 (a) A version of the correlation model using a square operation instead of the multiplication (Poggio, unpublished internal report, 1973). It is almost identical to the model more recently proposed by Adelson & Bergen (1985). The square operation may be slightly more plausible from the biological point of view than the multiplication. The trick of implementing a multiplication through linear combinations and squares is often used in analog electronics. (b) The model shows another obvious way of implementing a product: exponentiation of the sum of the logarithms of the input signals.

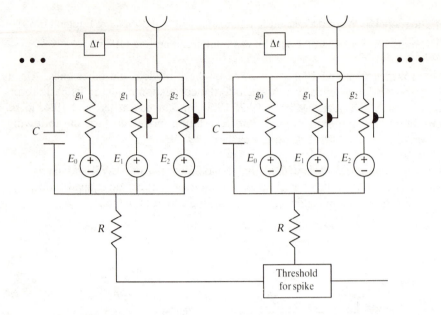

Figure 19.4 The biological model proposed by Torre & Poggio to account for direction selectivity in retinal ganglion cells. The electrical circuit is the equivalent of a patch of membrane of a direction-selective cell receiving two inputs from two photoreceptors or groups of photoreceptors mediated by other pre-synaptic cells. E_0 is the resting battery, E_1 is the excitatory battery with an equilibrium potential much more positive than the resting battery, E_2 is the inhibitory battery which is very close to the resting potential. The effect of inhibition is to *veto* or *shunt* the effect of excitation. The model works even better when the cable properties of a branched structure such as a dendritic tree are taken into account (Koch & Poggio, 1987).

19.3.4   Shunting inhibition model

The shunting inhibition model proposed by Torre & Poggio (1978) defines an optical flow similar to the correlation models. It is likely to be the scheme implemented by direction selective ganglion cells in the vertebrate retina (Amthor & Grzywacz, in preparation). The model is shown in Figure 19.4 (Torre & Poggio, 1978). A 2D array of such cells is required. The scheme seems to account well for the main properties of direction selective ganglion cells in the vertebrate retina. It can be shown that it is under certain conditions an approximation of the correlation model (Torre & Poggio, 1978).

Figure 19.4 illustrates how a non-hyperpolarizing synapse can shunt excitatory currents in one branch of a cell's dendritic tree to inhibit its responses. The excitatory conductance g_1 has a corresponding battery that injects, upon activation, a positive current into the cell. For motions in the preferred direction, the signal from the photoreceptor arrives before the signal g_2 and the current flows towards the soma. However, for motions in the null direction the signal activates g_1 and g_2 simultaneously, and the current is shunted by g_2 before reaching the soma. Shunting inhibition may account for the locality of directional selectivity. This is because the shunting inhibition of a given dendritic branch barely affects other branches. The circuit equations corresponding to Figure 19.4 show that the effect of a shunting synapse is a divisive inhibition of the cell's response, similar to a veto operation and also with some of properties of multiplication. Strong evidence for shunting inhibition in direction-selective retinal ganglion cells stimulated with moving stimuli has been provided in the turtle as well as in the frog (Marchiafava, 1979; Watanabe & MuraKami, 1984).

19.4 The second step: regularization and smoothing

All these definitions of optical flow require a prior regularization of the image data E because of the explicit or implicit (in the correlation model) spatial derivatives that are needed. In this case, regularization is equivalent to low pass filtering of E, through a blurry function such as a Gaussian or a Gabor filter. As a second step, the optical flow itself must be regularized because the detector data may be (i) noisy, (ii) sparse (locally, the $det[Hessian\ E]$ may be singular) and (iii) non-unique. Regularization of the optical flow may be done by Gaussian blurring. However, this is not ideal since the data may be sparse and effectively *not* on a regular lattice. It can also be done by standard regularization (Bertero *et al.*, 1986). The Horn & Schunck (1981) minimization scheme, the scheme suggested by Hildreth (1984) and the scheme of Yuille & Gryzwacz (1988) are all examples of standard regularization. It would be better, however, to regularize while integrating motion discontinuities. This can be done by using Markov Random Fields (MRFs) with coupled line process, especially if intensity edges are used to help find the motion discontinuities (as suggested by Gamble & Poggio, 1987, and Poggio *et al.*, 1988, and used subsequently by Hutchison *et al.*, 1987).

It is also interesting to note that the optical flow as defined by Equation 19.2 can be shown to be a partially regularized solution of Equation 19.1. By approximating the differential operator as a discrete difference between neighboring points, Equation 19.2b can be rewritten as the difference of the Fennema-Thompson equations at three neighboring points, (i, j), $(i - 1, j)$, and $(i, j - 1)$. Clearly, Equation 19.2 is more susceptible to noise than Equation 19.1, because of the higher order of derivatives involved. A subsequent regularization step is therefore even more important, though not for uniqueness:

$$\nabla \frac{\partial E}{\partial x} \cdot \mathbf{u} + \frac{\partial^2 E}{\partial x \partial t} = \left[\nabla E_{(i,j)} - \nabla E_{(i-1,j)} \right] \cdot \mathbf{u} + \left[\frac{\partial E}{\partial t}_{(i,j)} - \frac{\partial E}{\partial t}_{(i-1,j)} \right] = 0$$

$$\nabla \frac{\partial E}{\partial y} \cdot \mathbf{u} + \frac{\partial^2 E}{\partial y \partial t} = \left[\nabla E_{(i,j)} - \nabla E_{(i,j-1)} \right] \cdot \mathbf{u} + \left[\frac{\partial E}{\partial t}_{(i,j)} - \frac{\partial E}{\partial t}_{(i,j-1)} \right] = 0$$

$$(19.4)$$

So the optical flow computed by Equation 19.2 can be seen to incorporate more global information and therefore be less susceptible to the strong aperture problem than Equation 19.1.

19.5 Implementations: analog networks

Analog networks are capable of both computing the optical flow and regularizing the solution. The Fennema-Thompson optical flow is non-unique, and therefore any implementation of Equation 19.1 will require extra regularization circuitry that will impose the 'smoothness' constraints in addition to computing the optical flow. In fact, the regularization principle used by Horn & Schunck is given by the minimization of:

$$\left\|\frac{\partial E}{\partial x}u_x + \frac{\partial E}{\partial y}u_y + \frac{\partial E}{\partial t}\right\|^2 + \lambda \left\|\nabla u_x \cdot \nabla u_x + \nabla u_y \cdot \nabla u_y\right\| \tag{19.5}$$

Notice that the first term, the data term, actually computes the initial values of optical flow rather than simply assuming these as given. Furthermore, this computation requires a multiplication of the solution **u** with data. This differs from the prototypical regularization principle of surface interpolation given by the minimization of:

$$\|A\mathbf{u} - \mathbf{y}\|^2 + \lambda\|P\mathbf{u}\| \tag{19.6}$$

where A, P and λ are constant, **y** is the data term and **u** is the solution. Implementation of the prototypical regularization principle is simpler since it does not require an explicit multiplication between two variables, the solution **u** and data **y**. Furthermore, implementation of early vision tasks might be simplified if a single type of regularization network could be used.

An implementation of a network that computes the optical flow as defined by Verri *et al.* is shown in Figure 19.5. By setting the input sources and resistances to the appropriate values and provided that the *Hessian E* is not singular, the solution is found by imposing Kirchoff's Laws. Figures 19.5a and 19.5b are current-voltage duals of each other and are equivalent implementations. Figure 19.5c is a simpler implementation that uses a voltage controlled current supply or transistor. In general, however, these networks will be unstable due to possible negative resistance values (that are implemented by active components). One way of overcoming this difficulty is by replacing the positive/negative resistors and DC input sources with inductors/capacitors and sinusoidal input sources. Another interesting way of stabilizing the network shown in Figure 19.5c is to implement an identical network with the opposite polarity resistances and input sources. If either half of the network shown in Figure 19.5c is unstable then the corresponding half of the opposite polarity network will be stable. So some combination of the networks will yield a stable computation of both components of the optical flow. The implementation of the correlation model also relies on multipliers or some approximation to them. Its most plausible neural implementation is the shunting inhibition model, which is of course only an approximation to the correlation model (Torre & Poggio, 1978).

The prototypical regularization principle in 1D can be easily implemented with an analog resistive network (Horn, 1986; Poggio & Koch, 1985). An MRF regularization stage can be implemented in terms of a hybrid network of digital components that block the smoothing performed by the resistive grid at the location of discontinuities (Poggio *et al.*, 1988). Other workers (Hutchinson *et al.*, 1988) have proposed implementing similar regularization principles using 2D analog non-linear resistive networks. The extension of the prototypical regularization principle to 2D using an analog resistive network is discussed in detail by Yang & Poggio (in preparation).

19.6 Implementations: cortical neurons

Cortical mechanisms for motion detection are likely to be independent from the retinal ones: motion is probably computed anew. It is also possible that the computation is somewhat different (but see Poggio, 1982). In this perspective, it is useful to observe more closely the equation:

$$\frac{d}{dt}\nabla E = 0 \tag{19.2a}$$

which can be explicitly written as:

$$\nabla\frac{\partial E}{\partial x}\cdot\mathbf{u}^{\text{VTG}} + \frac{\partial^2 E}{\partial x \partial t} = 0$$

$$\nabla\frac{\partial E}{\partial y}\cdot\mathbf{u}^{\text{VTG}} + \frac{\partial^2 E}{\partial y \partial t} = 0 \tag{19.2b}$$

The solution of Equation 19.2b is

$$u_x{}^{\text{VTG}} = \frac{\dfrac{\partial^2 E}{\partial x \partial y}\cdot\dfrac{\partial^2 E}{\partial y \partial t} - \dfrac{\partial^2 E}{\partial y^2}\cdot\dfrac{\partial^2 E}{\partial x \partial t}}{\dfrac{\partial^2 E}{\partial x^2}\cdot\dfrac{\partial^2 E}{\partial y^2} - \dfrac{\partial^2 E}{\partial x \partial y}\cdot\dfrac{\partial^2 E}{\partial x \partial y}} = \frac{\dfrac{\partial^2 E}{\partial x \partial y}\cdot\dfrac{\partial^2 E}{\partial y \partial t} - \dfrac{\partial^2 E}{\partial y^2}\cdot\dfrac{\partial^2 E}{\partial x \partial t}}{det[Hessian\ E]} \tag{19.7a}$$

$$u_y{}^{\text{VTG}} = \frac{\dfrac{\partial^2 E}{\partial x \partial y}\cdot\dfrac{\partial^2 E}{\partial x \partial t} - \dfrac{\partial^2 E}{\partial x^2}\cdot\dfrac{\partial^2 E}{\partial y \partial t}}{\dfrac{\partial^2 E}{\partial x^2}\cdot\dfrac{\partial^2 E}{\partial y^2} - \dfrac{\partial^2 E}{\partial x \partial y}\cdot\dfrac{\partial^2 E}{\partial x \partial y}} = \frac{\dfrac{\partial^2 E}{\partial x \partial y}\cdot\dfrac{\partial^2 E}{\partial x \partial t} - \dfrac{\partial^2 E}{\partial x^2}\cdot\dfrac{\partial^2 E}{\partial y \partial t}}{det[Hessian\ E]} \tag{19.7b}$$

It is evident that the direction of the optical flow, at a given location, does not depend on the value of the *det[Hessian E]*, since:

(a)

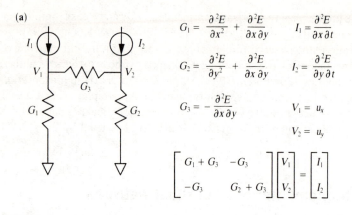

$$G_1 = \frac{\partial^2 E}{\partial x^2} + \frac{\partial^2 E}{\partial x\,\partial y} \qquad\qquad I_1 = \frac{\partial^2 E}{\partial x\,\partial t}$$

$$G_2 = \frac{\partial^2 E}{\partial y^2} + \frac{\partial^2 E}{\partial x\,\partial y} \qquad\qquad I_2 = \frac{\partial^2 E}{\partial y\,\partial t}$$

$$G_3 = -\frac{\partial^2 E}{\partial x\,\partial y} \qquad\qquad V_1 = u_x$$

$$V_2 = u_y$$

$$\begin{bmatrix} G_1 + G_3 & -G_3 \\ -G_3 & G_2 + G_3 \end{bmatrix} \begin{bmatrix} V_1 \\ V_2 \end{bmatrix} = \begin{bmatrix} I_1 \\ I_2 \end{bmatrix}$$

(b)

$$R_1 = \frac{\partial^2 E}{\partial x^2} + \frac{\partial^2 E}{\partial x\,\partial y} \qquad\qquad V_1 = \frac{\partial^2 E}{\partial x\,\partial t}$$

$$R_2 = \frac{\partial^2 E}{\partial y^2} + \frac{\partial^2 E}{\partial x\,\partial y} \qquad\qquad V_2 = \frac{\partial^2 E}{\partial y\,\partial t}$$

$$R_3 = -\frac{\partial^2 E}{\partial x\,\partial y} \qquad\qquad I_1 = u_x$$

$$I_2 = u_y$$

$$\begin{bmatrix} R_1 + R_3 & -R_3 \\ -R_3 & R_2 + R_3 \end{bmatrix} \begin{bmatrix} I_1 \\ I_2 \end{bmatrix} = \begin{bmatrix} V_1 \\ V_2 \end{bmatrix}$$

(c)

$$G_1 = \frac{\partial^2 E}{\partial x^2} \qquad\qquad I_1 = \frac{\partial^2 E}{\partial x\,\partial y}$$

$$G_2 = \frac{\partial^2 E}{\partial y^2} \qquad\qquad I_2 = \frac{\partial^2 E}{\partial y\,\partial t}$$

$$G_3 = \frac{\partial^2 E}{\partial x\,\partial y} \qquad\qquad V_1 = u_x$$

$$V_2 = u_y$$

$$\begin{bmatrix} G_1 & G_3 \\ G_3 & G_2 \end{bmatrix} \begin{bmatrix} V_1 \\ V_2 \end{bmatrix} = \begin{bmatrix} I_1 \\ I_2 \end{bmatrix}$$

Figure 19.5 Analog resistive networks that solve for the optical flow. If the conductances and current sources in (a) are set to the proper values, the voltages V_1 and V_2 will be the x and y components of the optical flow. The current-voltage dual of (a) is (b). Similarly, if the resistances and voltage sources in (b) are set to the proper values then the currents I_1 and **(Cont. opposite)**

$$\frac{u_x^{VTG}}{u_y^{VTG}} = \frac{\dfrac{\partial^2 E}{\partial x \partial y} \cdot \dfrac{\partial^2 E}{\partial y \partial t} - \dfrac{\partial^2 E}{\partial y^2} \cdot \dfrac{\partial^2 E}{\partial x \partial t}}{\dfrac{\partial^2 E}{\partial x \partial y} \cdot \dfrac{\partial^2 E}{\partial x \partial t} - \dfrac{\partial^2 E}{\partial x^2} \cdot \dfrac{\partial^2 E}{\partial y \partial t}} \tag{19.8}$$

but the sign of the optical flow is also determined by $det[Hessian\ E]$. However, the key features of Equations 19.7a and 19.7b, which determine the direction of the optical flow and avoid the aperture problem are products of terms, such as $\dfrac{\partial^2 E}{\partial x^2} \cdot \dfrac{\partial^2 E}{\partial y \partial t}$, $\dfrac{\partial^2 E}{\partial x \partial y} \cdot \dfrac{\partial^2 E}{\partial x \partial t}$ etc.

A biological implementation suggests itself (see Figure 19.6): terms such as $\dfrac{\partial^2 E}{\partial x^2}$, $\dfrac{\partial^2 E}{\partial y^2}$ and $\dfrac{\partial^2 E}{\partial x \partial y}$ can be directly implemented by visual neurons with an elongated receptive field with two excitatory lobes and a central inhibitory area. The axes of receptive fields of these cells have different orientations (0, 45 and 90°). These units are sustained units, while the units implementing $\dfrac{\partial^2 E}{\partial x \partial t}$ and $\dfrac{\partial^2 E}{\partial y \partial t}$ are transient with an elongated receptive field with only two lobes, one excitatory and one inhibitory.

Neurons with these spatial and temporal properties are indeed present in the primary visual cortex of most mammals. The approximate computation of the optical flow in terms of Equation 19.7a and 19.7b requires terms like $\dfrac{\partial^2 E}{\partial x^2} \cdot \dfrac{\partial^2 E}{\partial y \partial t}$, that is, a multiplication between a sustained and a transient unit with different orientations. Interestingly, a multiplication between a transient and a sustained unit is also present in all models of direction-selective units and seems a recurrent theme in motion analysis in the brain. The cortical implementation of multiplication between sustained and transient units is an open question: it may be based on shunting inhibition or on some more exotic mechanism, such as NMDA receptors. In the latter case, the depolarization produced by one of the input synapses would enhance the effectiveness of a nearby NMDA synapse. Still other mechanisms could be used, such as exponentiation of the sum of the logs of the inputs (see Figure 19.2). An approximation of the log operation (within certain input ranges) may be achieved at the level of the transduction between pre-synaptic voltage and post-synaptic current; the sum would then be what one expects in a roughly passive

---

(Fig. 19.5 cont.) I_2 will be the components of the optical flow. (c) is a simplified network that utilizes a voltage controlled current source, a transistor. By setting the conductances and current sources properly, the optical flow is similarly computed. In addition, by making an identical network to (c) except with opposite polarity resistances and current sources, there are guaranteed to be stable voltages representing both components of the optical flow.

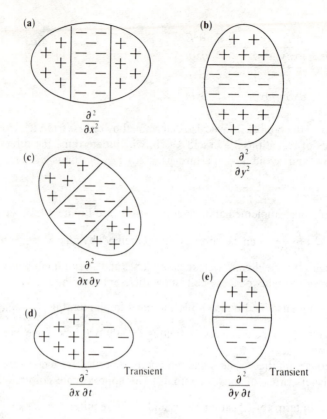

Figure 19.6 Receptive fields of cortical cells needed to compute spatial and temporal derivatives required for approximation of the optical flow.

cable, and the exponentiation may be provided (again only in a limited range) by the non-linear characteristic of the voltage-spike rate transduction.

Conclusions

This paper tries to summarize some recent results in the computational theory of optical flow: given the changing image how can motion be extracted from it? New definitions of the optical flow have been suggested and compared to previous ones. Thus we can now look at engineering and biological implementations from a new point of view. We sketch very briefly some examples of this different perspective. In particular, we show that there are many different definitions of the optical flow and corresponding motion detectors that are computationally reasonable. The question of which ones are biologically *correct* depends ultimately on the constraints of the wetware and, of course, on the vagaries of natural evolution.

References

Adelson E.H. & Bergen J.R. (1985) Spatiotemporal energy models for the perception of motion. **J. Opt. Soc. Am.** 2(2), pp. 284-299

Amthor F.R. & Grzywacz N. M. in preparation.

Bertero M., Poggio T. & Torre V. (1987) Ill-posed problems in early vision. **AI Memo No. 924**, AI Laboratory, MIT Also **Proc. IEEE**, in press.

Fahle M. & Poggio T. (1980) Visual hyperacuity: Spatiotemporal interpolation in human vision. **Proc. R. Soc. Lond. B 213**, pp. 451-477

Fennema C.L. & Thompson W.B. (1979) Velocity determination in scenes containing several moving objects. **Comp. Graphics Image Process.** 9(4), pp. 301-315

Gamble E. & Poggio T. (1987) Visual integration and detection of discontinuities: The key role of intensity edges. **AI Memo No. 970**, AI Laboratory, MIT

Hassenstein B. & Reichardt W. (1956) Systemtheoretische Analyse der Zeit-, Reihenfolgen- und Vorzeichenauswertun bei der Bewegungsperzeption des Rüsselkäfers *Chlorophanus*. **Z. Naturforsch. IIb**, pp. 513-524

Hildreth E.C. (1984) The computation of the velocity field. **Proc. Roy. Soc. Lond. B 221**, pp. 189-220

Horn B.K.P. (1986) **Robot Vision**. MIT Press, Cambridge, Mass.

Horn B.K.P. & Schunck B.G. (1981) Determining optical flow. **Artif. Intel.** 17, pp. 185-203

Hutchinson J., Koch C., Luo J. & Mead C. (1988) Computing motion using analog and binary resistive networks. **IEEE Computer Magazine 21**, pp. 52-64

Koch C. & Poggio T. (1987) Biophysics of computational systems: Neurons, synapses, and membranes. In: **Synaptic Function**. pp. 637-697, G.M. Edelman, W.E. Gall & W.M. Cowan (eds.) John Wiley & Sons, NY.

Longuet-Higgins H.C. & Prazdny K. (1980) The interpretation of moving retinal images. **Proc. R. Soc. Lond. B. 208**, pp. 385-387

Marchiafava P.L. (1979) Directional selectivity of retinal ganglion cells. **Vision Res. 19**, pp. 1203-1211

Marr D. & Ullman S. (1981) Directional selectivity and its use in early visual processing. **Proc. Roy. Soc. Lond. B 211**, pp. 151-180

Poggio T. (1982) Visual algorithms. In: **Physical and Biological Processing of Images**. pp. 128-153, O.J. Braddick & A.C. Sleigh (eds.) Springer-Verlag, Berlin.

Poggio T. & Koch C. (1985) Ill-posed problems in early vision: from computational theory to analog networks. **Proc. Roy. Soc. Lond. B 226**, pp. 303-323

Poggio T., Little J., Gamble E., Gillett W., Geiger D., Weinshall D., Villalba M., Larson N., Cass T., Bülthoff H., Drumheller M., Oppenheimer P., Yang W. & Hurlbert, A. (1988) The MIT vision machine. In: **Proc. Image Understanding Workshop**, Cambridge, MA. Morgan Kaufmann, San Mateo, CA.

Poggio T. & Reichardt W. (1973) Considerations on models of movement detection. **Kybernetik 13**, pp. 223-227

Reichardt W., Schlögl R.W. & Egelhaaf M. (1988) Movement detectors of the correlation type provide sufficient information for local computation of 2-D velocity field. **Die Naturwissenschaften**, in press.

van Santen J.P.H. & Sperling G. (1985) Elaborated Reichardt detectors. **J. Opt. Soc. Am. 2(7)** pp. 300-321

Torre V. & Poggio T. (1978) A synaptic mechanism possibly underlying directional selectivity to motion. **Proc. R. Soc. Lond. B 202**, pp. 409-416

Verri A., Girosi F. & Torre V. (1988) The mathematical properties of the 2D motion field: from singular points to motion parameters. **J. Opt. Soc. Am.**, submitted.

Verri A. & Poggio T. (1987) Against quantitive optical flow. **Proc. Int. Conf. Computer Vision**, London England. IEEE, Washington, DC pp. 171-180

Watanabe S. & MuraKami M. (1984) Synaptic mechanisms of directional selectivity in ganglion cells of frog retina as revealed by intracellular recordings. **Japan J. Physiol. 34**, pp. 497-511

Watson A.B. & Ahumada A. J. (1985) Model of human visual-motion sensing. **J. Opt. Soc. Am. 2(7)**, pp. 322-342

Yang W. & Poggio T. in preparation.

Yuille A. & Grzywacz N.M. (1988) A computational theory for the perception of coherent visual motion. **Nature 333**, pp. 71-74

20

Computing Optical Flow in the Primate Visual System: Linking Computational Theory with Perception and Physiology

Taichi Wang, Bimal Mathur, Andrew Hsu & Christof Koch

Summary

Computing motion on the basis of the time-varying image intensity is a difficult problem for both artificial and biological vision systems (for reviews on motion see Ullman, 1981; Nakayama, 1985; Horn, 1986; Hildreth & Koch, 1987). We show how one well-known gradient-based computer algorithm for estimating visual motion (Horn & Schunck, 1981) can be implemented within the primate's visual system. The algorithm computes the optical flow field in two steps. In the first stage, local motion is measured, while in the second stage spatial integration occurs by minimizing a variational functional of a form commonly encountered in early vision (Poggio et al., 1985). We use an implicit population representation of velocity, such that each neuron only codes for motion in one particular direction. The resulting network maps onto the magnocellular pathway of the primate visual system, in particular onto cells in the primary visual cortex (V1) as well as onto cells in the middle temporal area (MT). We explain a number of psychophysical observations and illusions as well as the single cell recordings of Movshon et al. (1985) and Albright (1984). We argue that the primate visual system implements an optical flow algorithm incorporating some measure of smoothness as well as explicit labeling of discontinuities in the optical flow.

20.1 Computational theory

One prominent school of thought holds that information processing systems, whether biological or man-made, should follow essentially similar computational strategies when solving complex perceptual problems, in spite of their vastly different hardware (Marr, 1982). However, it is not apparent how algorithms developed for machine vision or robotics can be mapped in a plausible manner onto nervous structures, given their known anatomical and physiological constraints. In this chapter, we show how one well-known computer algorithm for estimating visual motion could be implemented within the early visual system of primates.

The basic tenet underlying Horn & Schunck's (1981) analysis of the problem of computing the optical flow field $(\dot{x}, \dot{y})$ from the time-varying image intensity $I(x, y, t)$ falling onto a retina or a phototransistor array, is that the total derivative of the image intensity between two image frames separated by the interval dt is zero: $dI(x, y, t)/dt = 0$. In other words, the image intensity seen from the point-of-view of an observer located in the image plane and moving with the image, does not change. This conservation law is only strictly satisfied for translation of a rigid Lambertian body in planes parallel to the image plane. Thus, under rotation, $dI/dt = 0$ will break down (for a detailed error analysis see Kearney *et al.* (1987); Verri & Poggio (1987) discuss the principal limitations of this type of algorithm). Using the chain rule of differentiation, $dI/dt = 0$ can be reformulated as $I_x\dot{x} + I_y\dot{y} + I_t = 0$ where $\dot{x}$ and $\dot{y}$ are the x and y components of velocity $\mathbf{V}$, and I_x, I_y and I_t the spatial and temporal image gradients which can be measured from the image. We now have a single linear equation with two unknowns ($\dot{x}$ and $\dot{y}$). Additional constraints are needed to unambiguously compute the optical flow field. Measuring at n different locations does not help in general, since we are then faced with n linear equations in $2n$ unknowns. The fact that we are unable to measure both components of the velocity vector is also known as the 'aperture' problem. Any system with a finite viewing aperture and the rule $dI/dt = 0$ can only measure the component of motion $-I_t / |\nabla I|$ along the spatial gradient ∇I. The motion component perpendicular to the local gradient remains invisible. In addition to the aperture problem, the initial motion data is usually noisy and may be sparse. That is, at those locations where the local visual contrast is weak or zero, no initial optical flow data exists (thus, a perfectly featureless rotating sphere would be perceived as stationary), thereby complicating the task of recovering the optical flow field in a robust manner. Horn & Schunck's method belongs to a broad class of motion algorithms, collectively known as gradient algorithms. These exploit the relation between the spatial and the temporal intensity gradient at a given point to estimate the motion field (Limb & Murphy, 1975; Fennema & Thompson, 1979; Marr & Ullman, 1981; Hildreth, 1984; Yuille & Grzywacz, 1988). The aperture problem can be by-passed using a different definition of optical flow, as discussed in Chapter 19 (see also Uras *et al.*, 1988). However, even in this case, smoothness is still required to deal with unavoidable image noise.

Horn & Schunck (1981) first introduced a 'smoothness constraint' to solve this problem. The underlying rationale for this constraint is that nearby points on moving objects tend to have similar three-dimensional velocities; thus, the projected velocity field should reflect this fact. The algorithm then computes an optical flow field which is as compatible as possible with the measured motion components as well as varying smoothly almost everywhere in the image. The final optical flow field is determined by minimizing:

$$L(\dot{x}, \dot{y}) = \int \int (I_x\dot{x} + I_y\dot{y} + I_t)^2 + \lambda\left[\left(\frac{\partial\dot{x}}{\partial x}\right)^2 + \left(\frac{\partial\dot{x}}{\partial y}\right)^2 + \left(\frac{\partial\dot{y}}{\partial x}\right)^2 + \left(\frac{\partial\dot{y}}{\partial y}\right)^2\right] dx \, dy \quad (20.1)$$

where the parameter λ controls the compromise between the smoothness of the desired solution and its closeness to the data. This variational functional is quadratic in $\dot{x}$ and $\dot{y}$ and has a unique minimum. With the appropriate boundary conditions, this area-based optical flow algorithm computes the qualitative correct optical flow field for real images (Horn & Schunck, 1981). The smoothness constraint also stabilizes the solution against the unavoidable noise in the measured data.

It has been shown previously that this type of quadratic variational functional - common in early vision (Poggio *et al.*, 1985) - can be solved using simple electrical networks (Poggio & Koch, 1985). The key idea behind this mapping is that the power dissipated in a linear electrical network is quadratic in the currents or voltages; thus, if the values of the resistances are chosen appropriately, the steady-state voltage distribution in the network corresponds to the minimum of L in Equation 20.1. The resistive network for computing optical flow is shown in Figure 20.1. Here, the voltage in the top part of the network corresponds to the x component of the velocity, while the voltage in the bottom grid corresponds to the y component (Hutchinson *et al.*, 1988). The measured temporal and spatial intensity gradients determine the values of the resistances and batteries. The value of the horizontal conductances within both grids is given by λ. Efforts are now underway (see, in particular, Luo *et al.*, 1988) to build such resistive networks for various early vision algorithms in the form of miniaturized circuits using analog, subthreshold CMOS VLSI technology of the type pioneered by Mead (1989).

20.2 Implementation in a neuronal network

We will now turn towards a possible neurobiological implementation of this computer vision algorithm. Specifically, we will show that a reformulated variational functional equivalent to Equation 20.1 can be evaluated within the known anatomical and physiological constraints of the primate visual system and that this formalism can explain a number of psychophysical and physiological phenomena.

The resistive networks described above use *analog* or *frequency* coding (Ballard *et al.*, 1983): the x and y components of velocity are given directly by the voltages at the two nodes in the resistive grid (Figure 20.1). If the voltage at any one node doubles, the appropriate component of the velocity doubles. However, neurons in the visual cortex of mammals represent the direction of motion in a very different manner, using many neurons per location such that each neuron codes for motion in one particular direction (Figure 20.3). In this representation, the velocity vector $V(i, j)$ is not coded explicitly but is computed across a population of n such cells, each of which codes for motion in a different direction (given by the unit vector Θ_k), such that:

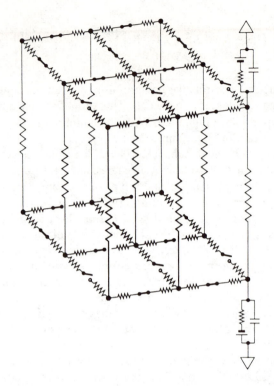

Figure 20.1 Computing motion in resistive networks. Hybrid network, computing the optical flow in the presence of discontinuities, by finding a local minimum of the functional in Equations 20.1 or 20.12. The voltages in the top grid correspond to the x components of the flow field, $\dot{x}$, and the voltages in the bottom grid to $\dot{y}$. The degree to which voltage spreads depends on the value of the horizontal conductances, given by λ. The values of the 'vertical' conductances connecting both grids as well as the values of the conductances and batteries connected to ground (for clarity, only two such elements are shown) depend on the measured intensity gradients I_x, I_y and I_t. Binary switches, which make or break the resistive connections between nodes, implement motion discontinuities, since an arbitrary high voltage (velocity) will not affect the neighboring site across the discontinuity. Adapted from Hutchinson *et al.* (1988).

$$\mathbf{V(i,j)} = \sum_{k=1}^{n} V(i,j,k)\Theta_k \qquad (20.2)$$

To mimic neuronal responses more accurately, the output of all our model neurons is half-way rectified; in other words, $f(x) = x$ if $x > 0$ and 0 if $x < 0$. We then require at least $n = 4$ neurons to represent all possible directions of movement. Note that in this representation the individual components $V(i, j, k)$ are *not* the projections of the velocity field $\mathbf{V(i, j)}$ onto the direction Θ_k (except for $n = 4$).

Let us now consider a two stage model for extracting optical flow field (Figure 20.2). In a preliminary stage, we assume that the image $I(i, j)$ is projected onto the image plane and relayed to the first processing stage via two sets of cells:

$$S(i,j) = \nabla^2 G * I(i,j) \tag{20.3}$$

and

$$T(i,j) = \frac{\partial \left(\nabla^2 G * I(i,j) \right)}{\partial t} \tag{20.4}$$

where G is the 2-D Gaussian filter (with $\sigma^2 = 4$ pixels; Marr & Hildreth, 1980; Marr & Ullman, 1981).

In the first processing stage, the local motion information (the velocity component along the local spatial gradient) is measured using n ON-OFF orientation- and direction-selective cells $U(i, j, k)$, each with preferred direction indicated by the unit vector Θ_k (here the V neurons and the U neurons have the same number of directions and the same preferred directions for the sake of simplicity, even though it is not necessary):

$$U(i,j,k) = \frac{-T(i,j)\nabla_k S(i,j)}{\left| \nabla S(i,j) \right|^2 + \varepsilon} \tag{20.5}$$

where ε is a constant and ∇_k the spatial derivative along the direction Θ_k. This derivative is approximated by projecting the convolved image $S(i, j)$ onto a 'simple' type receptive field, consisting of a 1 by 7 pixel positive (ON) subfield next to a 1 by 7 pixel negative (OFF) subfield. Because of the Gaussian convolution in the S cells, the resulting receptive field has an ON subfield of 3 by 9 pixels next to an OFF subfield of the same size (Figure 20.5a shows such a subfield). Such receptive fields are common in the primary visual cortex of cats and primates (Hubel & Wiesel, 1962). We assume that at each location n such receptive fields, each with preferred axis given by Θ_k ($k \in \{1..n\}$) exist. The cell $U(i, j, k)$ responds optimally if a bar or grating oriented at right angles to Θ_k moves in direction Θ_k; furthermore, its output is proportional to the magnitude of velocity. Our definition of U differs from the standard gradient model $U = -T/\nabla_k S$, by including a gain control term, ε, such that U does not diverge if the visual contrast of the stimulus decreases to zero; thus, $U \to -T \nabla_k S$ as $\nabla_k S \to 0$. Under these conditions of small stimulus contrast, our model can be considered a second-order model, similar to the correlation or spatio-temporal energy models (Hassenstein & Reichardt, 1956; Poggio & Reichardt, 1973; Adelson & Bergen, 1985; Watson & Ahumada, 1985). The value of ε is set to a fixed fraction (5%) of the square of the maximal magnitude of the gradient $\nabla_k S$ for all values of i, j. More sophisticated schemes, such as replacing ε by a term depending on the local peak magnitude of the gradient and a gradient independent term, are possible.

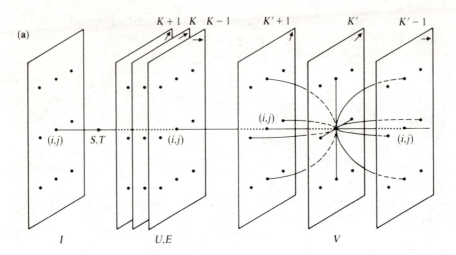

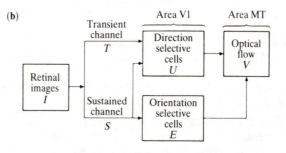

Figure 20.2 Computing motion in neuronal networks. (a) Simple scheme of our model. The image I is projected onto the rectangular 64 by 64 retina and sent to the first processing stage via the S and T channels. Subsequently, two sets of $n = 16$ ON-OFF orientation- (E) and direction-selective (U) cells code local motion in n different directions. Neurons with overlapping receptive field positions i,j but different preferred directions Θ_k are arranged here in n parallel planes. The ON subfield of one such U cell is shown in Figure 20.5a. The output of both E and U cells is relayed to a second set of 64 by 64 V cells where the final optical flow is computed. The final optical flow is represented in this stage, on the basis of a population coding $\sum_{k=1}^{n} V(i,j,k)\Theta_k$, with $n = 16$. Each cell $V(i, j, k)$ in this second stage receives input from cells E and U at location i,j as well as from neighboring V neurons at different spatial locations. (b) Block model of a possible neuronal implementation. The T and S streams originate in the retina and enter primary visual cortex in layer 4Cα and 4Cβ. The output of V1 projects from layer 4B to the middle temporal area (MT). We assume that the ON-OFF orientation- and direction-selective neurons E and U are located in V1 or in the input layers of MT, while the final optical flow is assumed to be represented by the V units in area MT.

Finally, we also require a set of ON-OFF, orientation- but not direction-selective neurons:

$$E(i,j,k) = \left| \nabla_k \, S(i,j) \right| \tag{20.6}$$

To recapitulate, we have now progressed from registering and convolving the image in the retina to representing the spatial and temporal image brightness gradients within the first stage of our network.

In the second processing stage, we determine the final optical flow field by computing the activity of a second set of cells, V. The state of these neurons - coding for the final optical flow field - is evaluated by minimizing a reformulated version of the functional in Equation 20.1. The first term expresses the fact that the final velocity field should be compatible with the initial data, i.e. with the velocity component measured along the local spatial gradient ('velocity constraint line'). In other words, the final velocity field

$$\mathbf{V(i,j)} = \sum_{k=1}^{n} V(i,j,k)\Theta_k$$

should be compatible with the local motion term U:

$$L'_0 = \sum_{i,j,k} \left(\sum_{k'} V(i,j,k')cos(k' - k) - U(i,j,k) \right)^2 \cdot E_T(i,j,k) \tag{20.7}$$

where $cos(k' - k)$ represents the *cosine* of the angle between $\Theta_{k'}$ and Θ_k and E_T the winner-take-all orientation-selective neurons. The E_T cells are defined as $E_T(i, j, k) = 1$ if $E(i, j, k)$ is the unit with highest activity at location i, j (and above a given threshold), otherwise, $E_T(i, j, k) = 0$. Although a winner-take-all approach is convenient on computational grounds and simple to build in VLSI, we feel that orientation-selective neurons E_T acting in such a manner are unlikely to be implemented in the nervous system. A more physiologically plausible approximation to Equation 20.7 could take the following form:

$$L_0 = \sum_{i,j,k} \left(\sum_{k'} V(i,j,k')cos(k' - k) - U(i,j,k) \right)^2 \cdot E^m(i,j,k) \tag{20.7a}$$

where $E(i, j, k)$ is the output of an orientation-selective neuron raised to the mth power ($m > 1$). This term ensures that the local motion components $U(i, j, k)$ only have an influence when there is an appropriate oriented local pattern; in other words, E^m prevents velocity terms incompatible with the measured data from contributing significantly to L_0. Thus, we require that the neurons $E(i, j, k)$ do not respond significantly to directions differing from Θ_k. If they do, L_0 will increasingly contain contributions from other, undesirable, data terms. A large exponent m is advantageous on computational grounds, since it will lead to a better selection of the velocity constraint line. For our model neurons (with a half-width tuning of approximately 60°), $m = 2$ gave satisfactory responses*.

The second term in Equation 20.1 can be reformulated in a straightforward manner by replacing the partial derivatives of $\dot{x}$ and $\dot{y}$ by their components in terms of $V(i, j, k)$ (for instance, the x component of the vector $\mathbf{V(i, j)}$ is given by $\sum_k V(i,j,k')cos\Theta_k$).This leads to:

$$L_1 = \sum_{i,j,k,k'} [4V(i,j,k) - V(i-1,j,k) - V(i+1,j,k) - V(i,j-1,k) - V(i,j+1,k)]$$
$$\cdot cos(k' - k)V(i,j,k') \tag{20.8}$$

We are now searching for the neuronal activity level $V(i, j, k)$ that minimizes the functional $L_0 + \lambda L_1$. Similar to the original Horn & Schunck's functional Equation 20.1, the reformulated variational functional is quadratic in $V(i, j, k)$, so we can find this state by evolving $V(i, j, k)$ on the basis of the steepest descent rule:

$$\frac{\partial V(i,j,k)}{\partial \tau} = \frac{\partial (L_0 + \lambda L_1)}{-\partial V(i,j,k)} \tag{20.9}$$

The contribution from the L_0 term to the right hand side of this equation has the form:

$$\sum_{k'} cos(k - k')E^m(i,j,k')\left(U(i,j,k') - \sum_{k''} cos(k' - k'')V(i,j,k'')\right) \tag{20.10}$$

while the contribution from the L_1 term has the form:

$$\lambda\sum_{k'} cos(k - k')[V(i-1,j,k') + V(i+1,j,k') + V(i,j-1,k')$$
$$+ V(i,j+1,k') - 4V(i,j,k')] \tag{20.11}$$

The terms in Equations 20.10 and 20.11 are all linear either in U or V. This enables us to view them as the linear synaptic contributions of the U and V neurons towards the activity of neuron $V(i, j, k)$. The left hand term of Equation 20.9 can be interpreted as a capacitive term, governing the dynamics of our model neurons. In other words, in evaluating the new activity state of neuron $V(i, j, k)$, we evaluate expressions 20.10 and 20.11 by summing all the contributions from the U and V of

---

* Notice that since any particular orientation-selective cells $E(i, j, k)$ and $E_T(i, j, k)$ correspond to motion in both Θ_k and the opposite direction, Equations 20.7 and 20.7a contain a contribution from the correct direction of motion as well as from the associated null direction. This second term can be suppressed by rectifying one of the *cos* functions in Equation 20.10.

the same location i, j as well as neighboring V neurons and subsequently using a simple numerical integration routine, such as $V_{t+\Delta t} = V_t + \Delta t(\partial V/\partial \tau)$, to arrive at the new state. The appropriate network carrying out these operations is shown schematically in Figure 20.2a. Solving the partial differential Equation 20.9 requires a boundary condition. All simulations reported here assume that the velocity along the image boundary must be zero (Dirichlet boundary condition). Alternatively, we could require that the slope of the velocity at the image boundary should be zero (von Neumann boundary condition).

This neuronal implementation converges to the solution of the Horn & Schunck algorithm as long as the correct constraint line is chosen in Equation 20.7, that is as long as the E^m term is selective enough to suppress velocity terms incompatible with the measured data. In the next two sections, we will illustrate the behavior of this algorithm by mimicking a number of perceptual and electrophysiological experiments.

20.3 Correspondence to cortical anatomy and physiology

The neuronal network we propose to compute optical flow (Figure 20.2) maps directly onto the primate visual system. Two major visual pathways, the parvo- and the magno-cellular, originate in the retina and are perpetuated into higher visual cortical areas. Magnocellular cells appear to be those specialized to process motion information (for reviews see Livingstone & Hubel, 1988; DeYoe & van Essen, 1988). Both pathways project into layer 4C of primary visual cortex. Here the two pathways diverge, magnocellular neurons projecting to layer 4B (Lund *et al.*, 1976). Cells in this layer are orientation- as well as direction-selective (Dow, 1974). Layer 4B cells project heavily to a small but well-defined visual area in the superior temporal sulcus called the middle temporal area (MT; Allman & Kass, 1971; Baker *et al.*, 1981; Maunsell & van Essen, 1983a). All cells in MT are direction-selective and tuned for the speed of the stimulus; the majority of cells are also orientation-selective. We assume that the orientation- and direction-selective E and U cells corresponding to the first stage of our motion algorithms are located in layers 4B or 4C in primary visual cortex or possibly in the input layers of area MT, while the V cells are located in the deeper layers of area MT. Inspection of the tuning curve of a V model cell in response to a moving bar reveals the similarity with the superimposed experimentally measured tuning curve of a typical MT cell of the owl monkey (Figure 20.3).

The structure of our network is indicated schematically in Figure 20.2a. The strengths of synapses between the U and the V neurons and among the V neurons are directly given by the appropriate coefficients in Equations 20.10 and 20.11. Equation 20.10 contains the contribution from neurons U and E in primary visual cortex as well as from MT neurons V at the same location i, j but with different oriented receptive fields k''. No spatial convergence or divergence occurs between our U and V modules, although this could be included. The first part of

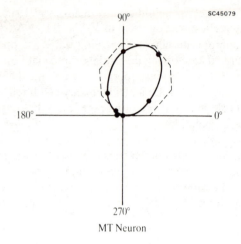

MT Neuron

Figure 20.3 Polar plot of the median neuron (solid line) in the medial temporal cortex (MT) of the owl monkey in response to a field of random dots moving in different directions (Baker *et al.*, 1981). The tuning curve of one of our model *V* cells in response to a moving bar is superimposed (dashed line). The distance from the center of the plot is the average response in spikes per second. Both the cell and its model counterpart are direction-selective, since motion towards the upper right quadrant evokes maximal response while motion towards the lower left quadrant evokes no response. Figure courtesy of J. Allman & S. Petersen.

Equation 20.10 gives the synaptic strength of the U to V projection $(cos(k - k')E^m(i, j, k')U(i, j, k'))$. That is, if the preferred direction of motion of the pre-synaptic input $U(i, j, k')$ differs by no more than $\pm 90°$ from the preferred direction of the post-synaptic neuron $V(i, j, k)$, the $U \rightarrow V$ projection will depolarize the post-synaptic membrane. Otherwise, it will act in a hyperpolarizing manner since the $cos(k - k')$ term will be negative. Note that our theory predicts neurons from all orientation columns k' projecting onto every V cell, a proposal which could be addressed using anatomical labeling techniques. The synaptic interaction contains a multiplicative nonlinearity (UE^m). This veto term can be implemented using a number of different biophysical mechanisms, for instance 'silent' or 'shunting' inhibition (Koch *et al.*, 1982). The smoothness term L_1 results in synaptic connections among the V neurons, both among cells with overlapping receptive fields (same value of i, j) and among cells with adjacent receptive fields (e.g. $i-1, j$). The synaptic strength of these connections act in either a de- or a hyper-polarizing manner, depending on the sign of $cos(k - k')$ as well as their relative locations (see Equation 20.11).

If two identical sine or square gratings are moved past each other, human observers perceive the resulting pattern as a coherent plaid, moving in a direction different from the motion of the two individual gratings (Adelson & Movshon, 1982). The direction of the resultant plaid pattern is given by the 'velocity space combination rule' (Adelson & Movshon, 1982; Hildreth, 1984). One such

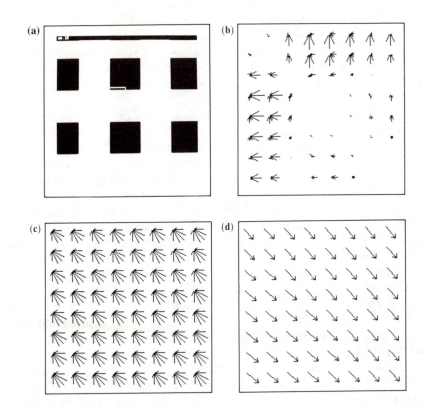

Figure 20.4 Mimicking perception and single cell behavior. (a) Two superimposed square gratings, oriented orthogonal to each other, and moving at the same speed in the direction perpendicular to their orientation. The amplitude of the composite is the sum of the amplitude of the individual bars. (b) Response of the direction-selective simple cells U to this stimulus. The output of all 16 cells is plotted in a radial coordinate system at each location where the response is significantly different from zero; the lengths are proportional to the magnitudes. (c) The output of the V cells using the same needle diagram representation after 2.5 time-constants. (d) The resulting optical flow field, extracted from (c) via population coding, corresponding to a plaid moving coherently towards the lower right hand corner, similar to the perception of human observers (Adelson & Movshon, 1982) as well as to the response of a subset of MT neurons in the macaque (Movshon *et al.*, 1985). $\lambda = 50$.

experiment is illustrated in Figure 20.4. A vertical square grating is moved horizontally at a right angle over a second horizontal square grating moving at the same speed vertically. The resulting coherent pattern is seen to move coherently to the lower right corner (Adelson & Movshon, 1982), as does the output of our algorithm. Note that the smoothest optical flow field compatible with the two local motion components (one from each grating) is identical to the solution of the 'velocity space combination rule'. Thus, for rigid planar motion as occurs in the plaid experiments, this rule and the 'smoothness constraint' lead to identical solutions, even when the velocities of the two gradients differ (see Wang *et al.*, 1989). Furthermore, we predict that as the contrasts of the two gratings making up the plaid differ, the final component velocity is biased towards the direction of motion of the grating with the higher contrast, a prediction borne out by recent psychophysical experiments (Stone *et al.*, 1988).

Movshon *et al.* (1985) repeated Adelson & Movshon's plaid experiments while recording from neurons in striate and extrastriate macaque cortex (see also Albright, 1984). All neurons in V1 and about 60% of cells in MT only responded to the motion of the two individual gratings (component selectivity; Movshon *et al.*, 1985), similar to our $U(i, j, k)$ cell population, while about 30% of all recorded MT cells responded to the motion of the coherently moving plaid pattern (pattern selectivity), mimicking human perception. As illustrated in Figure 20.4, our V cells behave in this manner and could be identified with this subpopulation.

An interesting distinction arises between direction-selective cells in V1 and MT. While the optimal orientation in V1 cells is always perpendicular to their optimal direction, this is only true for about 60% of MT cells (type I cells; Albright, 1984; Rodman & Albright, 1988). 30% of MT cells respond strongly to flashed bars oriented parallel to the cells' preferred direction of motion (type II cells). These cells also respond best to the pattern motion in the Movshon *et al.* (1985) plaid experiments. Based on this identification, our model predicts that type II cells should respond to an extended bar (or grating) moving parallel to its edge. Even though, in this case, no motion information is available if only the classical receptive field of the MT cell is considered, motion information from the trailing and leading edges will propagate along the entire bar. Thus, neurons whose receptive fields are located away from the edges will eventually (i.e. after several tens of *milliseconds*) signal motion in the correct direction, even though the direction of motion is parallel to the local orientation. This neurophysiological prediction is illustrated in Figure 20.5.

Cells in area MT respond well not only to motion of a bar or grating but also to a moving random dot pattern (Albright, 1984; Allman *et al.*, 1985), a stimulus containing no edges or intensity discontinuities. Our algorithm responds well to random-dot motion, as long as the spatial displacement between two consecutive frames is not too large (Figure 20.5).

The 'smooth' optical flow algorithms we are discussing only derive the exact velocity field if a rigid, Lambertian object moves parallel to the image plane. If an object rotates or moves in depth, the derived optical flow only approximates the underlying velocity field (Verri & Poggio, 1986). Is this constraint reflected in V1 and MT cells? No cells selective to true motion in depth have been reported in primate V1 or MT. Cells in MT do encode information about position in depth, e.g. whether an object is near or far, but not about motion in depth, e.g. whether an object is approaching or receding (Maunsell & van Essen, 1983b). The absence of cells responding to motion in depth supports the thesis that area MT is involved in extracting optical flow using a smoothness constraint, an approach which breaks down for 3-D motion. Cells selective to expanding or contracting patterns, caused

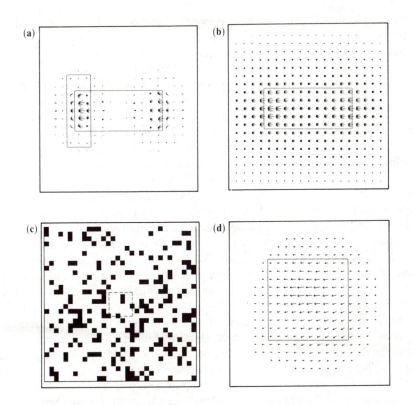

Figure 20.5 Simulated single-cell behavior. A dark bar (outlined in both images) is moved parallel to its orientation towards the right. (a) Those U neurons whose receptive field only 'see' the trailing or leading edges of the bar - and not a corner - will fail to respond to this moving stimulus, since it remains invisible on the basis of purely local information. The ON subfield of the receptive field of a vertically oriented U cell is superimposed for comparison purposes. (b) It is only after information has been integrated, following the smoothing process inherent in the second stage of our algorithm, that the V neurons respond to this motion. We predict that the type II cells of Albright (1984) in MT will respond to this stimulus while cells in V1 will not. (c) The first frame of two random-dot stimuli. The area outlined was moved by 1 pixel to the left. (d) The final population coded velocity field, signaling the presence of a blob, moving toward the right. $\lambda = 10$.

by motion in depth, or to rotations of patterns within the frontoparallel plane were first reported by Saito *et al.* (1986), in a cortical area surrounding MT, termed the medial superior temporal area (MST).

20.4 Psychophysics

We now consider the response of the model to a number of stimuli which generate strong psychophysical percepts. We have already discussed the plaid experiments (Section 20.3), in which our smoothness constraint lead to the correct, perceived interpretation of coherent motion.

In 'motion capture' (Ramachandran & Anstis, 1983; Ramachandran & Inada, 1985), the motion of randomly moving dots can be influenced by the motion of a superimposed low-spatial-frequency grating such that the dots move coherently with the larger contour, that is they are 'captured'. As the spatial frequency of the grating increases, the capture effect becomes weaker. As first demonstrated by Bülthoff *et al.* (1988), algorithms that exploit local uniformity or smoothness of the optical flow can explain, at least qualitatively, this optical illusion since the smoothness constraint tends to average out the motion of the random dots in favor of the motion of the neighboring contours (see also Yuille & Grzywacz, 1988). However, using the constraint line as formulated in Equation 20.7a did not lead to capture because the orientation-selective cells E failed to respond in a significant manner to the low-frequency grating (since their receptive fields are too small relative to the width of the grating). The winner-take-all version of Equation 20.7 did work and is illustrated in Figure 20.6. We believe that to properly explain this illusion, a version of our algorithm which works at multiple spatial scales is required (to perceive both the high-frequency random dots as well as the low-frequency grating).

Yuille & Grzywacz (1988) have shown how the related phenomenon of 'motion coherence' (in which a cloud of 'randomly' moving dots is perceived to move in the direction defined by the mean of the motion distribution; Williams & Sekuler, 1984) can be accounted for using a specific smoothness constraint. Our algorithm also reproduces this visual illusion quite well (Figure 20.7). In fact, it is surprising how often the Gestalt psychologists use the words 'smooth' and 'simple' when describing the perceptual organization of objects (for instance in the formulation of the key law of *Prägnanz*; Kofka, 1935; Köhler, 1969). Thus, one could argue that these psychologists intuitively captured some of the constraints used in today's computer vision algorithms.

Our algorithm is able to mimic another illusion of the Gestalt psychologists: γ motion (Lindemann, 1922; Kofka, 1931; for a related illusion in man and fly, see Bülthoff & Götz, 1979). A figure which is exposed for a short time appears with a motion of expansion and disappears with a motion of contraction, independent of the sign of contrast. Our algorithm responds in a similar manner to a flashed disk (Figure 20.6). This illusion arises from the initial velocity measurement stage and does not rely on the smoothness constraint.

20.5 Motion discontinuities

The major drawback of our, and all other motion algorithms, is the degree of smoothness required, smearing out any discontinuities in the flow field, such as those arising along occluding objects or along a figure-ground boundary. A powerful idea to deal with this problem was proposed by Geman & Geman (1984; see also Blake & Zisserman, 1987) by introducing the concept of binary line

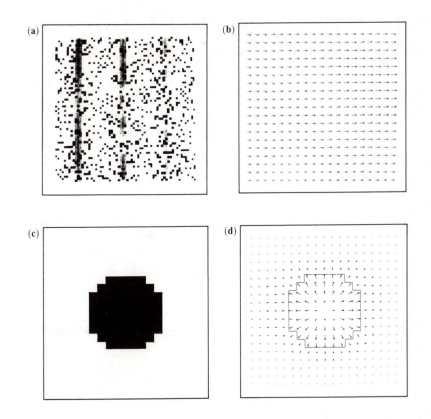

Figure 20.6 Psychophysical illusions. (a) The motion of a low-spatial-frequency grating superimposed onto a random-dot display 'captures' the motion of the random dots. (b) The entire display seems to move towards the right. Human observers suffer from the same optical illusion (Ramachandran & Anstis, 1983). We used the winner-take-all version of our algorithm in Equation 20.7 to compute the final optical flow. $\lambda = 50$. (c) If a stimulus, such as the one shown, is briefly flashed onto a white screen, it appears to expand. It will disappear with a motion of contraction (γ-motion; Lindemann, 1922; Kofka, 1931). (d) Our algorithm perceives a similar expansion when the stimulus is flashed onto the screen in the second image frame. The final population coded velocity field is shown for $\lambda = 10$.

processes which explicitly code for the presence of discontinuities. We adopt the same approach for discontinuities in the optical flow (as first proposed in Koch *et al.*, 1986) by introducing binary horizontal l^h and vertical l^v line processes representing discontinuities in the optical flow. If the spatial gradient of the optical flow between two neighboring points is larger than some threshold, the flow field is 'broken' and the appropriate motion discontinuity at that location is switched on ($l = 1$), and no smoothing is carried out. If little spatial variation exists, the discontinuity is switched off ($l = 0$). This approach can be justified rigorously using Bayesian estimation and Markov Random Fields (Geman & Geman, 1984). In such

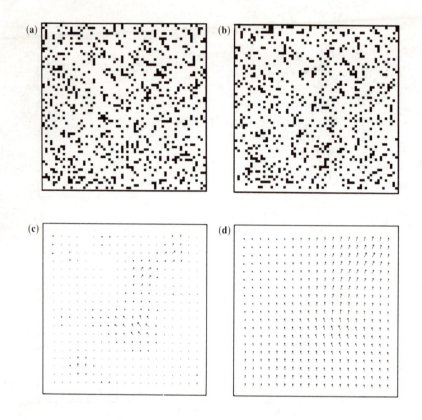

Figure 20.7 Motion coherence. (a) The upper left image shows a random-dot display. (b) In the second frame (upper right image) all dots move one pixel toward the top. In addition to this motion component common to all points, all dots have a random horizontal motion component which varies in a uniform manner between ± 2, ± 1 and 0 pixels. (c) With a weak smoothness constraint ($\lambda = 0.5$), the random motion is apparent. (d) If smoothness is increased ($\lambda = 10$), the final velocity field only shows the motion component common to all dots. Humans observe the same phenomenon (Williams & Sekuler, 1984).

a probabilistic formulation, the maximum *a posteriori* estimate of the solution is computed on the basis of observations and *a priori* constraints, such as smoothness, by minimizing:

$$\sum_{ij} (I_x \dot{x}_{ij} + I_y \dot{y}_{ij} + I_t)^2 + \lambda \sum \left(1 - l_{ij}^h\right)\left((\dot{x}_{i+1j} - \dot{x}_{ij})^2 + (\dot{y}_{i+1j} - \dot{y}_{ij})^2\right)$$

$$+ \lambda \sum \left(1 - l_{ij}^v\right)\left((\dot{x}_{ij+1} - \dot{x}_{ij})^2 + (\dot{y}_{ij+1} - \dot{y}_{ij})^2\right) + V_C(l^h, l^v) \qquad (20.12)$$

Notice that if all line processes are switched off, this cost function corresponds to the discrete version of Equation 20.1. The line potential $V_C(l^h, l^v)$ (defined on a given neighborhood C) contains terms explicitly encouraging the formation of discontinuities along continuous contours and along intensity discontinuities, that is edges (Geman & Geman, 1984; Gamble & Poggio, 1987). These domain-independent constraints capture some important aspect of natural scenes; thus, motion discontinuities usually do coincide with intensity edges (as for instance in the case of a figure moving over a background of different texture). As we have illustrated elsewhere (Hutchinson *et al.*, 1988), motion discontinuities lead to a much improved performance of the motion algorithm.

We have not yet implemented motion discontinuities into the neuronal model. It is known, however, that the visual system uses motion to segment different parts of the scene. A number of authors have studied the conditions under which discontinuities (in either speed or direction) in motion fields can be detected (Baker & Braddick, 1982; van Doorn & Koenderink, 1983; Hildreth, 1984). Van Doorn & Koenderink (1983) concluded that perception of motion boundaries requires that the magnitude of the velocity difference be larger than some critical value, a finding in agreement with the notion of processes that explicitly code for motion boundaries. Recently, Nakayama & Silverman (1988) studied the spatial interaction of motion among moving and stationary waveforms. A number of their results could be re-interpreted in terms of our motion discontinuities.

What about the possible cellular correlate of line processes? Allman *et al.* (1985) first described cells in area MT in the owl monkey whose 'true' receptive field extended well beyond the classical receptive field as mapped with bar or spot stimuli (see Tanaka *et al.*, 1986, for such cells in macaque MT). About 40 - 50% of all MT cells have an antagonistic direction-selective surround, such that the response of the cell to motion of a random dot display or an edge within the center of the receptive field, can be modified by moving a stimulus within the surrounding region that is 50 to 100 times the area of the center. The response depends on the difference in speed and direction of motion between the center and the surround, and is maximal if the surround moves at the same speed as the stimulus in the center but in the opposite direction. In brief, these cells become activated if a motion discontinuity exists within their receptive field. Thus, tantalizing hints exist as to the possible neuronal basis of motion discontinuities.

20.6 Discussion

The principal contribution of this article is to show how a well-known algorithm for computing optical flow, based on minimizing a quadratic functional via a relaxation scheme, can be mapped onto the early visual system of primates. Note that this 'neuronal network' implementation has some properties very different from the resistive network implementation. While two nodes per location suffice to represent the velocity in the resistive network, at least $n = 4$ half-way rectifying neurons are required in our neuronal model. Note also that the robustness of the latter representation to errors in the individual hardware components increases as n increases. If one of the resistances in the circuit shown in Figure 20.1 is grounded, the voltage at the associated node will be zero, while a missing 'synapse' in the neuronal implementation will at worst lead to a small deviation in the represented velocity (as long as n is large). This distributed and coarse population coding scheme is similar to the coding believed to be used in the system controlling eye movements in the mammalian superior colliculus (Lee *et al.*, 1988). Detecting the most active neuron at each location (winner-take-all scheme), as in the Bülthoff *et al.* (1988) model, is not required.

Recently, two studies have further refined our understanding of gradient based optical flow methods (Yuille & Grzywacz, 1988; Uras *et al.*, 1988). The principal idea behind the motion coherence theory of Yuille & Grzywacz is that a higher degree of smoothness has a number of desirable properties, in particular that the interactions between point measurements falls off to zero at large distances. They thus lead to the use of higher derivatives in the second term of the variational functional (Equation 20.1) imposing smoothness. Our network can be simply adapted to their form by increasing the range of the spatial interactions among our presumed MT neurons V (Figure 20.2). Uras *et al.* (1988) show that the aperture problem can be avoided by exploiting a different definition of optical flow: $d \nabla I/dt = 0$. This results in the use of second order spatial and temporal derivatives of the image brightness pattern to yield a dense optical flow field, in addition to the conventional smoothness term. Their algorithm can be mapped onto our representation by changing the definition of the local motion detecting cells U in Equation 20.5. Even-symmetric receptive fields (e.g. a central ON field with adjacent OFF subfields on both sides) to implement the required second spatial derivative are needed. It is presently a topic of active research whether these schemes give rise to different psychophysical or electrophysiological predictions (e.g. Nakayama & Silverman, 1988). All of these schemes can, however, be implemented at the neuronal level using the type of representation we have outlined above.

Acknowledgement

We acknowledge many fruitful discussions with Ted Albright, John Allman, David van Essen and Alan Yuille. Graeme Mitchison helped make the manuscript palatable to the non-initiated.

References

Adelson E.H. & Bergen J.R. (1985) Spatio-temporal energy models for the perception of motion. **J. Opt. Soc. Am. A2**, pp. 284-299

Adelson E.H. & Movshon J.A. (1982) Phenomenal coherence of moving visual patterns. **Nature 200**, pp. 523-525

Albright T.L. (1984) Direction and orientation selectivity of neurons in visual area MT of the macaque. **J. Neurophysiol. 52**, pp. 1106-1130

Allman J.M. & Kass J.H. (1971) Representation of the visual field in the caudal third of the middle temporal gyrus of the owl monkey (*Aotus trivirgatus*). **Brain Res. 31**, pp. 85-105

Allman J., Miezin F. & McGuinness E. (1985) Direction- and velocity- specific responses from beyond the classical receptive field in the middle temporal area (MT). **Perception 14**, pp. 105-126

Ballard D.H., Hinton G.E. & Sejnowski T.J. (1983) Parallel visual computation. **Nature 306**, pp. 21-26

Baker C.L. & Braddick O.J. (1982) Does segregation of differently moving areas depend on relative or absolute displacement? **Vision Res. 7**, pp. 851-856

Baker J.F., Petersen S.E., Newsome W.T. & Allman J.M. (1981) Visual response properties of neurons in four extrastriate visual areas of the owl monkey (*Aotus trivirgatus*): a quantitative comparison of medial, dorsomedial, dorsolateral and middle temporal areas. **J. Neurophysiol. 45**, pp. 397-416

Blake A. & Zisserman A. (1987) **Visual Reconstruction**. MIT Press, Cambridge, Mass.

Bülthoff H.H. & Götz K.G. (1979) Analogous motion illusion in man and fly. **Nature 278**, pp. 366-368

Bülthoff H.H., Little J.J. & Poggio T. (1988) Parallel computation of motion: computation, psychophysics and physiology. **Nature**, in press.

DeYoe E.A. & van Essen D.C. (1988) Concurrent processing streams in monkey visual cortex **TINS 11**, pp. 219-226

van Doorn A.J. & Koenderink J.J. (1983) Detectability of velocity gradients in moving random-dot patterns. **Vision Res. 23**, pp. 799-804

Dow B.M. (1974) Functional classes of cells and their laminar distribution in monkey visual cortex. **J. Neurophysiol. 37**, pp. 927-946

Fennema C.L. & Thompson W.B. (1979) Velocity determination in scenes containing several moving objects. **Comput. Graph. Image Proc. 9**, pp. 301-315

Gamble E. & Poggio T. (1987) Integration of intensity edges with stereo and motion, **AI Lab. Memo No. 970**, MIT, Cambridge, MA.

Geman S. & Geman D. (1984) Stochastic relaxation, Gibbs distribution and the Bayesian restoration of images. **IEEE Trans. Pattern Anal. Machine Intell. 6**, pp. 721-741

Hassenstein B. & Reichardt W. (1956) Systemtheoretische Analyse der Zeit-, Reihenfolgen- und Vorreichenauswertung bei der Bewegungsperzeption des Rüsselkäfers *Chlorophanus*. **Z. Naturforschung 11b**, pp. 513-524

Hildreth E.C. (1984) **The measurement of visual motion**. MIT Press, Cambridge, Mass.

Hildreth E.C. & Koch C. (1987) The analysis of visual motion. **Ann. Rev. Neurosci. 10**, pp. 477-533

Horn B.K.P. (1986) **Robotic Vision**. MIT Press, Cambridge, Mass.

Horn B.K.P. & Schunck B.G. (1981) Determining optical flow. **Artif. Intell. 17**, pp. 185-203

Hubel D.H. & Wiesel T.N. (1962) Receptive fields, binocular interactions and functional architecture in the cat's visual cortex. **J. Physiol. (Lond.) 160**, pp.106-154

Hutchinson J., Koch C., Luo J. & Mead C. (1988) Computing motion using analog and binary resistive networks. **IEEE Computer 21(3)**, pp. 52-61

Kearney J.K., Thompson W.B. & Boley D.L. (1987) Optical flow estimation: an error analysis of gradient-based methods with local optimization. **IEEE Trans. Pattern Anal. Machine Intell. 9**, pp. 229-244

Koch C., Marroquin J. & Yuille A.L. (1986) Analog neuronal networks in early vision. **Proc. Natl. Acad. Sci. USA 83**, pp. 4263-4267

Koch C., Poggio T. & Torre V. (1982) Retinal ganglion cells: a functional interpretation of dendritic morphology. **Phil. Trans. R. Soc. Lond. B 298**, pp. 227-264

Kofka K. (1931) Die Wahrnehmung von Bewegung. In: **Handbuch der normalen und pathologischen Physiologie**, A. Bethe *et al.* (eds) Vol. II, Springer, Berlin.

Kofka K. (1935) **Principles of Gestalt Psychology**. Harcourt, Brace & World.

Köhler W. (1969) **The task of Gestalt Psychology**. Princeton University Press, Princeton.

Lee C., Rohrer W.H. & Sparks D.L. (1988) Population coding of saccadic eye movements by neurons in the superior colliculus. **Nature 332**, pp. 357-360

Limb J.O. & Murphy J.A. (1975) Estimating the velocity of moving images in television signals. **Comput. Graph. Image Proc. 4**, pp. 311-327

Lindemann E. (1922) **Psych. Forsch. 2**, pp. 5-60

Livingstone M. & Hubel D. (1988) Segregation of form, color, movement, and depth: anatomy, physiology and perception. **Science 240**, pp. 740-749

Lund J.S., Lund R.D., Hendrickson A.E., Bunt A.H. & Fuchs A.F. (1976) The origin of efferent pathways from the primary visual cortex, area 17, of the macaque monkey as shown by retrograde transport of horseradish peroxidase. **J. Comp. Neurol. 164**, pp. 287-304

Luo J., Koch C. & Mead C. (1988) An analog VLSI circuit for two-dimensional surface interpolation. **Proc. IEEE Conf. Neural Inf. Proc. Systems**, Denver, November 28-30.

Marr D. (1982) **Vision**. Freeman, San Francisco, CA.

Marr D. & Hildreth E.C. (1980) Theory of edge detection. **Proc. R. Soc. Lond. B 297**, pp. 181-217

Marr D. & Ullman S. (1981) Directional selectivity and its use in early visual processing. **Proc. R. Soc. Lond. B 211**, pp. 151-180

Maunsell J.H.R. & van Essen D. (1983a) Functional properties of neurons in middle temporal visual area of the macaque monkey. I. Selectivity for stimulus direction, speed and orientation. **J. Neurophysiol. 49**, pp. 1127-1147

Maunsell J.H.R. & van Essen D. (1983b) Functional properties of neurons in middle temporal visual area of the macaque monkey. II. Binocular interactions and sensitivity to binocular disparity. **J. Neurophysiol. 49**, pp. 1148-1167

Mead C. (1989) **Analog VLSI and Neural Systems.** Addison-Wesley, Reading, Mass.

Movshon J.A., Adelson E.H., Gizzi M.S. & Newsome W.T. (1985) The analysis of moving visual patterns. In: **Pattern Recognition Mechanisms.** pp. 117-151, C. Chagas, R. Gattass, & C. Gross (eds.) Exp. Brain Res. Suppl. II, Springer, Heidelberg.

Nakayama K. (1985) Biological motion processing: a review. **Vision Res. 25**, pp. 625-660

Nakayama K. & Silverman G.H. (1988) The aperture problem. II. Spatial integration of velocity information along contours. **Vision Res. 28**, pp. 747-753

Poggio T. & Koch C. (1985) Ill-posed problems in early vision: from computational theory to analog networks. **Proc. R. Soc. Lond. B 226**, pp. 303-323

Poggio T. & Reichardt W. (1973) Considerations on models of movement detection. **Kybernetik 13**, pp. 223-227

Poggio T., Torre V. & Koch C. (1985) Computational vision and regularization theory. **Nature 317**, pp. 314-319

Ramachandran V.S. & Anstis S.M. (1983) Displacement threshold for coherent apparent motion in random-dot patterns. **Vision Res. 12**, pp. 1719-1724

Ramachandran V.S. & Inada V. (1985) Spatial phase and frequency in motion capture of random-dot patterns. **Spatial Vision 1**, pp. 57-67

Rodman H. & Albright T. (1988) Single-unit analysis of pattern-motion selective properties in the middle temporal area (MT). **Exp. Brain Res.**, in press.

Saito H., Yukie M., Tanaka K., Hikosaka K., Fukuda Y. & Iwai E. (1986) Integration of direction signals of image motion in the superior sulcus of the macaque monkey. **J. Neurosci. 6**, pp. 145-157

Stone L.S., Mulligan J.B. & Watson A.B. (1988) Neural determination of the direction of motion: contrast affects the perceived direction of motion. **Neurosci. Abstr. 14**, 502.5

Tanaka K., Hikosaka K., Saito H., Yukie M., Fukuda Y. & Iwai E. (1986) Analysis of local and wide-field movements in the superior temporal visual areas of the macaque monkey. **J. Neurosci. 6**, pp. 134-144

Ullman S. (1981) Analysis of visual motion by biological and computer systems. **IEEE Computer 14**, pp. 57-69

Uras S., Girosi F., Verri A. & Torre V. (1988) A computational approach to motion perception. **Biol. Cybern.**, in press.

Verri A. & Poggio T. (1987) Against quantitative optical flow. **AI Lab. Memo No. 917**, MIT, Cambridge, MA.

Wang H.T., Mathur B. & Koch C. (1989) Computing optical flow in the primate visual system. **Neural Computation**, in press.

Watson A.B. & Ahumada A.J. (1985) Model of human visual motion sensing. **J. Opt. Soc. Am. A2**, pp. 322-342

Williams D. & Sekuler R. (1984) Coherent global motion percepts from stochastic local motions. **Vision Res. 24**, pp. 55-62

Yuille A.L. & Grzywacz N.M. (1988) A computational theory for the perception of coherent visual motion. **Nature 333**, pp. 71-73

21
Models for the Development of the Visual Cortex
Alan Yuille & Daniel Kammen

21.1 Introduction

Mathematical and geometrical models of the emergence of neural structure in the visual cortex must explain not only the development of orientation-specific simple cell receptive fields but also the organization of these cells into assemblies with an orderly progression of orientation preference. In this paper we begin with a review of a number of candidate models for the maturation of cortical cells that exhibit well developed orientation selectivity in their response to retinal images. Current debate, and theoretical studies, in this area center on the importance of the orientation sensitivity in pre-cortical stages (i.e. in retinal ganglion and lateral geniculate nucleus, LGN, relay cells) of the visual pathway on the development of receptive fields in the visual cortex (Area 17) and on the role of intracortical interactions ('interneurons') in defining or accentuating the degree of orientation selectivity.

The visual cortex consists of orientation-selective cells (Figure 21.1) arranged by orientation preference. The classical description of this organization was in terms of regular hypercolumns and grew out of the pioneering electrode penetration experiments of Hubel & Wiesel (1962, 1974). These suggested that the orientations are arranged in rigid columns broken only by semi-periodic reversals in the direction of orientation increment or large, semi-regular (typically 90°or 180°) jumps in orientation. Later experiments (Blasdel & Salama, 1986), however, did not find such jumps and were consistent with computer simulations of a model by Swindale (1982). In summary, the precise organization of the full three-dimensional cortical map is still somewhat unclear (Swindale, 1985). Regardless of the detailed geometry of the hypercolumns, however, a large amount of information is required to specify the properties of such a large array of cells unless an orderly scheme or underlying developmental principle is responsible for the maturation of cortical neurons. We shall examine several variants of a developmental scenario that can produce biologically plausible cellular receptive fields and cortical hypercolumns. These models develop structure without recourse to coherent input signals and are thus consistent with the observation of orientation selectivity of cortical cells in prenatal animals. The motivation for these models is to discover how simple a set of

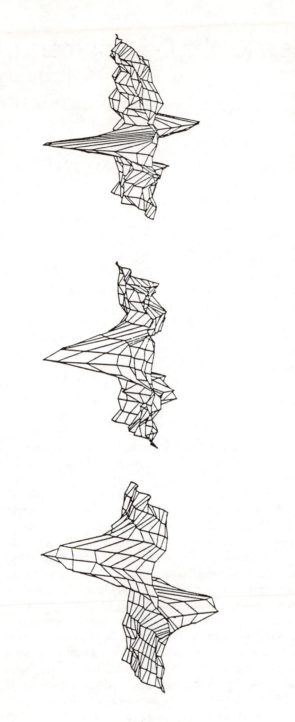

Figure 21.1 Two dimensional orientation selective receptive field profiles from simple cells in the cat primary visual cortex (recorded by Jones & Palmer, 1987). The figure is reproduced from Daugman (1985).

biologically plausible developmental rules is required for the genesis of an accurate model of the neural structure of the visual cortex.

Efforts to model and understand the function of the hypercolumnar cell assemblies and the other Area 17 cell layers are severely hampered by the lack of data on the intracortical, 'interneuron', neuronal network. Interneurons have been invoked in various models to do everything from providing the whole of the orientation tuning via inhibitory interactions, to merely communicating the activity of cells tuned to a particular orientation to those at another point in the hypercolumnar mosaic. Current investigations aimed at illuminating the prevalence and function of connections within Area 17 have led to various hypotheses concerning the role of the interneurons and more generally the *role* of the first few processing layers in the visual cortex. Building on the work of Levick & Thibos (1982), Leventhal (1983, 1985) and Schall *et al.* (1986a,b; Schall & Leventhal, 1987) have argued that cortical orientation tuning originates in the *retina* and the cortex acts merely to amplify the effect. We will compare these proposals to the self-organizing cortical models of Linsker (1986a,b,c), Kammen & Yuille (1988), and Yuille *et al.* (1988) that originate the orientation selectivity in networks with no initial orientation bias.

Models that simply mimic the morphology of the receptive fields and cell assemblies seen in Area 17 without serious consideration to what computational tasks are being performed are doomed to failure in enriching our understanding of the visual system. It is in this area that our understanding of the visual system, and in this case the early visual system, is weakest. In an effort to fill this void, researchers have begun to explore the connections between efficient information processing and the neuroanatomy of the visual system. Adaptive algorithms, such as back-propagation and feedforward network learning, are beginning to be used to naturally develop characteristics that resemble those found in real cortical neurons and seem to utilize computational approaches that are highly efficient from an information management perspective. We conclude this review with speculations on the relationship of promising models of cortical function to concepts from information theory.

21.2 Classical models of cortical organization

How do cortical cells develop orientation selectivity and how are these simple cells then organized into hypercolumns? Modern efforts to understand the organization and function of the visual cortex date back to the initial experiments of Hubel & Wiesel (1962). They suggested simply that the basically circular center/surround receptive fields of lateral geniculate nucleus cells project directly as excitatory input to comprise subfields that cortical simple cells then sum to produce spatially elongated weighting functions (1974). The orientation selectivity of cortical cells is therefore a 'geometric effect' resulting from the alignment of projected LGN fields in the cortex (the 'LGN-to-cortical map'). Many of the subsequent cortical models have been efforts to refine this basic scenario. A number of difficulties have developed in this model, primary among them the observation that cortical cells do not, in general, have elongated dendritic or receptive fields (Creutzfeldt *et al.*, 1974; Lund, 1981) and that *intracortical* interactions seem to play some role in orientation tuning (see e.g. Sillito, 1987).

A series of cortical models, proposed by Braitenberg & Braitenberg (1979), Schwartz (1980), Swindale (1982, 1985), Ferster (1987), Koch (1987), and Soodak *et al.* (1987) have explored increasingly sophisticated and essentially geometric ways of organizing non-oriented input from receptive fields in the LGN to produce hypercolumnar arrays of orientation-selective simple cells. These models are static in the sense that while they explain the structure of the cortex with varying degrees of success, no attempt is made to discuss the neurological development of the visual system. The models, for example, of von der Malsburg & Cowan (1973, 1982), Cooper *et al.* (1979), Bienenstock *et al.* (1982) and Edelman (1987) are distinct in that they do address the morphogenesis of the cortical system. In the von der Malsburg & Cowan model (1982), random activity in the developing cortex results in the spontaneous formation of periodic patterns of cellular activity. The cells interact via excitation of nearest neighbors and inhibition of next-nearest neighbors in a traditional center/surround relationship. Orientation inducing fibers (possibly from the retina) terminate in the developing cortex and bias the direction of the large-scale spontaneous pattern formation procedure. This model pertains to the development of large-scale structure and does not explicitly address the formation of individual simple cell receptive fields. The process is analogous to domain formation in magnetic spin systems. Sattinger (1979) has demonstrated formally that symmetry-breaking in two dimensional systems tends to produce linear structures which in this model aggregate into units that define the hypercolumnar cell mosaic. Von der Malsburg & Cowan (1982) discuss the possibility that input bias from LGN or retinal cells may act as the initial seed in the symmetry-breaking. We shall return to a discussion of the role of the pre-cortical visual pathway after considering two self-organizing models on the single neuron level that utilize biologically motivated learning algorithms.

21.3 Self-organizing neural network models of the cortex

The models we have considered so far predate the current interest in 'neural networks' and connectionism. In this section we present two variants of a model of cortical maturation and organization. The models considered below are distinct from the majority of recent network simulations in that they do not utilize the biologically unrealistic back-propagation algorithm but instead alter the synaptic weights through a feedforward, unsupervised, learning scheme.

Feedforward networks (Figure 21.2) typically alter the synaptic interconnection weights by application of some version of the Hebb (1949) learning rule. In the basic version of the Hebb rule the synaptic strength, or weight, from a pre-synaptic neuron A to a post-synaptic neuron B is increased if there is a

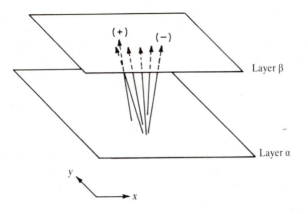

Figure 21.2 Schematic diagram of two layers in the multi-layer feedforward network. The arrows represent the synapse distribution (assumed to be a Gaussian function in Kammen & Yuille, 1988), from one layer to the next. The (+) and (–) signs indicate that the synaptic *weights*, Ø(x,y), may be of either sign and any intensity.

significant correlation between the activity of A and B. Feedforward networks have no enforced output condition akin to the supervised learning in delta rule networks. The dynamics (Meir & Domany, 1988) and self-organizational (Linsker, 1986a,b,c, 1988; Kammen & Yuille, 1988) capacities of feedforward networks have recently received considerable attention.

21.3.1 Hebb-rule learning: Linsker's model

In the feedforward network constructed by Linsker (1986a,b,c) the receptive fields, $Ø(x,y)$, measure the feedforward synaptic strength from cells in the ith layer to cells displaced by (x,y) in the $(i+1)^{th}$ layer (see Figure 21.2). The cells in the $(i+1)^{th}$ layer that receive input from the cell in the ith layer are determined by the dendritic arborization parameter, or feedforward window. Linsker's version of the Hebb rule can be expressed as:

$$\frac{dØ_i(x,y)}{dt} = k_1 + k_2 \sum_{(p,q)} (D_i(p-x, q-y) + k_3) Ø_i(p,q) \qquad (21.1)$$

where the k_a are constants, D_i is the auto-correlation function of the network activity in the ith layer. The $Ø_i(x,y)$ are hard limited to lie in a specified range, in this case between –0.50 and +0.50. Random noise is input to the network and spatial opponent and then orientation selective cells emerge after a few network layers. Further application of the unsupervised learning rule, with the addition of excitatory lateral connections, results in the cells organizing into groups with similar preferred orientation (Linsker, 1986c) like the cortical hypercolumns. The Linsker simulations are impressive in that they demonstrate that a relatively simple set of biologically plausible developmental rules are sufficient to generate such an accurate cortical model.

The Hebb rule used by Linsker can be shown to correspond to steepest descent in an energy space (Linsker, 1986a,b,c). More precisely, there is an energy function $E(\emptyset_i)$ such that:

$$\frac{d\emptyset_i (x, y)}{dt} = -\frac{\partial E}{\partial \emptyset_i(x, y)} \tag{21.2}$$

This feedforward network is thus guaranteed to converge, by steepest descent, to a stable state that corresponds to the minima of an energy function as was demonstrated by Hopfield (1984). The time derivative of a general energy function:

$$\frac{dE}{dt} = + \sum_{(x, y)} \frac{\partial E}{\partial \emptyset_i(x, y)} \cdot \frac{\partial \emptyset_i(x, y)}{dt} \tag{21.3}$$

which can be written as:

$$\frac{dE}{dt} = - \sum_{(x, y)} \left[\frac{\partial E}{\partial \emptyset(x, y)} \right]^2 \tag{21.4}$$

by the use of Equation 21.2. Equation 21.4 is clearly monotonically decreasing and we have the desired result.

Next we consider the analysis of a variant of this feedforward model in which it is explicitly shown that symmetry-breaking in an energy function governing the maturation of cortical cells gives rise to orientation selectivity.

21.3.2   Symmetry-breaking and neural development

In a closely related model, Kammen & Yuille (1988) showed that the occurrence of oriented cells could be explained in terms of the spontaneous symmetry breaking of an energy function governing the development of such cells. They demonstrated that symmetry-breaking can occur naturally in a network of feedforward neurons and is in no way an unnatural or complex mechanism for neuronal development. Simple cell response profiles (receptive fields) are generated using only center-surround antagonistic linear summation of receptive field profiles from one layer of the network to the next. We outline the mathematical construction of the model here; a complete description of the symmetry-breaking scenario can be found in Kammen & Yuille (1988). The basic model assumes random input to the first network layer (we assume the continuum limit for ease of presentation) and uses a modified Hebbian learning rule. The feedforward arborization is assumed to be a two-dimensional Gaussian, $G(x, y)$, from the neurons in layer i to a neuron in layer $(i+1)$. The feedforward network structure is depicted in Figure 21.2. Representing synapse strengths by $\emptyset(x, y)$ and the input to a layer by $I(x, y)$ we then use the linear output rule:

$$O(x, y) = \int G(x - w, y - z)\text{\O}(x - w, y - z)I(w, z) \, dw \, dz \qquad (21.5)$$

where $\text{\O}(x, y)$ is the receptive field profile of a cell and is the quantity that we expect to develop into an orientation-selective, bandwidth-limited, structure. Multiplying Equation 21.5 by $I(r, s)$ and time averaging to obtain a stochastic value yields:

$$O(x, y)I(r, s) = \int G(x - w, y - z)\text{\O}(x - w, y - z)\langle I(w, z)I(r, s)\rangle \, dw \, dz$$
$$(21.6)$$

The quantity $\langle I(w, z)I(r, s)\rangle$ is the correlation function for the ith layer, which we represent more generally as $D_i(w - r, z - s)$. Equation 21.6 thus becomes:

$$\langle O(x, y)I(r, s)\rangle = \int G(x - w, y - z)\text{\O}(x - w, y - z)D(w - r, z - s) \, dw \, dz$$
$$(21.7)$$

which we use as the increment for Hebbian learning.

The synapse modification rule used in the symmetry-breaking model is a simple continuum case of the Hebb rule:

$$\frac{d\text{\O}(x, y)}{dt} = -A - 2B\text{\O}(x, y) - 4C\text{\O}(x, y)^3$$

$$+ 2\int D(x - w, y - z)\text{\O}(w, z)G(w, z) \, dw \, dz \qquad (21.8)$$

where the first and fourth terms in Equation 21.8 are standard for Hebbian learning and correspond to a general inhibition and a positive correlation for neighboring synapses respectively. The second and third terms maintain synapse strengths in a bounded range, accomplished in other models by either setting fixed bounds (Linsker, 1986a,b,c, 1988) or using a strong saturation rule (Hopfield, 1984). The learning rule (Equation 21.8) is again (Equation 21.2) related to the minimum of an energy function by the update rule popularized by Hopfield (1984):

$$\frac{d\text{\O}(x, y)}{dt} = -\frac{dE[\text{\O}(x, y)]}{d\text{\O}(x, y)} \qquad (21.9)$$

The resulting energy function:

$$E[\emptyset(x, y)] = A \int \emptyset(x, y)G(x, y) \, dx \, dy \; + B \int \emptyset(x, y)^2 G(x, y) \, dx \, dy$$

$$+ C \int \emptyset(x, y)^4 G(x, y) \, dx \, dy$$

$$- \int \int \emptyset(x, y)G(x, y)D(x - w, y - z)\emptyset(w, z)G(w, z) \, dx \, dy \, dw \, dz$$

$$(21.10)$$

exhibits spontaneous symmetry-breaking as studied in physical (Coleman, 1985) and mathematical (Sattinger, 1979) systems. The main point is that although the minima of the energy function are symmetrically distributed (since the system is symmetric) any individual minimum is not symmetric. The system must settle into a unique minimum and in so doing breaks the symmetry.

As a quick introduction to symmetry-breaking consider the one dimensional 'Mexican hat' equation:

$$E(x) = A \, x^2 + Bx^4 \qquad\qquad (21.11)$$

which is plotted in Figure 21.3. For $A = 0$ the system has a single stable state at $x = 0$ (Figure 21.3a). For $A < 0$ the system is unstable at $x = 0$ (Figure 21.3b) and random perturbations will cause spontaneous symmetry-breaking to occur and the system will fall into one of the absolute minima (Figure 21.3c). Symmetry-breaking occurs in the neural system in essentially the same way as in this example. The symmetry-breaking parameter, A, is replaced by the correlation function, D, in the neural model.

To follow the development of receptive fields in this model only a knowledge of the variation of $D_i(x - r, y - s)$ from layer to layer is necessary. The correlation function, D_i, can be calculated in general from the stochastic auto-convolution of Equation 21.5. The details can be found in Kammen & Yuille (1988) with the result that:

$$D_{(i+1)} = G \, \emptyset_{i,i+1} * D_i * G \, \emptyset_{i,i+1} \qquad\qquad (21.12)$$

The correlation function in the first layer is simply a Dirac d-function because the input signal is assumed to be white noise. By repeated applications of Equation 21.12 we can calculate the correlation functions at any level (after the synapse strengths have been trained by Equation 21.8). Symmetry-breaking depends on the form of D. For early layers D remains roughly Gaussian and no symmetry-breaking is observed. For later layers the correlation function becomes positive for small distances and negative for large distances (Linsker, 1986a,b,c; Kammen & Yuille,

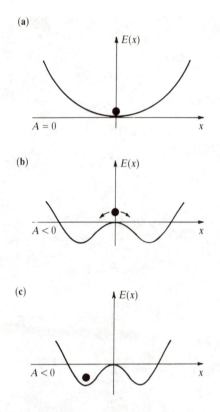

Figure 21.3 One-dimensional profile of the unbiased example system. In (a) we plot $E(x) = Ax^2 + Bx^4$ for $A = 0$ and note the single stable state at $x = 0$. With $A \neq 0$ (b) two minimum energy states exist - random fluctuations will drive the system into one of the two states. Symmetry has thus been broken and the system must lie in one of the two minima (c).

1988) and can be roughly approximated as the negative of the Laplacian of a Gaussian. As D develops into $-\nabla^2 G(x, y)$ symmetry-breaking will occur and orientation selectivity results. In Figure 21.4 we present several examples of the resulting two dimensional receptive field profiles and in Figure 21.5 we provide a one dimensional cross-section transverse to the major axis from one of the cells in Figure 21.4.

21.4 Neurophysiological data

The original Hubel and Wiesel model of the visual cortex assumed that retinal ganglion and LGN cells had circularly symmetric, center/surround receptive field profiles. The work of Levick & Thibos (1982), Leventhal (1983), and Schall *et al.* (1986a,b) has demonstrated that retinal ganglion cells are sensitive to the orientation

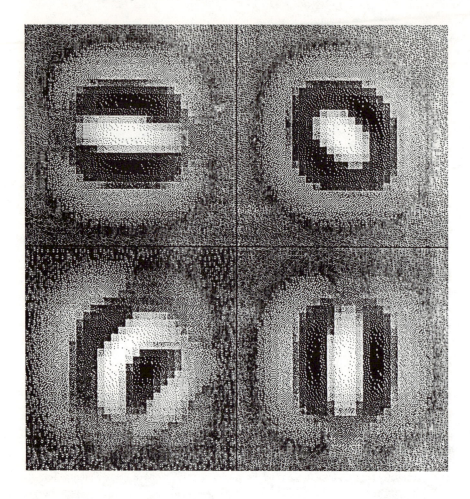

Figure 21.4 Examples of orientation-selective cells. Synapse field profiles, $\emptyset(x,y)$ calculated numerically with the symmetry-breaking model. Light and dark intensities represent positive and negative amplitudes respectively in the 2-dimensional profiles. Note the side-lobes of positive amplitude present in all cells.

of the visual stimuli. Similarly Vidyasagar & Urbas (1982), Reid *et al.* (1987), and Soodak *et al.* (1987) have demonstrated that LGN cells are orientation sensitive. The ratio of the response of LGN cells at the preferred to orthogonal orientations ranges from 1:1 to 1.5:1 (Soodak *et al.*, 1987).

While orientation sensitivity is certainly present early in the visual pathway there is no agreement on the role it plays in the orientation based organization of the cortex. Leventhal (1985) and Schall *et al.* (1987) have put forward the hypothesis, and corresponding model, that cortical orientation selectivity is no more than an amplification of the retinal orientation sensitivity. Sillito (1987) (see also Vidyasagar

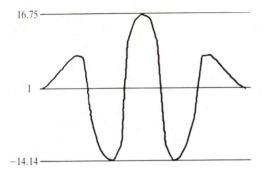

Figure 21.5 A one dimensional cross-section from a receptive field in Figure 21.4. The cross-section is transverse to the cell's major axis.

& Urbas, 1982), on the other hand, provides strong evidence that intracortical (interneuron mediated) inhibition is central to the orientation selectivity of cortical simple cells. They demonstrate that iontophoretic application of the GABA (gamma-aminobutyric acid) antagonist N-methyl-bicuculline to the cortex drastically reduced or even destroyed the orientation selectivity of simple cells. This suggested that orientation selectivity is generated *intra*-cortically and that pre-cortical orientation sensitivity may have no bearing on that in the cortex. The full effects of N-methyl-bicuculline on cellular function, however, may not be fully understood.

We have constructed a version of the symmetry-breaking model (Kammen, 1988) that incorporates the observed orientation sensitivity of pre-cortical cells as a bias to the development of cortical cells. Soodak *et al.* (1987) have constructed a model that accounts for LGN orientation sensitivity by a linear summation of retinal sensitivity. Instead of beginning with a Gaussian arborization window as in the basic symmetry-breaking model, we use elliptic Gaussians with the asymmetry taken directly from the neurological data. The asymmetry will bias the symmetry-breaking and neighboring cortical cells, which receive similar input from the LGN due to the overlap of the projecting synaptic fields, will tend to develop similar orientation preferences. We find that a bias of 20 to 30% is sufficient to yield a definite correlation between the cortical cell and its LGN inputs.

The orientation tuning curves for cortical cells have been extensively studied by many researchers (e.g. Hubel & Wiesel, 1974; Jones & Palmer, 1987; and Parker & Hawken, 1988) and must be accounted for by any viable model of striate cortex development. The symmetry-breaking model predicts that orientation selectivity is an *inherent* property of cortical cells developing in a feedforward network under the influence of a standard Hebbian learning rule. Intracortical effects, however, are required to sharpen the orientation tuning to its neurophysiologically observed values. Synaptic interconnections between hypercolumnar cells attuned to nearby spatial locations and orientations could mediate an inhibitory interaction between neighboring cells - perhaps in a way similar to the wiring proposals of Ferster & Koch (1987). This geometry would result in cells with sharper tuning than the basic symmetry-breaking scenario alone would predict (the full range of parameters in this scenario, however, has not yet been fully explored). This qualitative picture is in accordance with the bicuculline studies of Vidyasagar & Urbas (1982) and Sillito (1987) discussed above, which reveal significant loss of cellular selectivity when neurons are deprived of intracortical communication. In the final section we discuss an alternative model for the development of orientation selectivity which utilizes these results from neurophysiology.

21.5   Relation to information processing ideas

While models that mimic the form of the cortical architecture are a valuable step in our understanding of cortical function they tend to skirt the key question of the precise computational role of these cells in the function of the visual system. Current research on networks of neural processing units has enlivened research in information processing, subject to the limitations imposed by known neurological development and organization. While current models of neural input/output (transfer) functions, synaptic modification, and neuroembryological development are still somewhat simplistic, some algorithms for information manipulation are beginning to appear as natural consequences of self-organization in neural networks. In addition, models of self-organizing networks are beginning to develop computational subunits that strongly resemble biological structures such as cortical simple cell receptive fields (e.g. Linsker, 1988; Kammen & Yuille, 1988), cortical sensory maps (Edelman, 1987), and hypercolumns of orientation selective cells (Linsker, 1986c).

Barlow (1981), for example, has considered the information processing properties of a network designed to reproduce the input signal after passage through a variable number of internal or 'hidden' units. Consider the case of a network with *more* hidden than externally coupled units, as in the visual pathway where there is about a one hundred fold *increase* in the number of neurons between the retinal stage and layer IV in the visual cortex. The network might be expected to allocate the hidden units to tasks that result in infrequent firing of a given cell. In a network that conserves total information content from layer to layer this would result in a large information transmission when the cell *does* fire and hence a smaller number of cells are required to convey a *particular* fact about the image. The large number of cortical cells is necessary to perform a number of different information management tasks.

Very recently a number of self-organizing models have been invented, based on information processing principles, which have close similarities to the models described above and can also generate similar receptive field structures. The computational role of these new models, however, is far simpler to understand. These models are very promising and we briefly review them in the final section.

21.6 Self-organizing models performing principal component analysis

In a feedforward system Oja (1982) (also see Cooper *et al.*, 1979) and Linsker (1988) find that a particular version of the Hebb learning rule leads to a network that performs principal component analysis (PCA) on the input signal. PCA is a particularly useful statistical test for subdividing and managing large data sets based on correlations in the data - a task that the visual system must perform.

For a series of inputs f_i^μ, where the inputs are labelled by μ and their components by i, the principal components are defined to be the eigenvectors of the covariance, or auto-correlation matrix

$$F_{ij} = \frac{1}{N} \sum_{\mu=1}^{N} f_i^\mu f_i^\mu. \qquad (21.13)$$

The principal components can be ordered by the magnitude of their eigenvalues.

Yuille *et al.* (1988) describe a feedforward developmental layered model, using a modified Hebb rule, in which the receptive fields strengths converge to the largest principal component of the input signal. They use mathematical analysis and computer simulations to show that, when the correlation function D attains a certain form, small asymmetries in D (which could be due to small irregularities in the dendritic geometry) produce orientation selective cells. In addition, neighboring cells in the same layer of the network can interact via an inhibitory mechanism and develop quadrature phase relationships (receptive fields out of phase by 90 degrees, see Figure 21.6) like those observed by Pollen & Ronner (1981) in microelectrode recordings of cortical neurons. Sanger (1988) also describes a network using PCA ideas which can generate orientation selective cells.

Spiro (1987) constructed a back-propagation network (Rumelhart *et al.*, 1986) designed to maximize the information overlap between the input and output states, subject to the constraint that the signal passes through a reduced number of hidden units. The signal is therefore 'squeezed' through the intermediate neurons. Spiro found that the receptive fields of neighboring hidden units also exhibited the quadrature phase relationships. An analysis of this network (Kammen, 1988; Yuille *et al.*, 1988), using principal components, showed that it works in a similar manner to the feedforward networks doing PCA.

The self-organizing models using Hebb rules to perform PCA are very attractive due to their ability to mimic the development of the receptive fields of simple cells and their good computational properties. Together with recent experimental results (Carew *et al.*, 1984; Miles & Wong, 1987; Jahr & Stevens, 1987), which suggest that some variants of the Hebb rule may be biologically plausible, they give the promise of increased understanding of the development of the visual cortex.

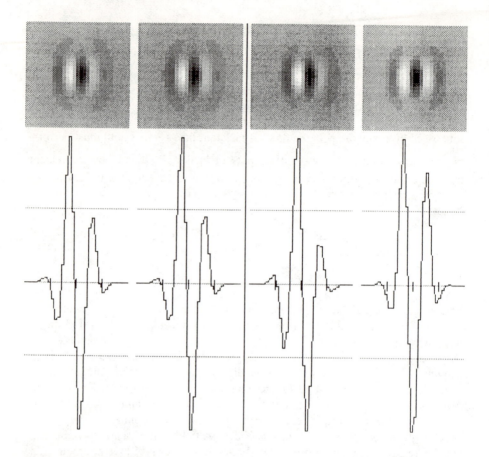

Figure 21.6 Cells exhibiting the quadrature phase relationship. The first two panels, and corresponding one dimensional profiles, are for cells developing independently under the Hebb rule. The third and fourth frames are the same two cells but *after* further development under the influence of the modified, inhibitory, Hebb rule. The one dimensional profiles, below, reveal the shift in the spatial phase of the second cell with respect to the first.

Acknowledgements

We would like to thank Dr. D. Kersten and David Cohen for interesting conversations and the editors for helpful comments on this paper. A.L.Y. was supported by the Brown, Harvard and MIT Center for Intelligent Control Systems with US Army Research Office grant DAAL03-86-C-0171.

References

Barlow H. (1981) Critical limiting factors in the design of the eye and visual cortex. **Proc. R. Soc. B 212**, pp. 1-34

Bienenstock E.L., Cooper L.N. & Munro P.W. (1982) Theory for the development of neuron selectivity: orientation specificity and binocular interaction in visual cortex. **J. Neurosci. 2**, pp. 32-48

Blasdel G.G. & Salama G. (1986) Voltage sensitive dyes reveal a modular organization in monkey striate cortex. **Nature 321**, pp. 579-585

Braitenberg V. & Braitenberg C. (1979) Geometry of orientation columns in the visual cortex. **Biol. Cybern. 33**, pp. 179-186

Carew T.J., Hawkins R.D., Abrams T.W. & Kandel E.R. (1984) A test of Hebb's postulate at identified synapses which mediate classical conditioning in *Aplysia*. **J. Neurosci. 4**, pp. 1217-1224

Coleman S. (1985) **Aspects of Symmetry**. pp. 113-184, Cambridge University Press, Cambridge.

Cooper L.N., Liberman F. & Oja E. (1979) A theory for the acquisition and loss of neuron specificity in visual cortex. **Biol. Cybern. 33**, pp. 9-28

Creutzfeldt O.D., Khunt U. & Benavento L.A. (1974) An intracellular analysis of visual cortical neurons to moving stimuli: responses in a co-operative neuronal network. **Exp. Brain Res. 21**, pp. 251-274

Daugman J.G. (1985) Uncertainty relation for resolution in space, spatial frequency, and orientation optimized by two dimensional visual cortical filters. **J. Op. Soc. Am. A 2**, pp. 1160-1169

Edelman G.M. (1987) **Neural Darwinism**. Basic Books, New York.

Ferster D. (1987) Origin of orientation-selective EPSPs in simple cells of cat visual cortex. **J. Neurosci. 7**, pp. 1780-1791

Ferster D. & Koch C. (1987) Neuronal connections underlying orientation selectivity in cat visual cortex. **TINS 10**, pp. 487-492

Hebb D.O. (1949) **The Organization of Behavior**. Wiley, NY.

Hopfield J.J. (1984) Neurons with graded response have collective computational properties like those of two-state neurons. **Proc. Nat. Acad. Sci. USA 81**, pp. 3088-3092

Hubel D.H. & Wiesel T.N. (1962) Receptive fields, binocular interactions, and functional architecture in the cat's visual cortex. **J. Physiol. 160**, pp. 106-154

Hubel D.H. & Wiesel T.N. (1974) Sequence regularity and geometry of orientation selectivity and binocularity in the monkey striate cortex. **J. comp. Neurol. 158**, pp. 267-294

Jahr C.E. & Stevens C.F. (1987) Glutamate activates multiple single channel conductances in hippocampal neurons. **Nature 325**, pp. 522-525

Jones J. & Palmer L. (1987) The two-dimensional spatial structure of simple receptive fields in cat striate cortex. **J. Neurophys. 58**, pp. 1233-1258

Kammen D.M. (1988) Self-organization in neural networks. Ph.D. Thesis, Harvard University, unpublished.

Kammen D.M. & Yuille A.L. (1988) Spontaneous symmetry-breaking energy functions for orientation selective cortical cells. **Biol. Cybern. 59**, pp. 23-31

Koch C. (1987) The action of the corticofugal pathway on sensory thalamic nuclei: a hypothesis. **Neurosci. 2**, pp. 399-406

Leventhal A.G. (1983) Relationship between preferred orientation sensitivity of cat retinal ganglion cells. **J. Comp. Neurol. 220**, pp. 476-483

Leventhal A.G. (1985) Retinal design of the striate cortex. In: **Models of the Visual Cortex.** D. Rose & V.G. Dobson (eds.) Wiley, NY.

Levick W.R. & Thibos L.N. (1982) Analysis of orientation bias in cat retina. **J. Physiol. (Lond). 329**, pp. 243-261

Linsker R (1986a) From basic network principles to neural architecture: Emergence of spatial-opponent cells. **Proc. Nat. Acad. Sci. USA 83**, pp. 7508-7512

Linsker R. (1986b) From basic network principles to neural architecture: Emergence of orientation-selective cells. **Proc. Nat. Acad. Sci. USA 83**, pp. 8390-8394

Linsker R. (1986c) From basic network principles to neural architecture: Emergence of orientation columns. **Proc. Nat. Acad. Sci. USA 83**, pp. 8779-9783

Linsker R. (1988) Self-organization in a perceptual network. **Computer**, March 1988, pp. 105-117

Lund J.S. (1981) Intrinsic organization of the primate visual cortex, area 17, as seen in Golgi preparations. In: **Organization of the Cerebral Cortex.** pp. 125-152, F.O. Schmidt *et al.* (eds.) MIT Press, Cambridge, MA.

von der Malsburg C. (1973) Self-organization of orientation sensitive cells in the striate cortex. **Kybernetik 14**, pp. 85-100

von der Malsburg C. & Cowan J.D. (1982) Outline of a theory for the ontogenesis of iso-orientation domains in visual cortex. **Biol. Cybern. 45**, pp. 49-56

Meir R. & Domany E. (1988) Iterated learning in a layered feed-forward network. **Phys. Rev. A 37**, pp. 2660-2668

Miles R. & Wong R.K.S. (1987) Latent synaptic pathways revealed after tetanic stimulation in the hippocampus. **Nature 329**, pp. 724-726

Oja E. (1982) A simplified neuron model as a principal component analyzer. **J. math. Biol.15**, pp. 267-273

Parker A.J. & Hawken M.J. (1988) Two-dimensional spatial structure of receptive fields in monkey striate cortex. **J. Op. Soc. Am. 5**, pp. 598-605

Pollen D. & Ronner S. (1981) Phase relationships between adjacent simple cells in the visual cortex. **Science 212**, pp. 1409-1411

Reid R.C., Soodak R.E. & Shapley R.M. (1987) Linear mechanisms of directional selectivity in simple cells of cat striate cortex. **Proc. Nat. Acad. Sci. 84**, pp. 8740-8744

Rumelhart D.E., Hinton G.E. & Williams R.J. (1986) Learning internal representations by error propagation. In: **Parallel Distributed Processing (vol. 1)**. D. E. Rumelhart & J.L. McClelland (eds.) MIT Press, Cambridge, MA.

Sanger T. (1988) Optimal unsupervised learning in a single-layer linear feedforward network. Submitted to Neural Networks

Sattinger DH. (1979) Group Theoretic Methods in Bifurcation Theory. In: **Lecture Notes in Math. 762**. Springer, Berlin.

Schall J.D., Perry V H. & Leventhal A.G. (1986a) Retinal ganglion cell dendritic fields in Old-World monkeys are oriented radially. **Brain Res. 368**, pp. 18-23

Schall J.D., Vitek D.J. & Leventhal A.G. (1986b) Retinal constraints on orientation specificity in cat visual cortex. **J. Neurosci. 6**, pp. 823-836

Schall J.D. & Leventhal A.G. (1987) Relationships between ganglion cell dendritic structure and retinal topography in the cat. **J. comp. Neurol. 257**, pp. 149-159

Schwartz E. (1980) Computational anatomy and functional architecture of striate cortex: a spatial mapping approach to perceptual coding. **Vision Res. 20**, pp. 645-669

Sillito A.M. (1987) Synaptic processes and neurotransmitters operating in the central visual system: A systems approach. In: **Synaptic Function**. pp. 328-371, G. Edelman, E. Gall & M. Cowan (eds.) Wiley Interscience.

Soodak R E., Shapley R.M. & Kaplan E. (1987) Linear mechanisms of orientation tuning in the retina and lateral geniculate nucleus of the cat. **J. Neurophys. 58**, 267-275

Spiro P. (1987) Receptive field shape as a function of dimensionality reduction and image statistics. B.S. Thesis, MIT, unpublished.

Swindale N.V. (1982) A model for the formation of orientation columns. **Proc. Roy. Soc. Lond. 215**, pp. 211-230

Swindale N.V. (1985) Iso-orientation domains and their relationship with cytochrome oxidase patches. In: **Models of the Visual Cortex**. D. Rose & V.G. Dobson (eds.) Wiley, NY.

Vidyasagar T.R. & Urbas J.V. (1982) Orientation sensitivity of cat LGN neurones with and without inputs from visual cortical areas. **Exp. Brain Res. 46,** pp. 157-169

Yuille A L., Kammen D.M. & Cohen, D. (1988) Quadrature and the development of orientation selective cortical cells by Hebb rules. Submitted to Biol. Cybern.

Index